Chi Nei Tsang

Internal Organ Chi Massage

Mantak Chia
and
Maneewan Chia

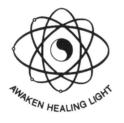

AWAKEN HEALING LIGHT

REVISED EDITION

HEALING TAO BOOKS/Huntington, New York

Editor/Revised Edition: Valerie Meszaros
Editor: David Flatley
Technical Editor: Gilles Marin
Contributing Writers: Valerie Meszaros, Larry Tupper,
            Shanti Barron, Ruth Carter, Ron Diana,
            David Flatley, Gilles Marin, Juan Li,
            and Rene Navarro
Illustrator: Juan Li
Cover Illustrator: Ivan Salgado
Graphics: Max Chia
Designer and
Desktop Publishing: Maneewan Chia

First Published in 1990 by
Healing Tao Books
P.O. Box 1194
Huntington, NY 11743

ISBN: 0935621-35-0
Library of Congress Catalog Card Number: 90-085548

Manufactured in the United States of America
Fifth Printing. 1997

10 9 8 7 6

Dedicated to Healers Everywhere

Table of Contents

  The Goal of the Taoist Practice
  International Healing Tao Course Offerings
  Outline of the Complete System of the Healing Tao
  Course Descriptions:
     Introductory Level 1: Awaken Healing Light
     Introductory Level II: Development of Internal Power
     Introductory Level III: The Way of Radiant Health
     Intermediate Level: Foundations of Spiritual Practice
     Advanced Level: The Realm of Soul and Spirit
  Healing Tao Books
  The International Healing Tao Centers

WORDS OF CAUTION

The meditations, practices, and techniques described herein are NOT to be used as an alternative to professional medical treatment. This book does not attempt to give any medical diagnosis, treatment, prescription, or suggestion for medication in relation to any human disease, pain, injury, deformity, or physical condition. Also if there are illnesses based on mental disorders, a medical doctor or psychologist should be consulted. Such problems should be corrected before you start training.

The practices described in this book have been used successfully for thousands of years by Taoists trained by individual instruction. Readers must not undertake the practice of Chi Nei Tsang without personal training by the Healing Tao since certain of these practices, if improperly done, may cause injury or result in health problems. This book is intended to supplement individual training by the Healing Tao and to serve as a reference guide for these practices. Anyone who undertakes these practices on the basis of this book alone does so entirely at his or her own risk.

Chinese medicine emphasizes balancing and strengthening the body so that it can heal itself. The meditations, internal exercises, and martial arts of the Healing Tao are basic approaches to this end. Follow the instructions for each exercise carefully, and do not neglect the supplemental exercises, particularly the Microcosmic Orbit Meditation. Also pay special attention to the warnings and suggestions in each chapter. People who have high blood pressure, heart disease, or a generally weak condition should proceed cautiously. Pregnant women should not practice Chi Nei Tsang. Those people with venereal disease should not attempt any practices involving sexual energy until they are free of the disease.

The Healing Tao is not and cannot be responsible for the consequences of any practice or misuse of the information in this book. If the reader undertakes any exercise without strictly following the instructions, notes, and warnings, the responsibility must lie solely with the reader.

Acknowledgements

We wish to thank the thousands of unknown men and women of the Chinese healing arts who developed many of the techniques and concepts presented in this book. We also wish to thank the Chi Nei Tsang teacher, Dr. Mui Yimwattana, and Taoist Master Yi Eng, both of whom worked so patiently to teach their students.

Without remembering our parents, teachers, and our son, Max, our continued efforts in presenting the Healing Tao System would be without joy or satisfaction. For their gifts, we offer our eternal gratitude and love.

We thank Juan Li for his beautiful illustrations. As always, his contribution has been crucial in presenting the concepts and techniques of the Healing Tao.

We wish to thank David Flatley for his editorial work and writing contributions on the first printing of this book, as well as his ideas for the cover. We appreciate his research and great labor.

We wish to thank Valerie Meszaros for her editorial contributions on the revised edition of this book, as well as thank our instructors, Renu Heisserer and Rene Navarro, for their insightful contributions to the revised version.

We thank Gilles Marin for his technical editing and clear writing throughout the book.

Thank you to Dan "Treelite" Reardon for his valuable information and writing regarding communicating with trees.

We also wish to express thanks to other contributing writers, some of whom have worked with us for many years to prepare this manuscript: Valerie Meszaros, Shanti Barron, Ruth Carter, Ron Diana, Juan Li, Rene Navarro, and Larry Tupper. We thank Dr. Nicole Tremblay for presenting Chapter 13.

We thank Ivan Salgado for the cover illustration and design.

Further, we wish to express our gratitude to all the instructors and students who have offered their time and advice to enhance this system, especially Larry Tupper, Ron Diana, Gilles Marin, Juan Li, and Dr. Angela C. Shen.

We thank Susan Aaron, Esq. and Gary Oshinsky, Esq. for their legal advice.

Finally, we thank the following people for their varied and helpful contributions: William Evans, Cecilia Caldas, Particia Capek, Linda

Hoffer, Jeeraporn Saeheng, Orathai Vudhisethakrit, Michael Winn, Dr. Alejandro Domingo, Dr. Louis Shen, Chong Mi Mueller, Oliver Pfeffer, Lisa Giglioli, Dr. John Cuadrado, Melinda Mills, Karl Danskin, Luis Nunez, Masahiro Ouchi, Renu Heisserer, Mary Beth Soares, Ming Chu Sim, Walter Beckley, Kyle Cline, Mary Anne Hilido, and Evelyn Ward of Dynamic Resources, San Francisco.

MASTER MANTAK CHIA AND MANEEWAN CHIA

MASTER MANTAK CHIA

Master Mantak Chia is the creator of the Healing Tao System and the director of the Healing Tao Center in New York. Since childhood he has been studying the Taoist approach to life as well as other approaches. His mastery of this ancient knowledge, enhanced by his study of other disciplines, has resulted in the development of the Healing Tao System which is now being taught in the United States, Canada, Europe, Australia, and Thailand.

Master Chia was born in Thailand to Chinese parents in 1944. When he was six years old, Buddhist monks taught him how to sit and "still the mind." While he was a grammar school student, he first learned traditional Thai boxing. He then was taught Tai Chi Chuan by Master Lu, who soon introduced him to Aikido, Yoga, and more Tai Chi.

Later, when he was a student in Hong Kong excelling in track and field events, a senior classmate named Cheng Sue-Sue introduced him to his first esoteric teacher and Taoist Master, Master Yi Eng. At this point, he began his studies of the Taoist way of life. He learned how to circulate energy through the Microcosmic Orbit, and, through the practice of Fusion of the Five Elements, how to open the other Six Special Channels. As he further studied Inner Alchemy, he learned the Enlightenment of the Kan and Li, Sealing of the Five Sense Organs, Congress of Heaven and Earth, and Reunion of Man and Heaven. It was Master Yi Eng who authorized Master Chia to teach and heal.

In his early twenties Mantak Chia studied with Master Meugi in Singapore, who taught him Kundalini, Taoist Yoga, and the Buddhist Palm. He was soon able to clear blockages to the flow of energy within his own body. He also learned to pass life-force energy through his hands to heal the patients of Master Meugi. He then learned Chi Nei Tsang from Dr. Mui Yimwattana in Thailand.

Later, he studied with Master Cheng Yao-Lun who taught him the Shao-Lin Method of Internal Power. He also learned from Master Yao-Lun the closely guarded secret of the organs, glands, and bone marrow exercise

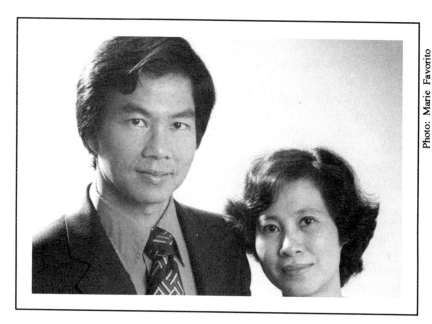

Photo: Marie Favorito

Mantak Chia and Maneewan Chia

known as *Bone Marrow Nei Kung* and the exercise known as *Strengthening and Renewal of the Tendons.* Master Cheng Yao-Lun's system combined Thai boxing and Kung Fu. At this time he also studied with Master Pan Yu, whose system combined Taoist, Buddhist, and Zen teachings. From Master Pan Yu he learned about the exchange of the Yin and Yang power between men and women, and also learned how to develop the *Steel Body.*

To understand the mechanisms behind healing energy better, Master Chia studied Western medical science and anatomy for two years. While pursuing his studies, he managed the Gestetner Company, a manufacturer of office equipment, and became well-acquainted with the technology of offset printing and copying machines.

Using his knowledge of Taoism combined with the other disciplines, Master Chia began teaching the Healing Tao System. He eventually trained other teachers to communicate this knowledge, and he established the Natural Healing Center in Thailand. Five years later, he decided to move to New York where, in 1979, he opened the Healing Tao Center.

Since then, centers have opened in many other locations including Boston, Philadelphia, Denver, Seattle, San Francisco, Los Angeles, San Diego, Tucson, and Toronto. Groups have also formed throughout Europe in England, Germany, the Netherlands, Switzerland, Austria, Australia, and Thailand.

Master Chia leads a peaceful life with his wife, Maneewan, and their young son, Max. (In 1990 Max, at age 11, became the youngest certified instructor in the Healing Tao System.) Master Chia is a warm, friendly, and helpful man who views himself primarily as a teacher. He presents the Healing Tao in a simple, practical manner while always expanding his knowledge and approach to teaching. He uses a word processor for writing and is very much at ease with the latest in computer technology. He has written and published eight Healing Tao Books: in 1983, *Awaken Healing Energy through the Tao*; in 1984, *Taoist Secrets of Love: Cultivating Male Sexual Energy*; in 1985, *Taoist Ways to Transform Stress into Vitality*; in 1986, *Chi Self-Massage: The Tao Way of Rejuvenation*, *Iron Shirt Chi Kung I*, and *Healing Love through the Tao: Cultivating Female Sexual Energy*; in 1989, *Bone Marrow Nei Kung*; and in 1990, *Fusion of the Five Elements I*. *Chi Nei Tsang: Internal Organ Chi Massage* is his ninth book.

Master Chia estimates that it will take twenty books to convey the full Healing Tao System. In June, 1990 at a dinner in San Francisco, Master Chia was honored by the International Congress of Chinese Medicine and Qi Gong [Chi Kung] who named him the Qi Gong Master of the Year. He is the first recipient of this annual award.

MANEEWAN CHIA

Born in China, Maneewan Chia was raised in Hong Kong and eventually moved with her parents to Thailand where she grew up to attend the University and earn a B.S. Degree in Medical Technology. Since childhood, Mrs. Chia has been very interested in nutrition and Chinese health food cooking. This she learned by assisting her mother, a very fine cook. Since her marriage to Mantak Chia, she has studied the Healing Tao System and currently assists him in teaching classes, including Taoist Five Element Nutrition, and managing the Healing Tao Center.

INTRODUCTION
WHAT IS CHI NEI TSANG?

A. The Causes of Sickness: Organ Obstructions and Congestion in the Abdomen

The Taoist sages of ancient China observed that humans often develop energy blockages in their internal organs that result in knots and tangles in their abdomens. These obstructions occur at the center of the body's vital functions and constrict the flow of *Chi* (energy), our life-force. The negative emotions of fear, anger, anxiety, depression, and worry cause the most damage. Problems can also be caused by overwork, stress, accidents, surgery, drugs, toxins, poor food, and bad posture.

Through meditative practices the sages learned to look within themselves. They discovered the internal organs connect with the Five Forces of the Universe and provide a link between the human microcosm and the universal macrocosm. The organs contain the essences of the spiritual force of a human being. They also provide the physical lines of force that hold the body together and give it structure.

When obstructed the internal organs store unhealthy energies that can overflow into other bodily systems and surface as negative emotions and sickness. Always in search of an outlet, these negative emotions and toxic energies create a perpetual cycle of negativity and stress. (Figure 1) If the negative emotions can't find an outlet, they fester in the organs or move into the abdomen, the body's "garbage dump." The abdomen can process some emotional garbage, but more often it can't keep up with the flow. The energetic center of the body located at the navel becomes congested and cut off from the rest of the body.

1

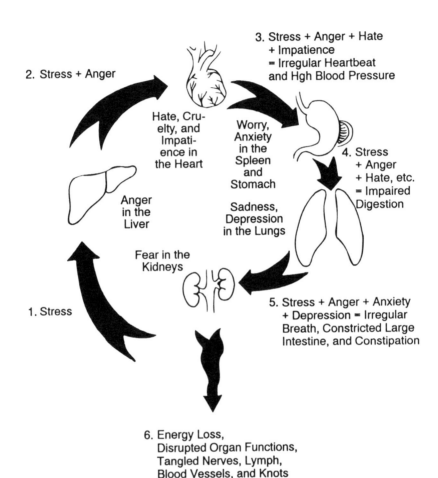

2. Stress + Anger

3. Stress + Anger + Hate
+ Impatience
= Irregular Heartbeat
and Hgh Blood Pressure

Hate, Cru-
elty, and
Impati-
ence in
the Heart

Worry,
Anxiety
in the
Spleen
and
Stomach

4. Stress
+ Anger
+ Hate, etc.
= Impaired
Digestion

Anger
in the
Liver

Sadness,
Depression
in the Lungs

Fear in the
Kidneys

1. Stress

5. Stress + Anger + Anxiety
+ Depression = Irregular
Breath, Constricted Large
Intestine, and Constipation

6. Energy Loss,
Disrupted Organ Functions,
Tangled Nerves, Lymph,
Blood Vessels, and Knots
in the Abdomen

**Figure 1. The negative energy cycle leads
to knots and tangles in the abdomen**

2

B. Chi Nei Tsang: A Method to Clear Blocked Energy

Chi, the life-force energy, moves through the body's internal channels, nervous system, blood vessels, and lymph glands. These systems concentrate and cross paths in the abdomen which acts as their control center. Tensions, worries, and stresses of the day, month, or year accumulate there and are seldom dispersed. These disturbances can cause physical tangling and knotting of the nerves, blood vessels, and lymph nodes. The result is the gradual obstruction of energy circulation.

The ancient Taoists realized that negative emotions cause serious damage to one's health, impairing both physical and spiritual functions. They understood that each human emotion is an expression of energy and that certain emotions could indicate the negative energy behind many physical ailments. They also identified a specific cycle of relationships between the emotions and the organs. For example, the experience of a "knot" in one's stomach indicated the presence of worry, the negative emotion that accumulates in the stomach and spleen.

The Taoists discovered that most maladies could be healed once the underlying toxins and negative forces were released from the body. They developed the art of *Chi Nei Tsang* to recycle and transform negative energies that obstruct the internal organs and cause knots in the abdomen. Chi Nei Tsang clears out the toxins, bad emotions, and excessive heat—or heat deficiencies—that cause the organs to dysfunction. (Figure 2)

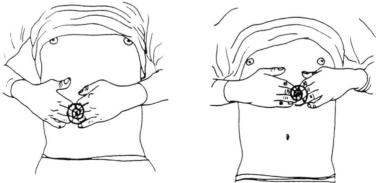

Figure 2. The ancient Taoists massaged their abdomens and organs to stay healthy

C. Chi Nei Tsang: A Complement to Other Disciplines

As an art and science, Chi Nei Tsang complements Reflexology, Psychology, Reiki, Shiatsu, Swedish Massage, and similar therapies. (Figure 3) However, unlike most practices which use indirect methods to contact the internal organs, Chi Nei Tsang directly massages the internal organs. Chi Nei Tsang is also the most comprehensive approach to energizing, strengthening, and detoxifying the internal system. It clears out negative influences and is particularly useful in relieving intestinal blockages, cramps, knots, lumps, scar tissue, headaches, menstrual cramps, poor blood circulation, back pain, infertility, impotence, and many other problems. Along with other disciplines, Chi Nei Tsang may help to eliminate the need for surgery.

D. The Healing Tao and Chi Nei Tsang

Other Healing Tao practices are useful for maintaining personal energy. Meditations such as the Inner Smile, the Microcosmic Orbit, and the Fusion of the Five Elements open channels and enable the flow of Chi to energize and cleanse the organs. Exercises such as the Six Healing Sounds prevent overheating and help to balance the internal system. (For a review of these meditations, refer to the Healing Tao books, *Awaken the Healing Light, Taoist Ways to Transform Stress into Vitality*, and *Fusion of the Five Elements I*.)

In fact, the most outstanding difference between a Chi Nei Tsang practitioner and those of other healing arts is the daily practice of the Healing Tao meditations. The meditations offer maximum physical and spiritual protection for instructors and their students.

E. What Every Chi Nei Tsang Practitioner Should Know

Society and religions throughout history have programmed people to give rather than to receive. Common sense is therefore ignored, and egos are gratified through self-denial beyond reasonable limits. Since the

4

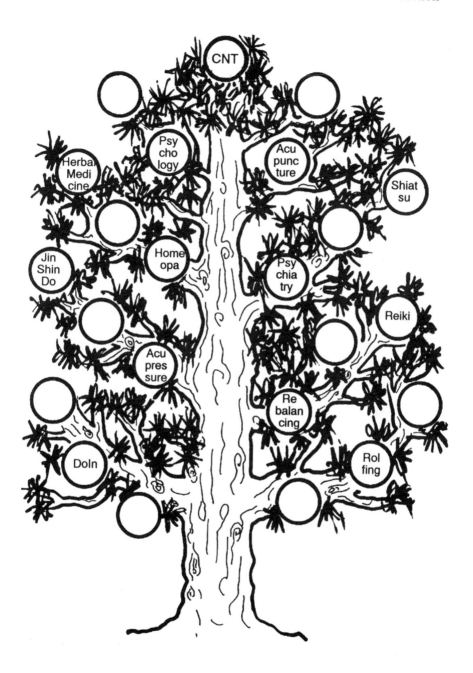

Figure 3. The Tree of Therapies

first concern of the practitioner must always be his or her own health, a few guidelines are offered.

1. Knowledge of the Human Body: Organs, Systems, and Tissues

It is necessary to have a working knowledge of the internal organs and their functions: the lymphatic, circulatory, and nervous systems, the energy channels, the muscles and fasciae (connective tissues), and the interrelationships among all of these facets of the body.

2. Understanding Chi

Understanding vital Chi and being able to distinguish the positive and negative qualities of it as a life-force are of the utmost importance. Without a clear working knowledge of Chi, the practitioners of healing arts have no means of protecting their own bodies and energies from the negative influences of others. They also may find themselves giving away more energy than they can spare. In time, Chi Nei Tsang practitioners may find themselves suffering from professional "burnout" because their own energies have been depleted. Once this happens they may not be able to continue to provide relief for others.

3. Developing the Proper Attitude

The most important requirement of Chi Nei Tsang is a proper attitude about yourself and others. This means that the practitioner needs to realize a few important facts. A practitioner should be aware that in seeking relief, people go to a healer fully loaded with sick energy and sick emotions. They expect to be able to unload all of their sicknesses onto the healer, thereby negating their responsibilities for their own healing. Initially, your ability to help people will gain their trust, but it is important never to allow them to become dependent on you. Learn to give them your attention, love, and care as you teach them how to get back on their feet through their own efforts. This means that you must teach them about their bodies and energetic systems. Explain their responsibilities so that you won't lose or pollute your own life-force.

F. Chi Nei Tsang Practitioners Educate Others to Heal Themselves

Chi Nei Tsang practitioners do not simply apply techniques, but are capable of generating and directing vital life-force through and around others. The main role of the Chi Nei Tsang practitioner, however, is educator not healer. The main philosophy and purpose of Chi Nei Tsang is to teach people how to heal themselves by providing insights into their own immense, internal healing powers. Chi Nei Tsang practitioners, therefore, never refer to their students as "patients" or "clients". A student who has awakened his or her own healing energy can continue the process by practicing at home and teaching family and friends. One must always remember that the most important healing energy comes from within oneself.

G. The Secret Technique of Chi Nei Tsang: Healing from the Heart

This book is full of brilliant and wonderful techniques that have the potential to significantly alter the basic way we care for ourselves and for each other. While the techniques are forceful and can relieve both chronic and acute illnesses, they will not work effectively unless they are activated and animated by a love and compassion that is given sincerely and abundantly from your heart. (Figure 4). Your fingers and hands can become healing hands only when you are full of good intentions.

When you touch others, touch them with all the love, care, and compassion that you can find within yourself. Connect yourself with the forces of the Universe, the Cosmic Particle or Human Plane, and the Earth and become a physical channel for these forces. Apply your hands with the tenderness of a mother touching her child. If your touch is from your center to theirs, they will open like the petals of a flower in the morning sun. Every life and body has a self-healing mechanism that you can help to awaken. Once the center at the navel is activated and freed and the organs are detoxified, the process of healing can be completed by your students through their own discipline.

Eventually you will learn to feel and "see" inside another. Those who come to you will do so because they are uncomfortable with their spirits and bodies. Your intention should be to help them become serene

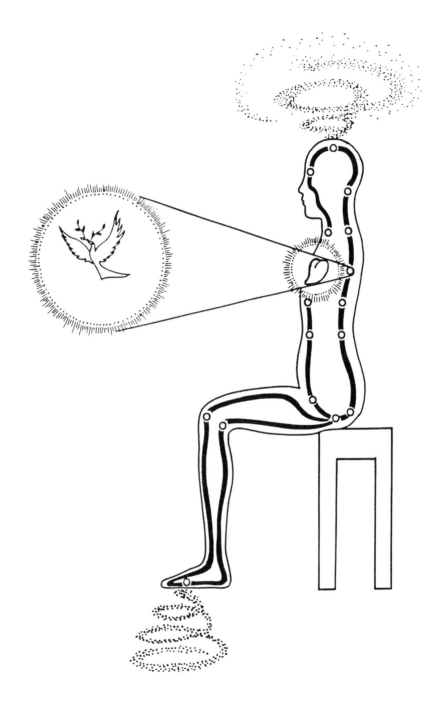

Figure 4. Healing with Love from the Heart

and peaceful within themselves. On the following pages you will be introduced to many ancient healing gifts from the Orient, born from the wisdom of the Taoists and perfected over many centuries. In time you can become a great healer and teacher. People will seek your guidance. Always remember the source of your real power. The secret touch has warmed bodies, spirits, and homes in every land throughout time. It is a touch of the heart when you freely give of yourself to another. You will find that the loving touch has enormous power to heal and renew lives and spirits.

Chi Nei Tsang

CHAPTER 1

WORKING IN
THE NAVEL CENTER

The ancient Taoists were confident that the human body and spirit could live forever. Those venerable men and women expressed this deft knowledge in the gentle poems, personal histories, social criticisms, and cryptic "how-to" formulas that comprise the five thousand volume history of Taoism known as the "Taoist Canon." Still largely untranslated, these books—sheaves of rice paper and wood block prints—now beckon us to explore a gifted culture of unsurpassed brightness and stunning human achievement.

The stories reveal that the ancients acquired and expressed such confidence only after centuries of testing and experimenting with the body's supple energetic systems in its swirling, surrounding energy environment. Depending only on their experiences and observations, these skilled, spiritual empiricists discovered the layout of the body's major and minor energy systems, its power sources, its "turbines," and its "transformers."

Moreover, they knew just where to go to get the right kind of energy to feed and balance those systems so that the body might proceed in a kind of perpetual motion. Had the energy not been right at hand, those agile adepts, having mastered the universal and Earthly laws of energy and matter, could cultivate and harvest the needed energy. Gathering the desired energy sometimes meant sitting in a certain meditation. At other times it meant swallowing a bitter brew strained from a mash of roots, bark, and assorted herbs. For more experienced Taoists stalking a potent restorative often meant gathering all their energies and essences and shooting themselves out of their earthbound bodies on exciting foraging journeys deep into space, to the edge of the Cosmos, to a place where they might pluck the perfect blend.

Whatever they did, wherever they went, the prized goal—a state of alertness—was to keep their organs free of emotional and environmental tensions and toxins, and to maintain a smooth and abundant flow of the acquired and balanced energies throughout their bodies. This was the secret of good health and long life, gifts that you can practice and master in the art of Chi Nei Tsang (often referred to in this book as "CNT").

This book is concerned with how to maintain the body's systems to live a full, healthy, and extended life. The Taoists were especially adept at knowing how to stay healthy. Whether you believe in or come to believe in their ideas of immortality, you will discover that because the Taoists pursued it, you are now the benefactor. They have passed down a treasure of many wonderful life-extending techniques. Their skills resulted from their understanding of energy and the discovery that all energy is part of one indivisible system. Once they knew how the body was programmed and how the system worked, it was easy to merge into or become the programming. They discovered that the body was a continuous process of energy becoming matter and of matter dissolving into energy. Having successfully perceived this ebb and flow, they could easily monitor their health and make any necessary adjustments. It is very certain that you can learn to do this as well.

Henry Maspero, a French scholar, was one of the first from the West to analyze and write about Taoism. His perception of the Taoist concept of energy, body, spirit, and immortality from "Taoism in Chinese Religion" is worth your consideration.

> "And if the Taoists, in the search for Long Life, conceived this not as a spiritual immortality but as a material immortality of the body itself, this is not a deliberate choice between the various possible solutions of the problem of immortality in the other world, it was because for them this was the only possible solution. In the Greco-Roman world, the habit of opposing Spirit to Matter was accepted early; and in religious beliefs this was translated into an opposition between a unique spiritual soul and a material body. For the Chinese...the world is a continuum which passes without interruption from void to material things, the soul did not take on this role as invisible and spiritual counterpart to the visible and material body."
> (p. 266)

When applied to your health this means that it is important to acquire the knowledge and techniques for the proper physical care of the body and its vital organs as well as for the spiritual or invisible energies that are involved. What Maspero's perceptiveness should mean to you is that if you want to stay healthy, you need to learn how to treat both the "Spirit and Matter" of the body, for they are One. Learning, applying, and teaching such skills comprise the heart of Chi Nei Tsang.

With enough faith in lore and myth and enough practical experience with these techniques as they apply to the internal energy systems, it is the Taoists' belief that one day masses of women and men will again discover they have the ability to live greatly extended lives. The most highly evolved can have the *choice* to live in their physical form for centuries, or until the Tao calls them to perform their services on a different plane of existence.

It is encouraging and inspirational to pursue such bold physical and spiritual achievements, not as much by ancient legends and dreams as by real successes. These successes are achieved by using both the beginning and advanced energy techniques used and passed down so long ago. By starting with the most basic techniques, you can begin to feel better and have greater, more positive energy. Learn to start each day by smiling inwardly to your vital organs and thanking them for sustaining your life. As you extend your meditations and techniques into more intricate alchemical procedures, you will discover that they work. You will develop the confidence that if you follow the processes handed down so carefully from one generation of Taoists to the next, they will do what the ancients said they would do.

This kind of internal work involves careful attention to all the body/spirit systems. Along with the stationary and moving meditations, such as Iron Shirt Chi Kung and Tai Chi Chi Kung, it is advisable that you learn Chi Nei Tsang. You will become more able to determine the great range of your body/spirit system and will learn how to play with it to make it "sing." You also can learn an extraordinarily effective means for sustaining the system in good running shape for a long time. Chi Nei Tsang is the best and only "hands-on" maintenance system known.

Whether any of us will live as long as storied ancients remains to be seen. Many people are less interested in the answer to this question than they would be in knowing how they could feel better right now, tomorrow, and next month. They would like to live out their average allotted life spans (60-80 years) in sustained good health. So while preparing for and pondering a long life, our experience and that of our students would easily allow us to handle such an everyday concern and you would receive the same advice you might have heard 5000 years ago. If you want to feel better, massaging the abdomen is a healthy practice

13

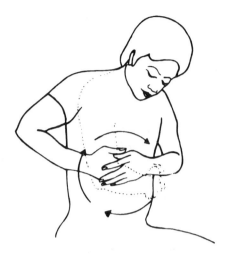

**Figure 1-1. Massaging the abdomen
is a healthy practice that anyone can do**

that anyone can do. (Figure 1-1) If you read no further that would be advice enough to keep you going in good shape for a long time. You can now begin the journey to the center of your navel.

A. The Taoist View of Nature and the Universe

The Taoists always tried to understand what was happening inside the body by comparing and contrasting it with what was happening outside in nature. They could always find exact counterparts. The Laws of Nature were identical on every level and in every situation. When they found an exact match between the body's internal system and a system in the universe, they had an energy match upon which they could depend.

The paired parts of these systems were known as the macrocosm (big—the universe) and microcosm (small—the human being). In effect they deduced, "Things are big out there and little in here. I'll bring it inside, make it small and master it in miniature, where my consciousness is, and then project it out." In order to understand the beginning of the universe and of existence itself, the Taoists chose to examine their own individual births and the proximity of the birth process to the navel center. Then they drew comparisons.

The Taoists said that the beginning of a human's life must be similar to the beginning of the life of the universe. Understand your body and you can understand the entire universe. Why not? The birth of a new human being is no less spectacular or less important than the birth of the universe. A birth is a birth. The Laws of Nature are the same for all births and conceptions. The microcosm is a mirror image of the macrocosm. The universe within is the same as the universe without. (Figure 1-2)

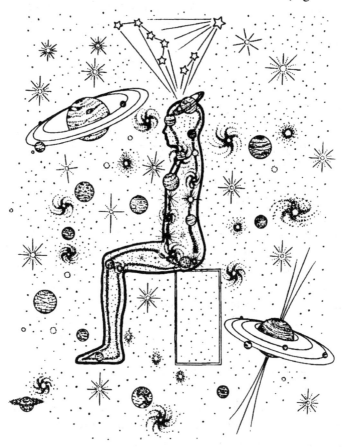

**Figure 1-2. The Microcosm and Macrocosm:
the Universe Within and Without**

1. The Wu Chi—Our Original Source

The Taoists noticed the effects of naturally occurring universal processes upon human nature. By observing nature and investigating the effects of its energy upon and within the human body, the Taoists traced nature's energy back to its source. They used meditation to make this "expedition." Their search led them to the discovery of a primordial void, a condition of nothingness. This void, recognized to have been the state of things at the beginning of all creation, was given the name *Wu Chi*.

The Wu Chi is depicted in Taoist art as an empty circle. Thus, the fountainhead of Taoism is the Wu Chi, the Great Emptiness, the beginning, nothingness—the Tao. You can compare this void to your own creation. Who knows or can say how you came to be? Trace yourself back as far as you can and you will come upon the same mystery that beguiled all of the ancients. Once you had the condition of "nothingness," and then you were born with all your splendor and force.

2. Your Original Energy

While the Tao was difficult to name and grasp, the ancients did describe primal forces emanating from it. The *Tao Te Ching* states,

> *"The Tao produced the One;*
> *The One produced the two*
> *The two produced the three;*
> *The three produced all the myriad beings. "*

The *One* is the highest unity, the primordial energy in the Cosmos. The well known Tai Chi symbol portrays this force in which Yin and Yang are perfectly balanced and still united. One can imagine it just about ready to burst out and create all the world. Yin and Yang separated and became the *Two*. Yin and Yang produced three elemental forces called the *Three Pure Ones*. The Three Pure Ones created the Five Elemental Energy Phases of the Universe. These Five Forces (often called the *Five Elements*) were powerful enough to generate the "all the myriad beings," that is, all the familiar forms of Nature and the Universe, including you. (Figure 1-3)

The energy born from the Wu Chi created the main energy forces that sustain our lives. They are: Universal Energy, Human Plane or Cosmic Particle Energy, and Earth Energy. These forces work together in harmony to sustain all existence. (Figure 1-4)

3. Universal Energy

The first force of nature is the Universal Force, also called *Heavenly Energy*. It manifests itself as the energy of the stars, planets, and galaxies. This vast, all-pervading force nourishes the mind, soul, and spirit of each individual and everything else in the universe. The organs of the human

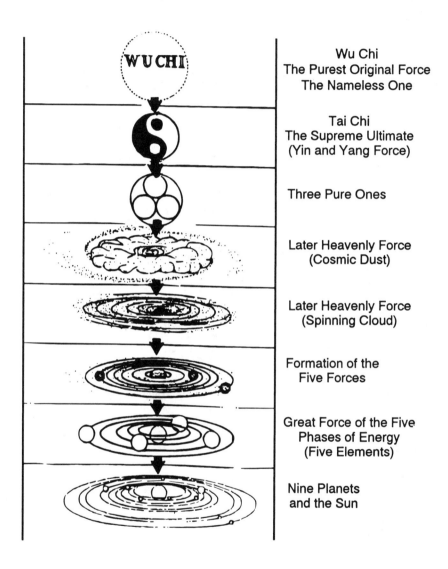

Wu Chi
The Purest Original Force
The Nameless One

Tai Chi
The Supreme Ultimate
(Yin and Yang Force)

Three Pure Ones

Later Heavenly Force
(Cosmic Dust)

Later Heavenly Force
(Spinning Cloud)

Formation of the
Five Forces

Great Force of the Five
Phases of Energy
(Five Elements)

Nine Planets
and the Sun

**Figure 1-3. The Creation of the Tai Chi,
the Five Phases of Energy, and the Solar System**

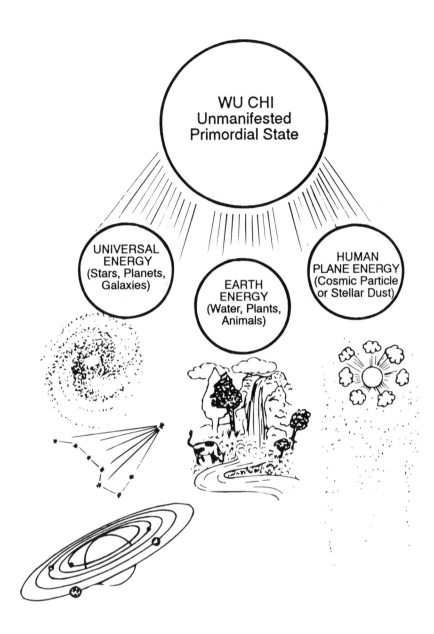

Figure 1-4. The Energy born from the Wu Chi created Universal Energy, Human Plane (Cosmic Particle) Energy, and Earth Energy. They sustain all that exists

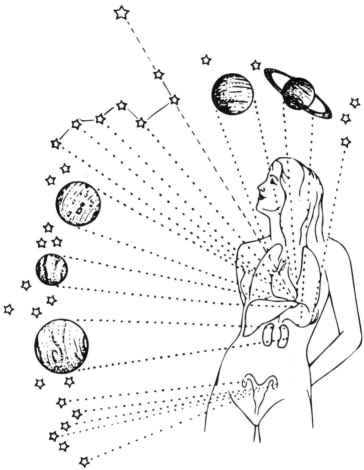

Figure 1-5. The organs are the essence of the stellar and planetary energies. They are also the connecting points between the microcosm and macrocosm

body are the essence of the stars' and planets' energies. They are also the connecting points between the microcosm and macrocosm. (Figure 1-5)

The Universal Force is concentrated on our planet because of the unique relationship between the Earth and its Moon. The combined forces of the Earth and the Moon create a very strong, magnetic power that attracts the energies of the stars in our galaxy. This force spirals down and energizes your body/mind/spirit. (Figure 1-6)

19

The Universal Force

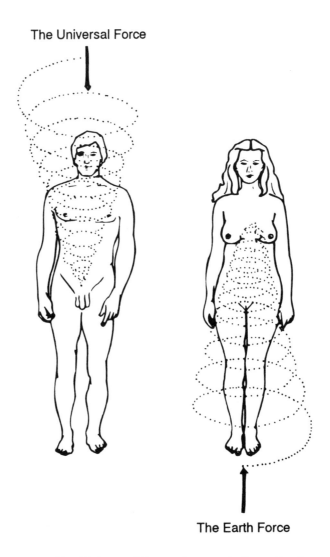

The Earth Force

**Figure 1-6. The Universal Force descends from the heavens
and the Earth Force rises from the Earth**

Many people have a hard time accepting the notion that the stars
and planets could affect our energy systems. Yet everyone is aware of
the power of the sun. If the sun were to burn out, life on Earth would
stop. Ignore its force and you are likely to end the day with a very bad
sunburn. The sun is a star—the personal star of our planetary system.

Many, especially women, also can feel the effect of the Moon. Because the other stars and planets are so remote, most people are not aware that they are projecting vital energy to us as well. Much of Taoist science and technique concerns itself with accessing and cultivating these additional beamed-down energies.

4. Human Plane or Cosmic Particle Energy

Human Plane or Cosmic Particle Energy is the second force of nature. Cosmic particles are part of the Original Energy that flows in space. The smallest are particles of light. Other particles resulted from exploded stars that have come to the end of their life cycles and are drifting in space as very fine particles. As the strong, magnetic power created by the Earth and Moon attracts many of these particles, they drift through the Earth's atmosphere as dust and eventually become topsoil.

It is a Taoists' belief that human flesh is formed by the falling cosmic dust of the universe. As the highest manifestation of Cosmic Particle Force, human beings breathe in its energy to nourish their organs, glands, and senses. You can gather this force easily during meditation.

5. Earth Energy

The Earth Force is the third force of nature. Yin in energy, it spirals up from the Earth (Figure 1-6) and mixes with Yang Universal Energy. The Cosmic Particle and Earth Forces form the human physique, and the Universal Force forms the soul and spirit that energize the physical body. (Figure 1-7)

6. Chi

Chi (sometimes spelled Qi, Ki, or Ch'i) is the unseen life-force, cosmic breath, or vital force that permeates and nurtures everything under the sun, as well as the sun itself. You can conceive of it as an electromagnetic force. In humans this energy cannot be seen in its smallest unit but can be felt; its effect on the body is noticeable. Within the human body Chi flows in interconnected pathways called channels. Chi activates all body processes. Normally, Chi is accumulated through prenatal parental energy, breathing, and eating. (Food is also transformed into this invisible force.) Those trained in the practices of the Healing Tao learn that they can concentrate to draw in Chi through the eyes, hair, fingertips, tips of the toes, perineum, and entire surface of the skin.

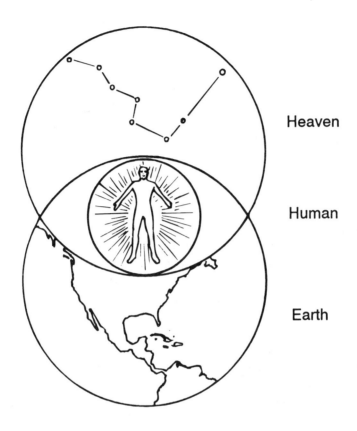

**Figure 1-7. A human being is a balance of
the Universal and Earth Forces**

Chi characteristics fluctuate back and forth from wave force to particle force, from having a frequency to having matter. Chi is both matter and energy. Chi is always revolving, condensing, and expanding.

Among many other things, Chi governs the mind and intention. It will do just about anything and go anywhere you ask. More than anything, its purpose is to be available to help generate life and love. As a CNT practitioner you need to know how to produce and circulate Chi in the body. You can help insure that its circulation is powerful and smooth.

If the Chi is not regulated and balanced, its control can be lost resulting in damage to the body. If the Chi cannot flow and becomes clogged, very hot or cold, or very weak, a person can become very ill.

The practice of CNT helps the Chi to flow and balance itself. Good Chi is properly flowing Chi. Bad Chi is stagnant Chi. Life is motion; death is lack of motion. Life is change and spontaneity; death is no change and rigidity.

In its full state of health and harmony, the body has the ability to monitor and regulate its Chi by itself. In CNT you try to bring the body and its Chi to a state of adaptability to any circumstance.

Similar to gold and diamonds, Chi has many different grades ranging from the very rare and ethereal to coarse. The coarsest Chi forms into matter. Another grade of Chi flows outside the channels of the body and on its surface, defending the body from sickness. The finest Chi nourishes the most delicate body systems as well as the spirit. The body is formed from a condensed mixture of Universal Chi (Yang) and Earth Chi (Yin).

There are many expressions of Chi. The most precious is the Chi accumulated while you are in the womb. This is the Original, Prenatal or Ching Chi inherited from your parents. All Healing Tao practices encourage you to conserve this type of Chi since it is so nourishing. This Chi is the Original Force.

7. Chi and Blood

Chi and blood are the fundamental circulating energies in the body. Their condition and movement form the theoretical and practical basis for all healing in the Chinese healing arts. Blood is formed by combining Chi energy from food, Prenatal Chi or Original Force, and Chi in the air. It is a very dense form of Chi. It circulates through the heart, arteries, capillaries, and veins. Its course and function have been well charted by modern medicine. The arterial blood carries nutriments, oxygen, and nutritious Chi to all the body's cells. Venous blood is blood that has given up its nutrition and oxygen to the tissues, returning to the heart through the veins and carrying carbon dioxide to be eliminated through the lungs.

Blood and Chi flow side by side throughout the body wherever energy channels and blood vessels are parallel to one another. Chi is the motor force in blood and makes it lively, energetic, and supplies the power that allows it to course through the body. A famous saying captures their relationship, "When the Chi moves, the blood flows; if the Chi stagnates, the blood congeals."

Blood and Chi have tremendous healing power when they are full of nutrition and energy and can flow naturally and abundantly throughout the body. Problems arise with both vital energies when they are energy deficient, too hot, too cold, stagnant, or not moving forcefully enough. In practicing and teaching Chi Nei Tsang, you particularly will be concerned with the condition and flow of blood and Chi.

8. Yin and Yang

Yin and Yang are the two great polarities that emerged from the Original Chi to form all matter, including the human body. To discuss and evaluate Chi energy in the human body, it is necessary to determine whether it is Yin or Yang.

Yin is expressed as emotional, passive, receptive, empty, cerebral, night, earth, interior, inertia, cold, water, dark, rest, and the moon. Yin usually contracts and flows downward and inward. Yin is hidden deep within the interior body. Intelligence is Yin in composition.

Yang is expressed as creative, full, active, day, motion, hot, exterior, fire, heaven, and the sun. Yang expands and flows upward and outward. Yang is superficial; it is what you see. It is the expression of intelligence.

Although opposite in characteristics, they are not separate forces. They exist in relation to each other, having a constant and continuing influence on each other. Each holds a seed of the other, developing and eventually changing into the other. They are the front and back of the same coin. Yin and Yang are like a bar magnet with two energy poles functioning in a single energy field.

Taoists describe and define everything by the degree or proportion of Yin and Yang. Humans are created by a harmonious balance of these forces. You can stay healthy and live for a long time by keeping them in harmony. Perfect harmony means perfect health. Chi Nei Tsang aims toward achieving perfect harmony.

9. The Five Phases of Chi

The Taoists observed that five basic energy transformations flow from the Yin and Yang interactions. They are the Five Movements or Five Elemental Phases of Energy, most commonly called the Five Elements. In Taoism the physical elements found in nature (wood, fire, earth, metal, and water) symbolically express the five tendencies of energy in motion.

Chi passes through these phases. Thus, wood represents energy that is developing and generating. Fire represents energy that is expanding and radiating. Earth represents energy that is stabilizing and centering. Metal represents energy that is solidifying and contracting. Water is energy that is conserving, gathering, and sinking. Each of the five energies simultaneously express the interaction of Yin and Yang that is continuously emanating from the Primordial Energy.

The Five Elemental Phases are expressions of energy that can be observed in nature and throughout the universe. In space they influence the motions of the stars, planets, and other cosmic phenomena. On Earth they manifest themselves as the four seasons: Winter, Spring, Summer, and Fall with the fifth mediating element of Earth itself represented as Late Summer. Within the human body they affect the five sets of organs: the kidneys/bladder (Water), the liver/gall bladder (Wood), the heart/small intestine (Fire), the lungs/large intestine (Metal), and the pancreas/spleen/stomach (Earth). The forces that influence the Cosmos are identical with those that affect nature and our bodies.

B. Prenatal Chi: A Human Being's Original Energy

Taoists believe that when a man and woman join to make a child, all their body's essences are condensed in the sperm (Yang) and egg (Yin). The orgasmic forces generated during the sexual union of the sperm and egg have the power to draw in and join the Universal, Human Plane (Cosmic Particle,) and Earth Energies. Taoists refer to this process as the *Reunion of Heaven and Earth*. When these forces unite, they can draw in higher forces. These forces create the Prenatal Force that has no form and is like the Tao. Every new life starts with an "eyedropper" full of Prenatal Energy from the Tao.

All of these forces unite to form the first part of the embryo's Original Chi. The formation of the human body mirrors the formation of the Universe. First there is nothing. Then a human being starts to grow from the joining of one cell of the mother and one cell of the father. This is a mirror of the Tai Chi—the Great Primal Beginning. This cell generates the two primary forces of Yin and Yang which, in turn, generate three energy centers. These three energy centers form the Five Phases of

25

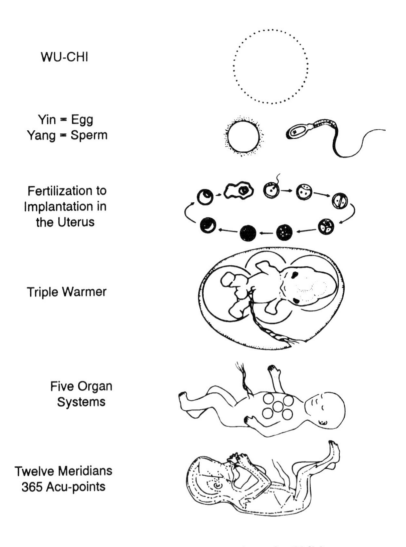

WU-CHI

Yin = Egg
Yang = Sperm

Fertilization to
Implantation in
the Uterus

Triple Warmer

Five Organ
Systems

Twelve Meridians
365 Acu-points

Figure 1-8. The Formation of a Child

Chi and the five paired organ systems whose energies extend throughout
the body creating all its myriad parts. (Figure 1-8)

From conception through the beginning of life at birth, the Original
Chi remains as the force of life. As a principal force, it continues to be a

dynamo of balanced Yin and Yang energy. If conserved and carefully cultivated, Taoists contend that it could empower you *forever*.

The Navel Center of the body constitutes the core of your Original Chi. All the functions of the body/mind/spirit revolve around the energetic Navel Center. It is the supplier of your energy, your "battery" or "power pack." It stores and transforms your most powerful energy. The area is known by the Taoists by many names. These names include the *Ocean of Chi*, the *Sea of Energy*, the *cauldron*, the *lower Tan Tien*, and the *Navel Center*. The Navel Center is the headquarters of our body and spirit. It is the main area you first will be concerned with and care for in Chi Nei Tsang. Later in your practice you will care for other centers.

C. The Navel Center or Tan Tien

Although the exact location of the Navel Center can vary with each individual, it is generally located in an area centrally behind the navel and in front of the point between Lumbar 2 and 3 of the spine. Occasionally it can be found as far as one to one and a half inches below the navel. If you dissect the physical body, you will not find a Tan Tien. It is located in what Taoists call the *subtle body*, so the location in the physical body is approximate.

The Tan Tien is considered to be the center of the body. It is both a generator and storage place for Chi energy. Also called the "Medicine Field," it has the curative power of the Original Chi or Prenatal Energy gathered there. In Chi Nei Tsang, the energy from this center is used to help the body function normally. For Taoist spiritual practice, the Tan Tien is the chief laboratory and center of internal alchemy.

The Lower Tan Tien Center is one of three "cauldrons" (energy centers) in the body that transform energy frequencies. The Middle Tan Tien is in the heart/solar plexus and the Upper Tan Tien is in the center of the brain. The importance of the Tan Tien, or Navel Center, stems from its role in the development of the embryo.

At conception, the embryo immediately begins to divide and soon attaches to the wall of the uterus. The umbilical cord develops and through it the developing fetus is nourished. The point where the umbilical cord attaches to the baby is the baby's navel. While a fetus is still in its mother's womb, energy enters the navel through the umbilical cord. It then travels through the left kidney, then the right kidney, then down to the sexual center, through the perineum, and up through the spine to

27

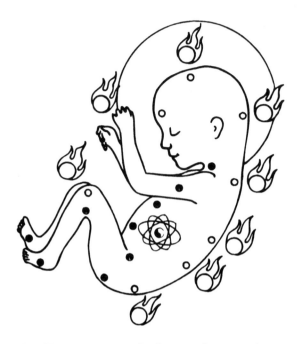

**Figure 1-9. Energy enters the human fetus at the navel
and circulates in the Microcosmic Orbit,
harmonizing Yin and Yang energies**

the head. Next it flows down through the tongue and back to the navel. This circulation route constitutes the Microcosmic Orbit which harmonizes the fetus' Yin and Yang energy. (Figure 1-9)

The fetus is nourished by navel energy. Also, waste is eliminated through the navel. After birth, as the child's body grows, the body continues to eliminate toxins into the navel area. Chi Nei Tsang has many techniques that will cause the toxins to leave the navel area and the body. The Navel Center balances all forces and is the center of physical gravity. The body moves around this center when sitting, standing, or practicing Tai Chi. The Navel Center processes and transforms the Universal, Human Plane or Cosmic Particle, and Earth Energies into life-force energy that is useful to the body. This function is similar to our physical digestive process. Taoists regard the navel as the place to transform, store, and receive the external forces. This area needs to be clear of congestion and tension so that energy can easily flow in and out. (Figure 1-10) The importance of the navel area cannot be overemphasized.

The Navel Center is where you can unify your body, mind, and spirit. This is the body's forceful Chi Energy Center. (Figure 1-11) If there is any problem with the energy in the Center, such as tangles, knots, blockages, or stagnation, then there may not be sufficient energy to feed the organs and their energy systems fully.

All Tao practices, including the Microcosmic Orbit, Tai Chi Chi Kung, Iron Shirt Chi Kung, and the higher practices, always end by bringing the energy back to the navel area. Energy is built up through the practices and exercises and stored in its storeroom—the Original Center. By keeping the center of the body filled with Chi and free of blockages, the energy can flow easily and powerfully, assuring good health, rejuvenation, and longevity.

D. The Body's Channels Circulate Healing Energy

Having cleared the toxins and emotional tensions that stagnate and congest Chi and blood, the Chi Nei Tsang process revitalizes the energy in the Navel Center. Knots, tangles, lumps, masses, fibroids, fat, swellings, and tumors can form, cluster, and accumulate in the abdomen, hindering the free and forceful flow of energy from the body's generator. After having cleared the area and infusing it with Cosmic, Universal, and Earth Energies, nature takes over to restore, renew, and revive the area. Once the energy can flow forcefully in its channels and vessels, the body/spirit is well on the way to healing itself.

When you allow the body/spirit free space to gather and circulate the three energies, you have taken a big step toward developing the immortal body/spirit. Human Plane (Cosmic Particle), Universal, and Earth Energies are the immortal energies. They have been around since time began. The more energies you can receive and integrate, the more like the energies you become. These energies are drawn into the Navel Center where they are mixed, "cooked," used to form an elixir, and circulated as combined energy throughout the body. The natural gestation of these energies stimulates the formation of white blood cells and T-cells that form the basis of the immune system. They can make the body disease resistant and enhance your health for a long life.

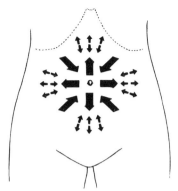

**Figure 1-10. The Navel Center collects and transforms
the Universal, Human Plane (Cosmic Particle), and Earth Forces
into life-force energy. It needs to be clear of emotional and environmental toxins so that energy can flow in and out**
Based on a drawing from *Emotional Anatomy* by Stanley Keleman, p.6.

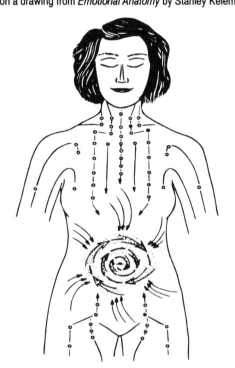

**Figure 1-11. The Navel Center is where you can unify
your body, mind, and spirit. It is impossible
to overemphasize its importance**

The immortal energies' mixture has the power to make new cells and tissues and replace toxic cells and tissues. Although this kind of cellular restoration is possible, it requires constant work since the health of new cells continuously deteriorates. If practiced regularly the Healing Tao process will allow you to gather and store enough energy to keep you well ahead of the day-to-day needs of cells and tissues. You will be able to provide for their needs and have energy left over. With these additional energies you can begin slowly to build a new body/spirit composed of immortal energies.

1. The Channels

The channels (often called *meridians* or *routes*) form an energy distribution network that connect and integrate all parts of the body. (Figure 1-12) Joined internally to the organs, the channels flow to the surface of the body and connect the limbs and sensory organs. Chi flows through the channels. Chi Nei Tsang work helps to provide the proper energy to the organs and their systems.

2. The Microcosmic Orbit

a. The Governor Channel

The Governor Channel moves the Yang Chi (Heavenly, Universal Energy) combining it with the Yin force that it channels up from the Earth. It runs from the perineum, up the spine, to the head. At the head it enters the brain, runs over the crown, down to the midpoint between the eyes, and ends at the roof of the mouth where it connects with the Functional Channel. (Figure 1-13) The Governor Channel, sometimes called the *Ocean of the Yang Channels,* can feed the combined energies to all six Yang channels that constantly reunite and flow in and out of it. This channel is closely associated with the brain, spinal fluid, and the reproductive system. Abundant energy flowing through this channel can help to strengthen and lengthen the spine. You will feel taller and stronger.

b. The Functional Channel

The Functional Channel moves the Yin Chi (Earth Energy) and helps channel the Yang force down from the Heavens to combine it with the Yin force. It normally runs up the front of the body from the perineum to the tip of the tongue. (Figure 1-13) When this channel is opened during the Microcosmic practice, its flow is reversed to run down the front of the body as it did when in the womb. Thus, the Taoists learned to restore

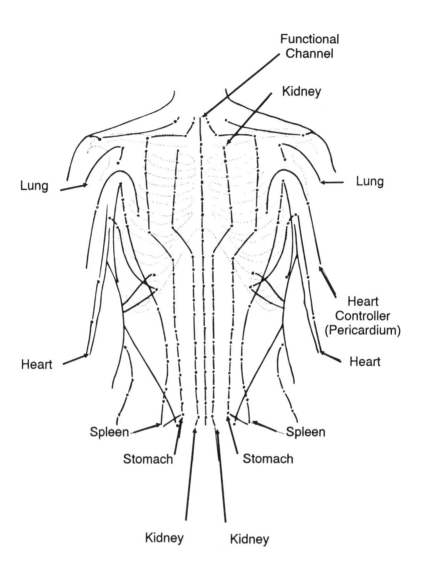

Figure 1-12. The meridians of the torso form part of the network of energy channels

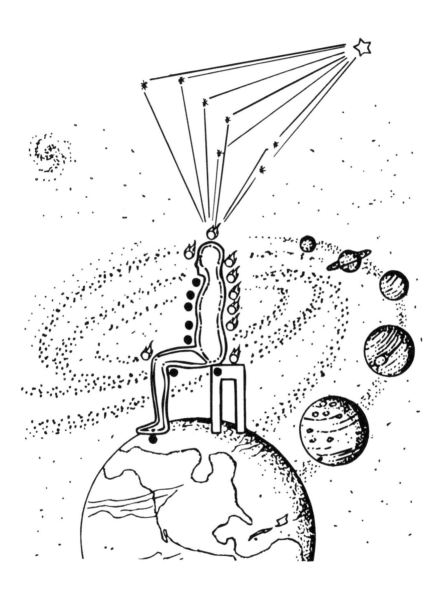

Figure 1-13. The Functional Channel (black dots—Yin) and Governor Channel (flaming balls—Yang) help absorb and circulate three basic energies

its prenatal flow. The Functional Channel, sometimes called the *Ocean of the Yin Channels,* can feed its combined energies to all six Yin channels that join it. This channel governs the fetus and the menstrual cycle.

3. The Thrusting Channels

The Thrusting Channels are very important and powerful energy routes in the body. They are in vertical alignment with the spine, and they most directly connect the Universal and Earth Energy's axes in men and women. If the energy from the Navel Center can flow powerfully through these routes, the organs and glands can be detoxified and energized.

Each channel is approximately one to one and a half inches wide. The Fusion II practice opens the Thrusting Channels to a much wider width. It also increases your awareness of these channels. Nonetheless, these channels are open and working to some extent in everyone.

Because the Thrusting Channels are connected to all the channels, they are considered a part of the *Sea of the Twelve Channels.* Thus, they can feed energy throughout the body.

Acupuncturists use the Middle Thrusting Channel, the *Chong-Mai,* to break up congested Chi and blood in the abdomen and chest. This channel is called the *Sea of Blood.* If you can clear out congestion in the abdomen and organs and vitalize the Navel Center, energy can flow freely through the Thrusting Channels to fortify the body.

The Thrusting Channels also extend down both legs to the feet and can be used to bring Earth Energy up into the lower cauldron. When practicing Chi Nei Tsang, you will be able to use the Thrusting Channels to draw in the Universal and Earth Energies and transfer them directly to your student.

a. The Left Thrusting Channel

The Left Thrusting Channel starts in the left testicle (in men), passes through the left perineum, left side of the anus, left ovary (in women), left kidney, spleen, heart, lung, left parathyroid and thyroid glands, left ear and eye, and left hemisphere of the brain. (Figure 1-14)

b. The Middle Thrusting Channel

The Middle Thrusting Channel starts at the middle of the scrotum (in men), passes through the perineum, middle of the anus, cervix (in women), prostate (in men), aorta, vena cava, pancreas, stomach, part of the liver, heart, thymus gland, throat, tongue, pituitary, hypothalamus and pineal glands, and crown. (Figure 1-15)

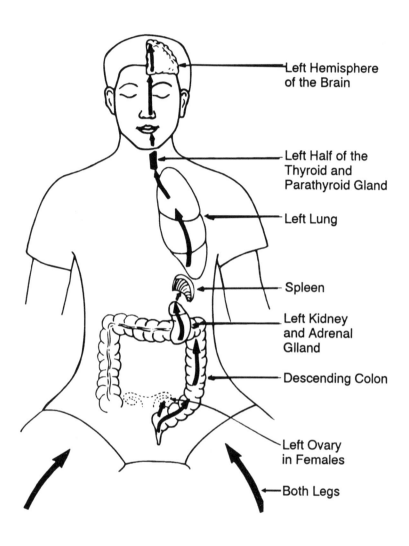

Figure 1-14. The Path of the Left Thrusting Channel

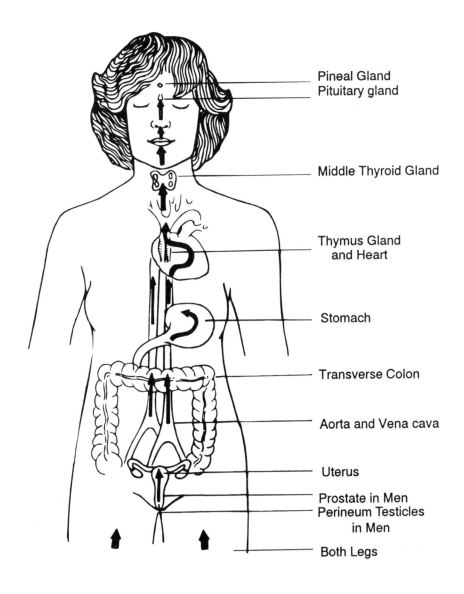

Pineal Gland
Pituitary gland

Middle Thyroid Gland

Thymus Gland
and Heart

Stomach

Transverse Colon

Aorta and Vena cava

Uterus

Prostate in Men
Perineum Testicles
in Men

Both Legs

Figure 1-15. The Path of the Middle Thrusting Channel

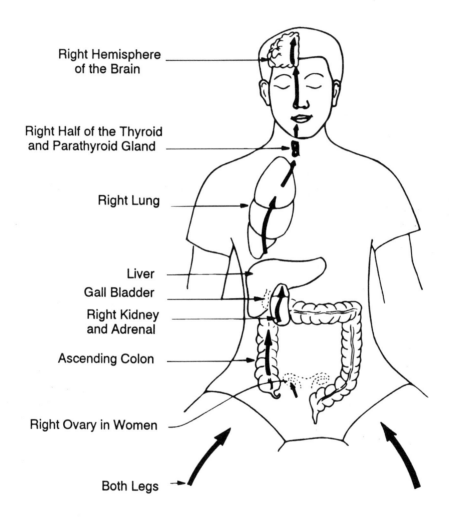

Right Hemisphere of the Brain

Right Half of the Thyroid and Parathyroid Gland

Right Lung

Liver

Gall Bladder

Right Kidney and Adrenal

Ascending Colon

Right Ovary in Women

Both Legs

Figure 1-16. The Path of the Right Thrusting Channel

c. The Right Thrusting Channel

The Right Thrusting Channel starts from the right testicle (in men), passes through the right perineum, right side of the anus, right ovary (in women), right kidney, liver, lung, right parathyroid and thyroid glands, right ear and eye, and right hemisphere of the brain. (Figure 1-16)

d. The Three Thrusting Channels

The three Thrusting Channels form a central energy route. The Universal and Earth Energies flow up or down them through the navel region. (Figure 1-17) They are interior to the Microcosmic Orbit.

4. The Belt Channel

The Belt Channel encircles the body with energy. Its circles protect and feed Chi to the surface of the body and help ward off negative energy from outside the body. Starting at the navel the Belt Channel crosses and encircles all the main energy centers of the torso, head, and legs. It

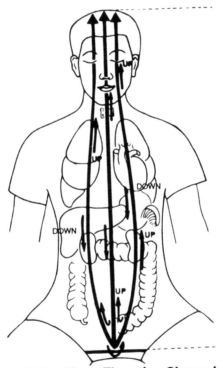

**Figure 1-17. The Three Thrusting Channels—
Chi energy can flow up or down**

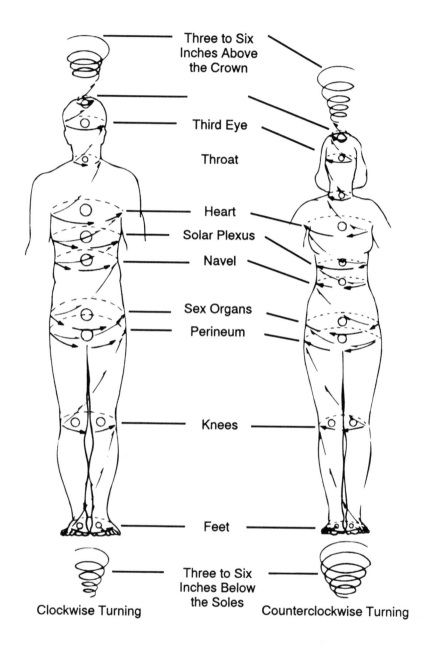

Three to Six Inches Above the Crown

Third Eye

Throat

Heart

Solar Plexus

Navel

Sex Organs

Perineum

Knees

Feet

Three to Six Inches Below the Soles

Clockwise Turning

Counterclockwise Turning

Figure 1-18. The Belt Channel encircles the body and feeds Chi energy to its surface

connects and binds all the channels that run up and down the body, including all the pathways passing through the abdomen. (Figure 1-18)

A cross section of the navel area shows that the Belt Channel connects all the vertical channels. At the front of the body, the Belt Channel connects with the Functional Channel. As the channel moves to the left side, it connects with the Left Thrusting Channel. In the back it connects with the Governor Channel. To the right it connects with the Right Thrusting Channel. Returning to the front, it completes the circle. (Figures 1-19, 1-20, and 1-21)

Energy traveling around the Belt Channel can move clockwise or counterclockwise. In addition, the vertical channels (Thrusting and Microcosmic) are also linked and bridged. Chi can flow up, down, in circles, right and left, and to the front or back.

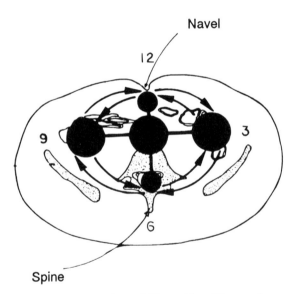

**Figure 1-19. The Belt and Thrusting Channels
at the Level of the Navel
These energy channels run throughout the body
and are interconnected by energy bridges permitting
energy to flow in many directions**

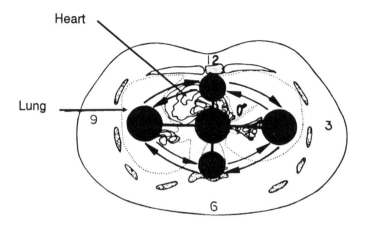

**Figure 1-20. The Belt and Thrusting Channels
at the Level of the Heart**

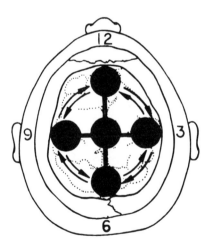

**Figure 1-21. The Belt and Thrusting Channels
at the Level of the Crown**

41

5. The Triple Warmer

The Triple Warmer is not recognized in Western medicine, but the Taoists believe it is Yang in quality and has three parts. The upper part includes the head, the heart, and the lungs. The middle part includes the digestive system. The lower part includes the kidneys, the lower intestines, and the reproductive system. (Figure 1-22) The Chinese believe that the Triple Warmer is also related to the hypothalamus, the part of the brain in charge of basic life functions including appetite, body temperature, and fluid balance. CNT "tunes up" the Triple Warmer by harmonizing its three parts, thereby maintaining its good working condition.

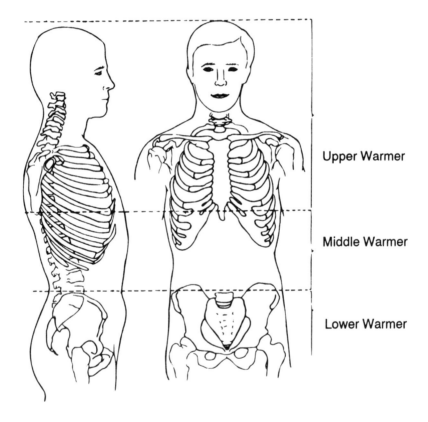

Upper Warmer

Middle Warmer

Lower Warmer

Figure 1-22. The Triple Warmer

The Triple Warmer is the body's thermostat, air conditioner, and heater for the energy that is flowing through it. When the heart is overheated, the Triple Warmer circulates heat down through the Middle Warmer to the lower area in the loins. There the hot energy is cooled and circulated back to the heart where it can help cool it. The descended warmth prevents the lower cool energies from becoming too cold.

6. Fasciae—Protective Layers of Chi

The fasciae are tissues that are the protective layers of every organ. They need to be moist to allow the free flow of energy. They are of varying thickness and strength and are found in all regions of the body surrounding the softer, more delicate organs. Medical books list 120 different types of fasciae. The deep and superficial fasciae hold our skin, muscles, bones, organs, and systems together, offering them a shield of protection and lubrication. (Figure 1-23)

Fasciae are structures for Chi. Large amounts of Chi can be packed into the fasciae to make them strong and keep them moist. When they

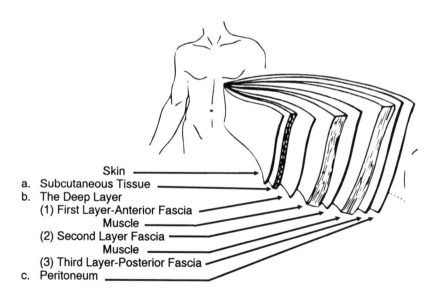

Skin
a. Subcutaneous Tissue
b. The Deep Layer
    (1) First Layer-Anterior Fascia
            Muscle
    (2) Second Layer Fascia
            Muscle
    (3) Third Layer-Posterior Fascia
c. Peritoneum

Figure 1-23. The Three Layers of the Fasciae of the Skin

are deficient in Chi, they become dry, hard, and brittle. The fasciae are the conduits of Chi flowing in the body. The organ channels pass through the fasciae. When the fasciae are dry, Chi cannot flow well and the body can feel stiff and hard. Movement can become painful.

Good Chi flow through the fasciae means good flow everywhere. Healthy fasciae means good energy, flexibility, and structural integrity. Healthy fasciae feel like taut sheets of strong, thin material offering a flexible shield of protection. As you practice Chi Nei Tsang, especially skin detoxification, you are improving the fasciae and the organ or system you are focusing on.

The abdomen has many levels of fasciae; in fact, it has the greatest concentration of fasciae in the body.

E. The Body's Energy Grid and Center

In combination all of these channels comprise the body's energy grid. The body is sufficiently well wired to send energy where it is

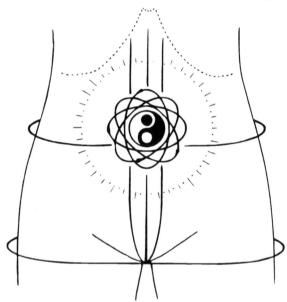

Figure 1-24. The Navel Center and the Energy Grid
This Center feeds energy to the body/mind/spirit
via the vertical and horizontal channels

needed. It is crucial that the abdominal region be clear so that pure energy coming from the energetic core is always free to flow. (Figure 1-24)

The Navel Center is the doorway between the physical body and the energy body. All energy channels that create and sustain the physical body emerge from there and return there. You can feel and experience it. The Tan Tien is the *Ocean of the Real Elixir* (Original Chi, the mother of the body's energies). Original Chi can heal the human body and restore it to its original wholeness. The water from the cosmic, mother womb which flows into your body through the doorway of the Navel Center restores health and purity and balances cells. If blockages build up around its passageways, this marvelous energy cannot get through. Chi Nei Tsang massage can open the way for it so it can help restore your vim and vigor.

F. The Taoist View of the Human Energy System

1. The Five Phases of Chi (the Five Elements)

The five energies that give birth to the Universe also form the organs and the personality. (Figure 1-25) Thus, each human being, as a microcosm of these same elemental energies, reflects the Universe and its interacting forces. At the human level these *Five Phases of Chi* are constantly energizing and returning to the primordial Chi within the body's three Tan Tiens (navel, heart, and head). This is why Taoists view human beings as a microcosmic copy of the macrocosmic forces.

The organs and bowels each emanate their special form of Chi. The variety of energy relationships among the Five Phases of Chi allows the skilled Chi Nei Tsang practitioners, using techniques described in Chapter 3, to figure out the strengths and weaknesses of the prevailing energies and to respond to them.

One way to perceive the state of the body, the mind, and the spirit is through constant observation of the Five Phases and of the Yin and Yang components of all processes in Heaven, on Earth, and in human beings. Although conditions are constantly changing, they do so according to the Laws of Nature which constantly repeat themselves. In observing the seasons you can, if you are keen, see what is coming. This is no easy task, but the tools are available. You can learn to use them.

Planet Venus
Autumn
Metal Force
Lungs/Large Intestine

Planet Mars
Summer
Fire Force
Heart/Small Intestine

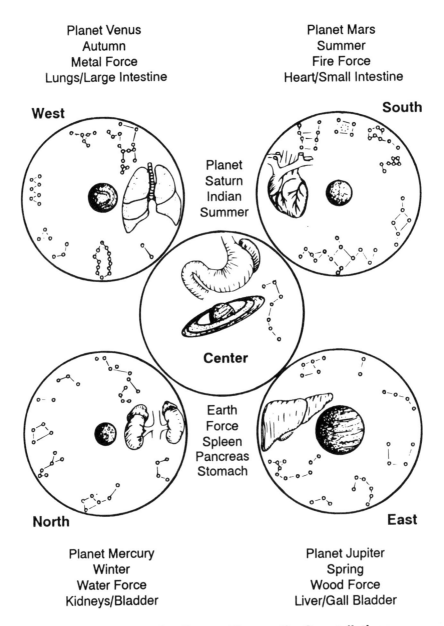

West

Planet
Saturn
Indian
Summer

South

Center

Earth
Force
Spleen
Pancreas
Stomach

North

East

Planet Mercury
Winter
Water Force
Kidneys/Bladder

Planet Jupiter
Spring
Wood Force
Liver/Gall Bladder

Figure 1-25. The Five Energy Phases, the Constellations, and the Organs Associated with Them

Author John Blofeld in his book, *The Quest for Immortality*, has captured the essence of the Taoists' understanding of these Five Phases as follows:

> "The Five Elements are not elements so much as activities. The sages who devised the science recognized five main types of natural processes whose interactions bear a certain resemblance to the inter-actions of wood, fire, earth, metal and water, the affinity being more allegorical than actual. They understood that nature's workings depend upon a system of fine balances among processes that may help, hinder or block one another according to the relative strength of each in a given situation. Having devoted much of their time to tranquil contemplation of nature, they had watched these sometimes conflict-ing forces at work and learnt to predict the outcome of such conflicts, or even to manipulate that outcome within certain narrow limits, as when one…diverts the water in a stream. Mastery of the five element science conferred a degree of foresight that amounted to divination and the power to divert the course of nature in ways that must often have seemed spectacular to the uninitiated." (p. 6)

a. The Wood Phase of Energy and the Liver/Gall Bladder

The liver is the general in charge of defending the body. It is in charge of the smooth, unhampered flow of Chi and blood to all parts of the body. Its Chi flows upward and outward and approaches from the planet Jupiter and the East. The liver is associated with the Spring season. This energy is most powerful between one and three a.m.

The liver provides a growing, generating, developing, warm, moist, and fertile type of energy. Wood energy recalls that of an equatorial morning sun, the promise and potentiality of a newborn child, the rising sap in a young tree, or the full, abundant energy of a swollen spring river.

The liver stores and filters the blood, regulates the blood supply, and produces proteins. It also stores toxins until it has the time to transform them into healthy energy.

If the liver's Chi and blood is healthy, balanced, and abundant, then the nails will be healthy, the vision clear, the nerves calm, and the sinews and tendons will have sufficient energy.

The positive quality of the emotion in Wood is kindness tempered with intelligence. One tends to be cool-headed, discreet, relaxed, clear minded, creative, progressive, constructive, conciliatory, and willing to work with others.

The negative qualities of the Wood phase's emotion are anger, violence, or making big plans without knowing what one is doing. One tends to be opportunistic, short-tempered, hot-headed, loud, tight, pressured, rough, obsessed, stubborn, pedantic, formalistic, competitive, and antagonistic.

The idea that anger can affect the liver is recognized in the English language as the word "liverish," meaning irascible or short-tempered and full of anger.

Once sober, many recovering alcoholics who spent years poisoning their livers (for the liver collects toxins) are able and embarrassed to see how rough and full of anger they once were. They are grateful and pleasantly surprised to discover that once they have stopped drinking, they are very gentle and solicitous about the feelings of others and are often overcome with many spontaneous acts of human kindness.

b. The Fire Phase of Energy and the Heart/Small Intestine

The heart is the ruler of the body/mind/spirit. It transforms Chi and blood and is in charge of the circulation of the blood. Its Chi flows upward to the brain and downward to balance the organs. This Chi approaches from the South and from the planet Mars. It is associated with the Summer season. It is most active from eleven a.m. to one p.m.

The heart is the home of the spirit. The spirit comprises the best energy from all the organs: joy, compassion, courage, fairness, gentleness, kindness. The presence (or absence) of these qualities determines the personality.

Although the energies of all the organs are important because they balance each other and allow us to live varied and interesting lives, the heart is the favorite organ in every culture. In Chinese medicine, the heart is known as the *Emperor of the Five Vital Organs*. Its function is to issue the *Imperial Fire Energy* of love and compassion.

English speaking people recognize the warmth and centrality of the heart in such expressions as heart-warming, heartthrob, heart of gold, heart-to-heart, hearten, hearty, heart and soul. Those humans with negative energy in the heart are called heartless or hard-hearted. Their callousness often causes others to feel heartsick.

Fire Chi is youthful but mature energy that is available at any age. It is expansive and vigorous. It is like the energy of the full bloom of Summer. It fuels art, inspiration, creativity, the force of genius, and many functions most vital to the person, family, and society.

Fire Chi feeds the face and eyes. It is easy to recall the face of an absent friend who has abundant heart Chi, for his or her face has a radiant, rosy, lustrous complexion and is bright, sparkling, and lively.

It is not surprising to learn that this energy also powers the will and feeds the hormones and the endocrine system. As you continue working with the Fire Force, you will become more familiar with its central role and can teach your students how they can protect their Spirit and kindle a steady Fire Chi and warm glow.

The positive qualities of emotion in Fire are joy, happiness, spirituality, lovingness, virtuosity, heartiness, warmth, patience, respect, politeness, refinement, brightness, and concern.

The negative aspects are cold, cruel, vicious, inconsiderate, obsequious, thoughtless, tasteless, impatient, dull, humorless, and hateful.

c. The Earth Phase of Energy and the Spleen/Pancreas/Stomach

The Earth Force approaches from Saturn and is associated with the center of all directions.

If Wood is the *infant* or growing Chi, and Fire is the maturing, *young adult* Chi, then the Earth Force is the fully mature, *adult* Chi. Earth Chi provides a stabilizing energy. If the body/spirit was all Fire, one can easily burn out. Like a beautiful fiery comet, one can present a startling and glowing display, but a display that is too short-lived. The opposing force of the Earth Force is Water, powerful as an iceberg or glacier. If the body/spirit was all Water energy, then one could be considered cold and withdrawn.

The Earth Force refracts all the other energies as they pass from one phase to another. In this way it introduces a mediating factor in our systems that helps to balance and blend the other energies. This fits in with the central location of the spleen, pancreas, and stomach. This Earth Energy controls thought and provides mental clarity. It allows the kind of energy that is necessary to evaluate and review our lives and make necessary adjustments.

The spleen, pancreas, and stomach are the organs through which the Earth element functions. Operating like a switchboard, it is in charge of absorbing, forming, and transporting the energy and Chi from food. The Earth produces food and, so, the Earth Energy is the energy of Indian Summer or harvest time. In almost every land and culture, this is the time for assessment, reflection, planning, and preparation. This is when we feel the first chill of Autumn, which usually makes us momentarily ground and stabilize ourselves so that we can make sure that we are prepared for the coming Winter.

The positive qualities of Earth Energy are associated with sensitivity to others and feeling spontaneous, fair, open-minded, genuine, harmonious, centered, rooted, balanced in desire and appetite, punctual, synchronized, sociable, and hospitable.

Being prejudiced, overly prepared (not spontaneous), and too worried are the negative qualities of Earth. Timing is always off and one is always too soon or too late. The person lacking abundant and balanced Earth Energy tends to be artificial, fake, awkward, disconnected, and imbalanced. Desire turns to envy. Any negative traits in the other four phases are amplified without the moderating influence of strong Earth Energy. The appetite turns into craving or there is no appetite at all. One becomes unfriendly and inconsiderate.

The English and French languages both contain a word that indicates that at one time people in the West were aware of the potential negative emotional content of the spleen, and the havoc its negative qualities of worry and anxiety could create. The words are *splenetic* and *spleneitique*, respectfully. Webster's dictionary defines splenetic as, "bad-tempered; irritable; peevish; spiteful; spleenful."

d. The Metal Phase of Energy and the Lungs/Large Intestine

The force of Metal is said to be linked with the planet Venus, approaches from the West, and is strongest during the Fall season. Its energy is most active between three and five a.m.

Metal is the energy of the lungs. The Chinese word for this energy is *gold* which implies the highest and most evolved quality of metal.

It is appropriate that the Taoists named this phase of Chi Metal for the lungs are the body's energy forge. In the lungs Chi from the air mixes with Chi from food and Prenatal Chi to produce blood and two refined Chi's: nutritious and defensive. These types of Chi combine with the Prenatal Chi stored in the kidneys.

Nutritious Chi is the hardest working Chi in the body. It travels with the blood and in the channels throughout the system. When you feel full of energy or need a burst of energy you are drawing upon your reservoir of nutritious Chi. When abundant, this Chi warms the feet and hands, moistens the skin, and grows luxuriant hair.

The lungs also control the skin, pores, and sweat, and brings into play defensive Chi. Defensive Chi travels from the lungs to the surface fasciae. It inhabits the cells of surface skin as well as beneath the skin. When the Taoists developed Iron Shirt and Golden Bell, two legendary kung fu forms, they mastered the development of defensive Chi. They could pack the fasciae and concentrate the Chi on the surface so that they were invincible and could absorb a punch or deflect a knife thrust.

Keeping defensive Chi plentiful and abundant works to your advantage because it protects you from outside germs and viruses that want to invade the body. These can include winds, dampness, flu, tuburculosis, and others.

The skin is also known as "the third lung" both in the East and West and helps the lungs eliminate carbon dioxide. In the Taoist exercises of Bone Marrow breathing, one learns to draw in Chi directly through the pores of the skin.

Good Metal Chi, like the Autumn air, helps one to experience clear, crisp, sharp, cool, and dry sensations and mental states.

Serious and sober, it is the energy of a steady gaze and heroic determination. This is the energy one can call upon to resolve any contradiction and get the job done. Metal energy fills one with courage, purity, rectitude, solidity, sharing, generosity, and forgiveness.

The negative qualities of Metal include hypocrisy, grief, sadness, depression, dishonesty, affectation, confusion, unreliability, irresponsibility, pettiness, stinginess, jealously, and resentment.

e. The Water Phase of Energy and the Kidneys/Bladder

Water, associated with the kidneys, is the foundation energy in the body which feeds energy to all the organs. When it is abundant, the body is balanced, beautiful, and powerful. It is crucial to keep the kidneys healthy, producing this vital energy. All the organs are vital. If any one of them became dysfunctional, you could become very ill. If matched according to the vitality of the energy they can produce, the kidneys would easily be the most powerful. The Water phase is also associated with the planet Mercury, approaches from the Northern direction, and corresponds to the Winter season.

The Winter is a time for gathering and conserving. External life is chilled or frozen, but life continues internally. This is the season of hibernation both for bears and humans snowbound in warm homes and cabins. Trees, seeds, animals, and people are all saving and conserving their energies until they can again welcome the Spring—the season of growth and renewal.

51

ELEMENT \ QUALITY	WOOD	FIRE	EARTH	METAL	WATER
YIN ORGAN	LIVER	HEART	SPLEEN/PANCREAS	LUNGS	KIDNEYS
YANG ORGAN	GALL BLADDER	SMALL INTESTINE	STOMACH	LARGE INTESTINE	BLADDER
POSITIVE EMOTIONS	KINDNESS	LOVE, JOY, RESPECT	FAIRNESS, OPENNESS	UPRIGHTNESS, RIGHTEOUSNESS, COURAGE	GENTLENESS
NEGATIVE EMOTIONS	ANGER	HATE, IMPATIENCE	WORRY, ANXIETY	SADNESS, DEPRESSION	FEAR
PLANET	JUPITER	MARS	SATURN	VENUS	MERCURY
DIRECTION	EAST	SOUTH	CENTER	WEST	NORTH
QUALITY OF ENERGY	GROWING, DEVELOPING, GENERATING	EXPANDING, RADIATING	STABILIZING	CONTRACTING	CONSERVING, GATHERING
GROWING CYCLE	SEED SPROUTING, LEAVES GROWING	BLOOM, FRUIT GROWING	FRUIT, RIPENING, HARVETST	SEED FALLING	DORMANSEED
SEASON	SPRING	SUMMER	INDIAN SUMMER	FALL	WINTER
PASSAGE ON EARTH	INFANCY	YOUTH	ADULT	OLD AGE	DEATH
BODY'S SOUND	SHOUTING	LAUGHING	SINGING	WEEPING	GROANING
TASTE	SOUR	BITTER	SWEET	SPICEY, PUNGENT	SALTY
NOURISHES THE:	NERVES, TENDONS	BLOOD VESSELS, VASCULAR SYSTEM	MUSCLES, FLESH,FASCIAE	SKIN	BONES, TEETH
OPENS INTO AND COMMANDS THE	EYES	TONGUE	LIPS,MOUTH	NOSE	EARS
TEMPERATURE	WARM & DAMP	HOT	MILD	COOL & DRY	COLD
PRODUCES	TEARS	SWEAT	SALIVA	MUCOUS	URINE
BODY SCENT	RANCID, GOATISH	BURNED, SCORCHED	FRAGRANT	RANK, FLESHY	ROTTEN, PUTRID

ELEMENT / QUALITY	WOOD	FIRE	EARTH	METAL	WATER
EXPANDS INTO	NAILS	FACIAL COLOR	LIPS	BODY HAIR	HAIR ON HEAD
COLOR	GREEN	RED	YELLOW,BROWN	WHITE	BLACK,DARK BLUE
SOUND	SHHHHHHHH	HAWWWWWWW	WHOOOOOOO (GUTTERAL)	SSSSSSSSS	WOOOOOOOO
FUNCTION	CONTROL & DECISIVENESS	WARMTH, VITALITY, EXCITEMENT	ABILITY TO INTEGRATE, STABLIZE, FEEL CENTERED & BALANCED	STRENGTH & STABILITY	AMBITION & WILL POWER
RELATIONHIP TO VITAL FUNCTION	NERVOUS SYSTEM	BLOOD, HORMONES ENDOCRINE SYSTEM	DIGESTION, LYMPHATIC & MUSCULAR SYSTEMS	RESPIRATORY SYSTEM	REPRODUCTIVE & URINARY SYSTEM
RELATIONSHIP WITH THE BLOOD	STORES & FILTERS THE BLOOD	CIRCULATES THE BLOOD	STORES & CLEANSES THE BLOOD	ELIMINATES CO_2 & OTHER TOXINS, OXYGENATES THE BLOOD	PRODUCES BLOOD IN THE BONE MARROW
RELATIONSHIP WITH THE DIGESTION OF FOOD	MANUFACTURES PROTEINS,RECYLES POISONS, DISTRIBUTES NUTRITION	ABSORPTION & SELECTION OF FOOD IN SMALL INTESTINE	MONITORING FOOD INTAKE, SENDS ENERGY TO EACH ORGAN ACCORDING TO TASTE	ELIMINATION THROUGH LARGE INTESTINE	MONITORING
RELATIONSHIP TO THE CHI	HAS A WARMING EFFECT	HAS A HEATING EFFECT	HAS A BALANCING EFFECT	HAS A COOLING & DRYING EFFECT	HAS A CHILLING EFFECT
ANIMAL SPIRITS	GREEN DRAGON	RED PHEASANT	YELLOW PHOENIX	WHITE TIGER	BLACK TORTISE
SPIRITUAL HOME	SPIRITUAL SOULS	SPIRIT	DECISION	ANIMAL SOULS	INTENTION
MENTAL ASPECT	MENTAL CLARITY	INTUITION	SPONTANEITY	EMOTIONAL SENSITIVITY	WILL POWER, CREATIVITY

Figure 1-26. Chart of Relationships of the Five Phases of Energy

Water means life. It is the element of birth, growth, purification, cleanliness, regeneration, and renewal. It is also the essence of the Earth. Life energy arises from the Water element. This follows most theories of evolution that portray the human being as a life form that emerged from the sea. The life that water gives also can be taken away by destructive floods or tidal waves.

The kidneys store the energy passed down from our ancestors and parents. The kidneys govern all the crucial functions of life including birth, growth, reproduction, sexuality, and aging. Taoists say the kidneys also store the energy that determines the length of your life.

The negative emotion of fear originating in the kidneys can adversely effect the kidneys and the bladder, its paired organ. One sometimes hears stories of soldiers or airmen frightened in battle who have lost control of their bladder.

If you are balding, and it is not due to congenital defects, it is because you have a problem with the kidneys. The kidneys determine the strength of the bones and the health of bone marrow. They can also affect brain matter and can influence whether you are smart or dull-witted. Beside controlling hearing they are also in charge of the urethra, bladder, urine, and sperm. One of the most vital function of the kidneys is their control of the uterus.

Water controls the will; a strong will means that Water energy is abundant. If the kidneys' energy is weak, you may lose the power to decide what happens to you in your future.

The positive emotions of the Water phase of Chi are connected with a prudent, sensuous, and persistent power of alertness. Strong kidneys' energy helps to create men and women who are cool, comfortable, and unafraid, as opposed to those who feel cold, wet, and terrified.

Gentleness is the positive quality associated with Water energy. It is implied in the smooth rhythms of a bubbling brook, the placid calm of a high mountain lake, or the gentle but powerful movement of waves arising from the oceans' great depths.

Fear, as a negative emotion of Water, is fast and constricting. Other negative emotions are lewdness, paranoia, impermanence, coldness, small-mindedness, scatteredness, stagnancy, and running in circles without getting anywhere.

2. The Chart of the Five Phases of Energy

A Chart of the Five Phases of Energy (Figure 1-26) presents the qualities and relationships of Wood, Fire, Earth, Metal, and Water. Study and refer to it often and learn to distinguish their differences.

G. The Laws of Creation and Control

1. The Law of Creation

The Law of Creation establishes a cycle and an engendering Mother and Child relationship among the Five Phases. Spring/Liver/Wood provides the nourishment and helps maintain its child, Summer/Heart/Fire. This energy engenders, mothers, nourishes, and maintains its child, the Harvest/Spleen/Earth. The Harvest bears and brings forth the Autumn/Lungs/Metal which fosters the coming of Winter/Kidneys/Water. Winter ends the cycle, but in the way that it has always been, Winter will soon awaken the Spring. (Figure 1-27)

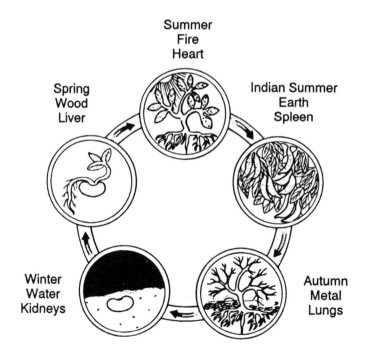

Figure 1-27. The Creation Cycle

55

For example, within the Law in the Creation, if an organ is weak, cold, and too Yin, or what Chinese medicine calls "deficient," then strengthen the Season/Organ that proceeds it in the Cycle. This would be the "mother" of the sick organ, the one from which the sick organ was born. The theory is that the Mother, when stronger, will pass on her excess energy to the child.

Similarly, if an organ has too much energy, is too hot, or too Yang, or has what Chinese medicine calls "excess" energy, you would take away some of the energy from the next organ, or child, in the cycle. This would give the excess energy in the troubled organ a place to go. Again, the mother will always give her excess energy to the child.

2. The Law of Control

This concept establishes a way for an organ to cross check, constrain, and temper an organ that is trying to overwhelm a weaker organ. The image of an adult abusing a child, as grim as it is, captures this relationship. In this case you may call in another member of the family,

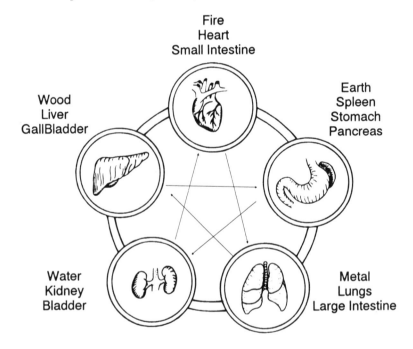

Fire
Heart
Small Intestine

Earth
Spleen
Stomach
Pancreas

Wood
Liver
GallBladder

Water
Kidney
Bladder

Metal
Lungs
Large Intestine

Figure 1-28. The Control Cycle

perhaps an aunt or sister (organ), to restrain the overbearing parent and rescue the child.

Under the Law of Control, the liver controls the spleen, the spleen controls the kidneys, the kidneys control the heart, the heart controls the lungs, the lungs control the liver. (Figure 1-28)

Chi Nei Tsang

CHAPTER 2

PREPARATION, TRAINING, AND PROTECTION

A. Adapting to the Healing Energy Environment

As a Chi Nei Tsang practitioner or instructor, you have the responsibility to maintain a clear, healthy body with a pure, strong blood and Chi flow. You are the standard of healthy energy and a healthy body to which you can compare the energy of your student. You then can distinguish any problems or foreign elements that may be blocking his or her energy flow. Remember that the process of Chi Nei Tsang involves not only direct channeling of the Universal, Cosmic Particle, and Earth Forces into your body, but also processing them within your body to make their energies suitable for others to use.

Any negative emotions that you may be feeling can be passed on to another person. Therefore, continually practicing Chi Nei Tsang on yourself is very important. Once you have cleared your abdominal area, you may find your emotional condition has changed and your attitude has improved. By releasing your blockages, you will be better equipped to help another release them.

In this chapter, many exercises are presented that will help you to keep your energy clear, balanced, and powerful. You do not need to do all the practices before working with someone. You can choose one practice and come back to the others later. Gradually, you can master them all.

1. Establishing a Strong Connection with Your Sources of Energy

Since it is important to maintain your energy, it is first necessary to establish a connection with your sources of energy. You can connect with the energies of the Universe, Human Plane, and Earth, and unify and blend them into one energy. When you connect with these energies, you will be strong and the energy flowing through you will be of the correct quality and quantity to help your student.

2. Practicing Meditation Daily

To maintain your energy, meditate every day to reconnect with the outer forces and burn out sick and undesired energy. Often, those who lose touch with these outer forces find their egos rising and expanding. In such a situation you may believe you have the power to heal others, but you really are not equipped and can easily pick up sick energy.

The Healing Hands Meditation, when practiced every day, increases the ability of your hands to channel the Universal, Human Plane (Cosmic Particle), and Earth Energies. You will be able to feel the energy emerging from your palms and fingers as you touch the student.

3. Preventing the Depletion of Your Energy

Most healing professionals inadvertently pick up sick energy from their students. Many discover they need to help themselves once they realize what has happened to them. The procedure followed in CNT is to channel the Universal, Human Plane Cosmic Particle, and Earth Forces and preserve your energy when possible.

4. Recognizing that Healing is a Gift of Nature

Everyone in good health can heal. The healing ability means having a powerful life-force. Having a powerful life-force means having a higher vibration, something that can be given to others to help them. When you send your life-force energy into another, your energy has to be greater or at a higher level to affect his or her energy.

Each person, however, has only a limited amount of energy. This is why it is important to connect with the Universal, Human Plane, and Earth Energies and let yourself become a channel through which the energy can flow. Your success will depend on your ability to open your channels and transform the energy.

Most people can transform outside energies into useful energy. Ordinarily, it takes one year for a person to absorb enough Universal Energy to be effective. That is the time it takes for the Earth to revolve around the Sun. (Figure 2-1) But with the practice of the Cosmic Particle Chi Circulation and the Tree exercises, you can quicken the process of energy absorption and transformation without overheating your system or creating a problem of cosmic energy indigestion. The energy is immediately useful.

5. Transforming Energy

You cannot destroy energy, but you can transform it. As you engage in healing someone, Chi Nei Tsang techniques help you locate the problem and boost their level energy. You help them to transform their energy. You start the fire, but the student has to maintain it and not let it die out. If you teach the student the Inner Smile, the Six Healing Sounds, and the Microcosmic Orbit, these techniques, along with the CNT training, will help them transform their sick, negative energy into good life-force energy.

6. Giving and Taking Energy

As you try to help a person and your life-force energy flows into him or her, be sure your energy is healthy. Otherwise any sick energy you send will create the same sickness in that person.

The reverse also holds true. As you send energy into a person, his or her energy passes to you. This means that this person's problems become your problems. There is no such thing as becoming involved with the healing without also becoming involved with the problem. This is how many people in the healing arts get sick. Their energy systems are not efficient enough to counteract the effects of the sick energy to which they have exposed themselves.

Young and healthy people who enter these professions can get by with no apparent ill effects because they have "energy to burn." However, they are depleting their energies and the sick energies they take on eventually do affect them. This is why it is important to think that you are not simply healing them, but you are a teacher and an adviser. Developing and maintaining an open channel to the Universal, Human Plane, and Earth Energies will help you avoid picking up sick energy and help you burn out the sick energy when it enters you.

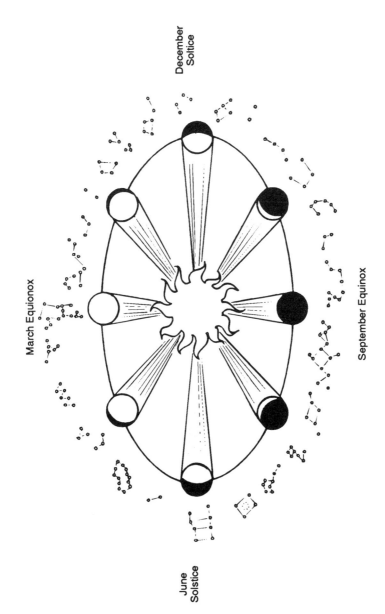

Figure 2-1. Ordinarily, it takes one year for a person to absorb enough Universal Energy to be an effective healer. Meditation can greatly quicken the absorption process.

7. Becoming a Channel for Powerful Forces

The more channels you open, the better off you are. Therefore, to receive energy, it is important to open at least the two major channels (Functional and Governor) of the Microcosmic Orbit. It is better still to add the Thrusting and Belt Channels. By doing so you will know firsthand the way your energy flows. Then you can direct and draw in healthy energy, and use it to burn sick energy out of your system. By first opening the energy channels within yourself, you become more efficient as a healer and can avoid succumbing to the illnesses that you are removing from another.

The quickest way to open your Microcosmic Orbit is to take a weekend workshop with a certified Healing Tao Instructor. You may also teach yourself by using the *Awakening the Healing Light* book or video. To open the Thrusting and Belt Channels, you could study with us, a certified instructor, or teach yourself by using the *Fusion of the Five Elements I* book and Fusion I, II, and III videos. Audio tapes are also available.

8. Restoring the Force after Each Session

It is important that after each practice session you sit and meditate. Be sure that you are free of sick energy before ending your meditation. You may feel coldness in the hands, itchy skin, and a lack of energy. Meditate until you feel warmth in your hands; it will burn out the sick energy. Use the Fusion I practice to get more energy into the navel and transform the sickness into positive life-force.

9. Protecting Your Body from Sick Energy

When helping someone it is possible to accumulate sick energy on the surface of the skin of the hands and arms. Do not allow it to go beyond the shoulders and enter the body. If you practice daily, your mind's power can hold back the encroachment of the sick energy.

There are many different theories on how to get rid of this unwanted energy. Some people advocate washing the hands. If you do this, make sure that you use cold, running water, or you can drive the energy into your body further.

One method is to place your hands on a surface conductive to Earth Energy and connected to a ground (e.g., a water pipe). Iron will do, as will a brick or cement wall that has a footing. It will pass the sick energy down to the earth. The earth can help neutralize sick energy.

With some sick energies this grounding method is not effective or powerful enough. Therefore, our advice is that you meditate as well so that you are sure to be clean.

10. Using the Earth and Trees for Healing

Trees, especially pines, are excellent for taking the sick energy into the Earth, as are other trees and plants. Houseplants, however, do not receive the direct energy of the Sun, nor are they directly connected with the Earth. They can only absorb limited quantities of sick energy.

The sick energy of other people can seep into your inner organs and accumulate there. It is a very dense, coarse energy and can feel both cold and biting. This is, by far, the worst way to experience sick energy. A tree can handle this energy by sending it into the healing Earth.

11. Handling with Care

When you help other heart-to-heart and center-to-center, permitting the sick energy to enter you, it is very easy to exhaust your energy. You are then of no use to anyone. Evil or sick energy needs an outlet. If it is not eliminated, it will stay with you. Therefore, meditating as soon as possible after a session is extremely important. Do not ignore this advice.

The previously mentioned Healing Hands Meditation, used to expand your aura, and Cosmic Chi Kung (to be described in a forthcoming book) are very important practices. They create a field of energy within and around you that will defend your body and spirit. This field of energy burns out and transforms the sick energy as it enters through your fingers before it has the chance to enter your organs. Iron Shirt Chi Kung is another very effective means of protecting your organs from another's sick energy.

Energies are very real and must be treated with respect. As your energy channels and aura become strong, you can control and have access to your energy. You can magnify your ability to sense what is happening in your hands. This will place you in a better position to deal with the presence of sick energies. You will learn a means of forcibly moving energy out through your fingertips, thereby strengthening all your energy systems.

A healer is knowledgeable and, above all, careful with his or her treatment of life-force energy. Only then can the healing experience be gratifying both for the teacher and the student. Risking affliction could be very costly.

12. Checking Your Energy Level

Upon arising in the morning, spend a few moments checking your energy level. If your energy level is not good, take time to raise its level.

Never overdo anything. If your energy is low, or if you do not feel well, do not attempt to give a session to anyone. The meditations mentioned or described above and below are very important to help you raise your energy to a higher level. The Microcosmic Orbit and Fusion exercises are very powerful means of checking and replenishing your energy level. Fusion II is very useful for warding off most ill effects by using the Thrusting Channels, and, especially, the Belt Channel.

At all times it is wise to take precautions and to know what you are doing. Advice and warnings about healing energy and sick energy are consistently given throughout this book. It is extremely important that you follow instructions carefully on how to care for yourself.

B. Preparing Yourself Physically

When creating the strong, healthy body necessary to practice CNT, bear in mind that energy flows to the place it is needed. If your energy is lower than your students, his energy will flow to you and he will become weaker. In emphasizing physical preparation, it is important to know that tendons, muscles, fasciae, channel systems, and bones draw in power that can be channeled to another.

1. Iron Shirt Chi Kung

The Iron Shirt Chi Kung exercises allow you to draw energy from the Earth, Cosmos, and Universe to strengthen the tendons and clean out and energize the fasciae. This provides protection and opens the channels so that they can receive more energy.

2. Tai Chi

By practicing Tai Chi you can learn to move the body in one unit using Chi instead of muscle power. You can build inner strength by circulating energy through the channels, muscles, tendons, bones, and fasciae. This ability is very important in CNT for protection and for storing and channeling energy. The Healing Tao's Tai Chi Chi Kung, which can be learned very quickly, is a short but powerful way of achieving such results.

3. Bone Marrow Breathing

The Healing Tao has published a book on the subject of bone marrow breathing entitled *Bone Marrow Nei Kung*. By studying and practicing bone marrow breathing, you can cleanse and grow bone marrow, refresh the blood, and develop enormous power. You can develop the ability to channel energy through breathing while using less muscular force and passing on more energy.

4. Diet

Whether or not you are familiar with cooking using the Five Phases of Energy theory, you may find it very interesting because it is so full of novelty and surprise. Culinary artists who incorporate the Five Phases of Energy (Five Element) theory in their cooking skills using the produce and foods of their countries or regions are quickly creating new and exciting trends in cooking.

The Five Element theory of cooking that pervades much of the world of Chinese cuisine is served in many wonderful restaurants. In fact, its cooking rules are a part of every Asian culture. Asian cooks balance their food in five ways, separating food according to five tastes, five colors, hot, cold, and PH balance. Then the foods are combined and beautifully prepared.

The stomach, spleen, and saliva sort out the food and distribute it to the organs according to taste and color. Each color and taste feeds energy to its own particular organ group. Each organ will only accept that energy designed for it by nature.

a. A Balanced Diet

A balanced diet is one that provides each organ with its own kind of energy. Each organ's energy also feeds primary energy to certain systems in the body. To nourish the body's various systems, you have to plan your meals accordingly. Thus, a balanced diet has equal parts of the following five tastes and colors:

The liver and gall bladder like food that is green and sour tasting. This food feeds the nerves.

The heart and small intestine like bitter tastes and food that is red. This food feeds the heart and its vessels.

The spleen, pancreas, and stomach like food that is sweet. This food feeds the muscles. This does not mean adding sugar or sweeteners, but refers to food that is naturally sweet.

The lungs and large intestine like food that is spicy and light colored. This food feeds the skin.

The kidneys and bladder like food that is dark and salty. This food feeds the bones. This does not mean adding salt, but refers to food that is naturally salty.

While food also has cold and hot, Yin/Yang properties that are important to understand and balance, many macrobiotic diets are incomplete because they only balance food according to Yin and Yang and do not include the Five Phases of Energy theory.

b. Chewing Well and Activating the Saliva

Another important aspect of diet is chewing. You should chew your food so that it becomes like liquid, because this starts the saliva flowing.

Saliva has tremendous power to help heal the intestines. First, the saliva determines the taste of the food. Then it sends a taste message along the channel or meridian to the stomach which begins to prepare the proper mixture of digestive fluids accordingly. You must, therefore,

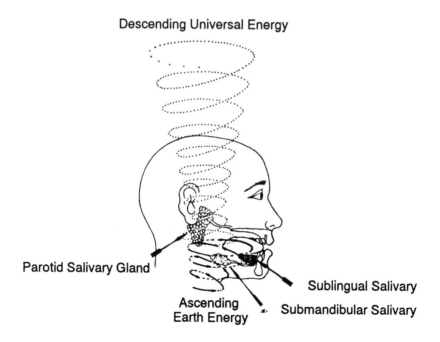

Descending Universal Energy

Parotid Salivary Gland

Ascending Earth Energy

Sublingual Salivary

Submandibular Salivary

Figure 2-2. The Universal and Earth Energies combine in the saliva

chew slowly. If you swallow too quickly, the stomach will not know what food is coming and will not be prepared. The food then travels to the stomach via the saliva where it can be sorted and easily assimilated. The spleen, meanwhile, has already figured out where it is going to assign the Chi of that particular food.

c. Combining the Heaven and Earth Forces in Saliva

In Taoism it is said that the Heaven and Earth forces combine to make saliva. (Figure 2-2) Saliva is a major energy force similar to the energy of semen or the ovum. The Taoists also believe saliva is a major food. If you chew well until you have a mouth full of saliva, your stomach will receive one part food and two parts saliva. This is the best condition for digestion. It is important, then, to be careful not to drink too much liquid while eating for it could dilute all the naturally pre-assigned tasks of the saliva and digestive juices. Food that is too spicy or salty often can cause one to drink too much liquid with meals.

C. Preparing Yourself Emotionally: the Fusion Practices

In addition to a strong, healthy body, you need to work from a clear emotional base to practice CNT. You cannot help anyone if you are full of negative emotional energy. You need to have balanced emotions if you a going to touch someone, especially if you expect to help balance their emotions.

The Fusion of the Five Elements practices will allow you to clear out your negative emotional energy and transform it into positive emotional energy.

This is a very powerful and effective meditation and formulation. It is one technique for balancing the emotions. If you practice Fusion I, you will learn how the Five Energy Phases and their related organs can interact with one another. This technique teaches you how to construct an internal system of turbines, transformers, and vortexes which can be used to cleanse the emotions. If you know how to engage this system, you can switch it on while you are massaging someone and any negative and sick energies trying to invade your body can be quickly neutralized.

Fusion II teaches additional methods for gathering the pure energy of the five organs. With this practice you can increase your positive energy. If you need to pass on some positive energy to your student, this practice will provide you with reserves that you may draw upon to replenish yourself.

Fusion II and III also open and widen channels all over the body. The idea, in part, is to clear congestion out of energy passageways so that you can deliver energy through these channels to your students.

D. Using the Inner Smile and the Microcosmic Orbit

1. The Inner Smile

The Inner Smile is a powerful relaxation technique which begins at the mid-eyebrow and eyes. It utilizes the expanding energy of happiness as a language to communicate with the internal organs of the body.

A genuine smile transmits loving energy that has the power to warm and heal. By learning to smile inwardly to the organs and glands, the whole body will feel loved and appreciated. You will feel the energy flow down the entire length of the body like a waterfall. This is a very powerful way to counteract stress and tension.

a. Sit on the edge of a chair with your hands clasped and eyes closed.

b. Begin the Inner Smile by picturing a radiant, smiling face in front of you. (Figure 2-3)

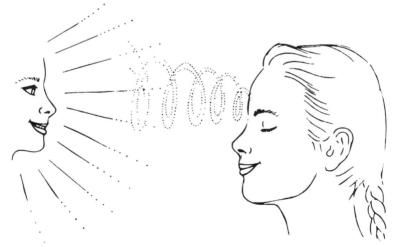

**Figure 2-3. Begin the Inner Smile
by picturing a radiant, smiling face in front of you**

c. Smile to activate the Cosmic Particle Energy. (Figure 2-4)

d. Slightly lift the corners of the mouth.

e. Sense a coolness in your eyes to attract and absorb the warm energy. Inhale the energy through the mid-eyebrow and spiral it.

f. Smile down to the thymus gland and the heart. Feel the heart open with love, joy, and happiness.

g. Smile down to all the organs: lungs, liver, pancreas, spleen, kidneys, and sexual organs and reproductive system. Thank them for their work.

h. Return your attention to your eyes. Create a big smile and draw in the Cosmic Particle Energy.

i. Smile down the intestinal tract: the esophagus, stomach, small intestine, large intestine, bladder, and urethra.

j. Return your attention to your eyes. Create a big smile and draw in the Cosmic Particle Energy.

k. Smile to the brain and the pituitary, thalamus, and pineal glands. Smile down the spinal column.

l. Return your attention to your eyes.

m. Smile down to the whole body.

n. Collect the energy in the Navel Center.

2. The Microcosmic Orbit

The Microcosmic Orbit meditation awakens, circulates, and directs Chi through the Functional Channel, which runs down the chest, and the Governor Channel, which ascends the middle of the back. (Figure 2-5) Dedicated practice of this ancient esoteric method eliminates stress and nervous tension, massages internal organs, restores health to damaged tissues, and establishes a sense of well-being.

a. Practice the Inner Smile; collect the energy in the Navel Center.

b. Let the energy flow down to the sexual center, the ovarian or sperm palace.

c. Move the energy from the sexual center to the perineum.

d. Draw the energy up from the perineum to the sacrum.

e. Draw the energy up to the Ming Men (Door of Life), located opposite the navel.

f. Draw the energy up to the T-11 vertebrae.

g. Draw the energy up to the base of the skull (Jade Pillow).

h. Draw the energy up to the crown.

i. Move the energy down from the crown to the mid-eyebrow.

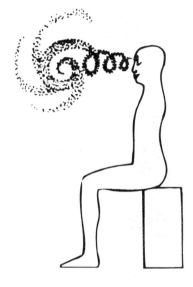

1. Smile to activate the Cosmic Particle Force
2. Slightly lift the corners of the mouth
3. Inhale through the mid-eyebrow and spiral

4. Smile down to the thymus gland and the heart. Feel the heart open with joy, love, and happiness

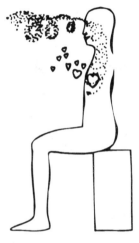

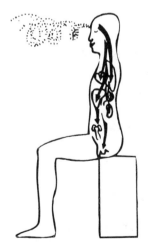

5. Smile down to all the organs (lungs, liver, pancreas, spleen, kidneys, and sexual organs)

Figure 2-4. The Inner Smile

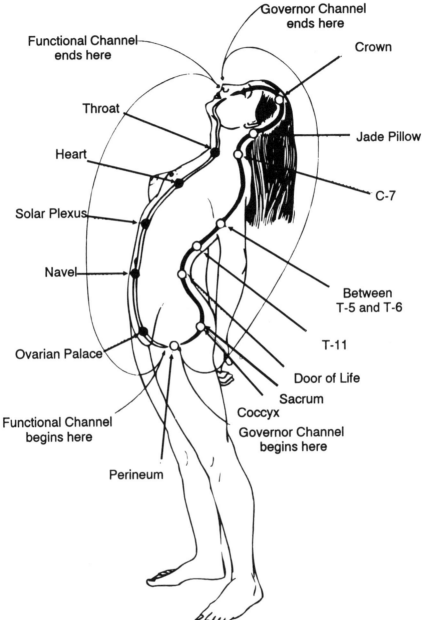

Figure 2-5. The Functional and Governor Channels and the Stations of the Microcosmic Orbit

j. Pass the energy down through the tongue to the Throat Center.

k. Bring the energy down from the throat to the Heart Center.

l. Bring the energy down to the solar plexus.

m. Bring the energy back to the navel.

n. Circulate the energy through this entire sequence at least nine or ten times.

o. Collect the energy at the navel.

MEN: Cover your navel with both palms, left hand over right. Collect and mentally spiral the energy outward at the navel 36 times clockwise, and then inward 24 times counterclockwise.

WOMEN: Cover your navel with both palms, right hand over left. Collect and mentally spiral the energy outward from the navel 36 times counterclockwise, and then inward 24 times clockwise.

E. Performing the Healing Hands Meditation

The more you are aware of your sources of energy, the more that energy will come to you from those sources. According to the wisdom of the ancient Taoists, the energy that you receive from meditating is superior to the energy that you obtain from food.

The Healing Hands Meditation will help to grow and strengthen the energy in your hands and fingers. Your hands will develop sensitivity and you will be able to feel the energy in your own and your student's organs and abdomen. You will find this to be very useful.

1. Meditating to Expand the Aura

a. Practice the Inner Smile down to the organs and glands.

b. Bring the energy to your Navel Center and practice the Fusion Meditations.

(1) Form the four pakuas and the collection points.

(2) Clean out negative emotions by transforming them into positive, healing forces.

(3) Form their energies into a pearl.

NOTE: Anyone who is not familiar with the Fusion practice of the Healing Tao System can substitute his or her practice for clearing undesirable emotional energy at this time. If you have not yet learned the Fusion Meditations, do the Microcosmic Orbit at this time.

c. Circulate the energy in the Microcosmic Orbit faster and faster until it expands outward from your body.

d. Feel the energy expanding outward from your navel as you visualize the sun shining in that area. Feel the energy filling your aura with a warm, pleasant sensation. (Figure 2-6)

e. Be aware of the North Star and Big Dipper above you and absorb their respective violet and red lights, the golden light of the Cosmic Particles, and the blue force of the Earth into the navel. (Figure 2-7)

f. When you feel your aura has expanded, maintain a distance of at least two square feet away from other people. If their auras are stronger than yours at this time, your aura may be squeezed and you will experience discomfort. After you have felt the outer forces strongly, proceed with the following meditation.

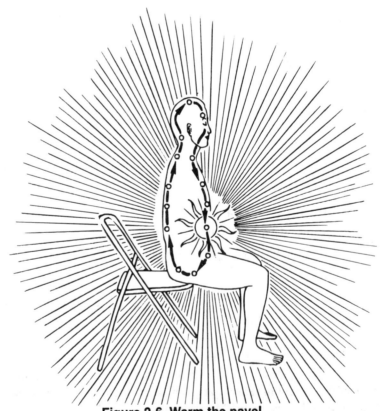

**Figure 2-6. Warm the navel
and feel the warmth radiate from the body**

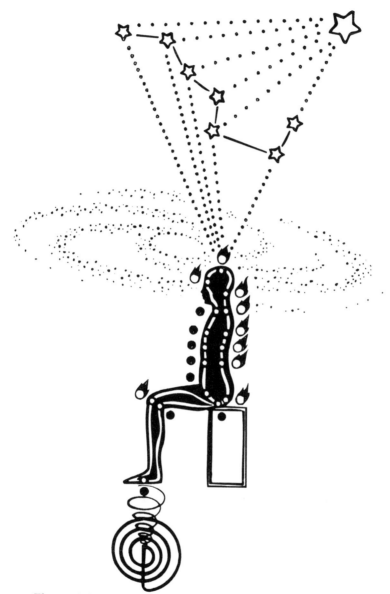

Figure 2-7. Absorb the violet light from the North Star, the red light from the Big Dipper, the golden light of the Human Plane, and the blue force from the Earth

2. Channeling the Force through the Palms

a. Hold both of your hands in front of your eyes and gaze at both palms. (Figure 2-8)

b. Focus on the middle of your palms by using the corners of both eyes to gaze at the palms' centers. The corners of the eyes have special

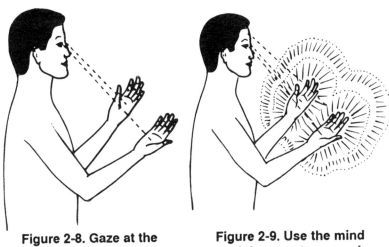

Figure 2-8. Gaze at the center of the palms

Figure 2-9. Use the mind and the eyes to expand the hand's aura

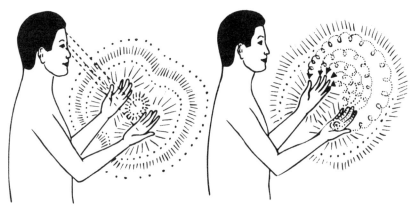

Figure 2-10 Feel an energy ball between the hands

Figure 2-11. Be aware of the fingers pulsing. Use the mind and eyes to send Chi from the right fingertips to the left. Repeat nine times

cells that can see in very dim light. Using your eyes to focus this way will help you develop the ability to see auras and movements in the dark. Using the combined power of the mind and the eyes, you can cause the aura of each palm to grow and expand. (Figure 2-9) The Chi can feel like it is contracting and absorbing, and the sensation can be of drawing the forces into the palms, or an expansion of the palms. You might see a ball of Chi or a ball of color between the palms through the corners of your eyes. (Figure 2-10)

c. Be aware of the fingers. Feel your fingertips pulsing. Use your mind and eyes to absorb the Cosmic Chi into the right palm. Send the Chi from the right palm and fingers across to the left palm and fingers. Repeat nine times. (Figure 2-11)

d. Next move the fingers of both hands until they nearly touch each other: thumb to thumb, index finger to index finger, etc. You can feel sensations like electric sparks traveling across from one fingertip to the other. (Figure 2-12) Some can feel pain, swelling, or simply expansion in their fingertips.

e. Gradually spread the hands apart, but not so far that you permit the Chi connection to diminish or break. (Figure 2-13) If this happens,

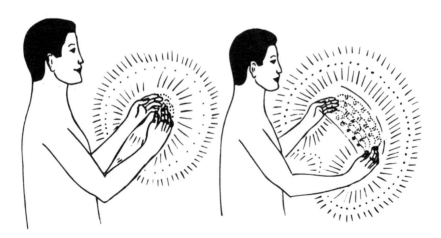

Figure 2-12. Bring the hands close together, with the fingertips nearly touching, and let the energy flow from one hand to the other

Figure 2-13 . Slowly move the hands apart while feeling the Chi connection

stop moving them and project more energy with the mind to re-establish the connection. Spread the hands from nine to eighteen times.

This practice will increase your sensitivity to energy and your healing ability. Transforming the Universal and Cosmic Particle Forces for immediate use will prevent drainage of your life-force. The energy can feel warm and pleasant.

3. Growing the Right Fingers' Auras

When your palms feel full of Chi, start to grow more Chi in the right hands' fingers.

a. With both hands' fingertips still raised in front of your eyes, begin by gazing at the right hand's fingers.

b. Use the corners of both eyes to gaze at the tips of the fingers. Focus on the tip of the index finger. Using the energy of your eyes, cause the aura of the index fingertip to grow and expand. (Figure 2-14) Feel that fingertip pulsing. Make the energy cool and pleasant.

c. Next grow the middle finger, thumb, fourth finger, and pinky finger auras. (Figures 2-15, 2-16, 2-17, and 2-18)

d. Choose your main healing finger(s) by observing and feeling which finger most noticeably permit(s) the energy to be absorbed in and passed out. Choose by comparing the length of the aura of each finger by the intensity of a tingling sensation or by any method that feels comfortable to you. Don't neglect the finger(s) that you do not select. Continue to practice with them as well.

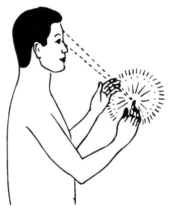

Figure 2-14. Focus on the right hand's index finger and let the aura grow

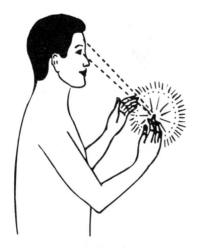

Figure 2-15. Focus on the right hand's middle finger, and let the aura grow

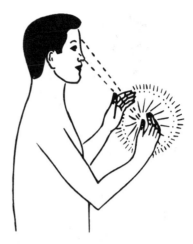

Figure 2-16. Grow the aura of the right hand's thumb

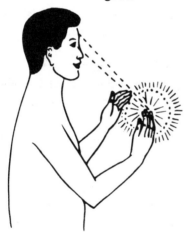

Figure 2-17. Grow the aura of the ring finger

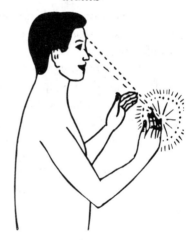

Figure 2-18. Grow the aura of the pinky finger

4. Growing the Left Fingers' Auras

    a. Inhale energy into the left hand and fingers.

    b. Grow the thumb aura beginning with the tip. (Figure 2-19)

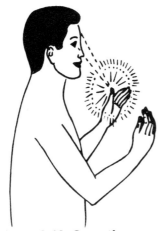

Figure 2-19. Grow the aura of the left thumb

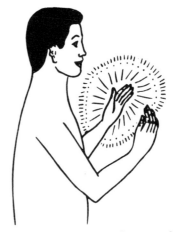

Figure 2-20. Grow and expand the auras of the left hand's index, middle, ring, and little fingers

c. Next, grow and absorb the auras of the index, middle, fourth, and little fingers. (Figure 2-20) Receive and feel the Universal and Cosmic Particle Energies.

d. Select the finger on the left hand with the strongest energy. Press that fingertip with the tip of the thumb, forming a circle. Keep the other fingers straight. Rest the left hand on your lap. This circle is the best way to receive Universe and Cosmic Particle Energies.

e. Curl the pinky and fourth fingers of the right hand and press them with the tip of the thumb, again forming a circle. Keep the index and middle fingers straight. (Figure 2-21)

f. Form these circles and use your mind and eyes to absorb the external Cosmic Particle Force through the fingers of the left hand. Send it up through the left hand, outside the left arm and the left shoulder, to the back side of the left ear, and across the crown. Blend this energy with the Universal Force entering through the crown. Then send their combined energy down to the right ear, the right shoulder, the outside right of the right arm, and the right hand to its index and middle fingers. Send it out through these fingers and receive it again through the extended fingers of the left hand. Continue this practice for nine, eighteen, or 36 cycles. (Figure 2-22)

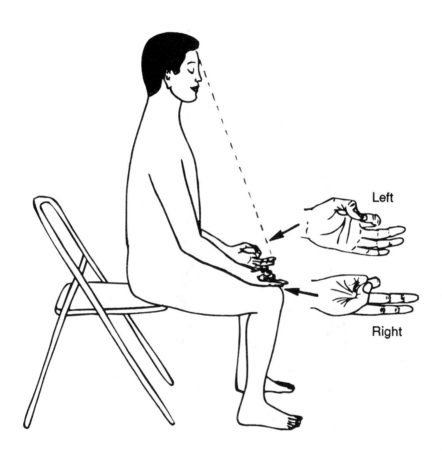

Figure 2-21. Choose which finger in the left hand has the strongest energy. Join the thumb with the strong finger, and place the left hand on the lap. Curve and join the right hand's little finger and ring finger with the thumb. Keep the other fingers straight

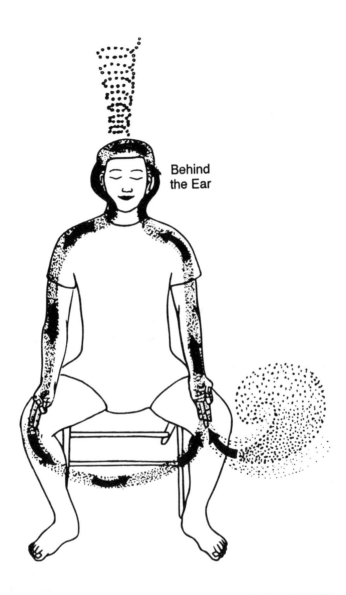

Behind
the Ear

Figure 2-22. Absorb the Human Plane (Cosmic Particle) Energy through the left fingers. Circulate it and blend it with the Universal Force at the crown. Circulate these energies down the right arm, out through the index and middle fingers, and back to the left fingers

5. Practicing Cosmic Chi Kung

Cosmic Chi Kung integrates both static and dynamic exercise forms to cultivate and nourish Chi. The Chi is accumulated in the organs, penetrates the fasciae, tendons, muscles, and bones and finally transfers itself out through the hands and fingers into your student. This is a higher level of practice that allows you to channel more Cosmic Particle and Universal Energies. The Cosmic Chi Kung practice is taught on video tape and is available at the Healing Tao Center.

F. Receiving the Universal and Earth Forces

1. Choosing a Personal Star Force

a. Picture a star over your head as your personal star, or choose the North Star and the Big Dipper constellation. Allow the energy from your star to flow into the top of your head.

b. Under your feet visualize a moon, which is symbolic of your connection with Mother Earth. Allow the energy of this moon to flow up your legs and into your body, mixing with the star energy in your navel, your heart, or your head. (Figure 2-23)

c. This mixing may occur at different places (navel, heart, mid-eye-brow) and at different times, depending on the quality of energy you may need for a particular task. The navel is best for beginners.

d. Next, circulate this blended energy in your Microcosmic Orbit three times. (Figure 2-24)

e. Then move the energy into your right arm channel. (Figure 2-25) Maintain the circuit and flow.

f. To end the meditation, draw your energy into your Tan Tien (behind the navel, one and one half inches inside), and condense it with 36 spirals outward, and 24 spirals back inward. Men spiral clockwise 36 times, then counterclockwise 24 times; women spiral counterclockwise 36 times, then clockwise 24 times. (Figure 2-26)

2. Healing with Love from the Heart's Center

When people come to you for healing, you should wish them well with all your heart. Give them your love, kindness, and openness, and you will feel your heart open. The healing force from the Universe will pour down to you and out to the people simultaneously.

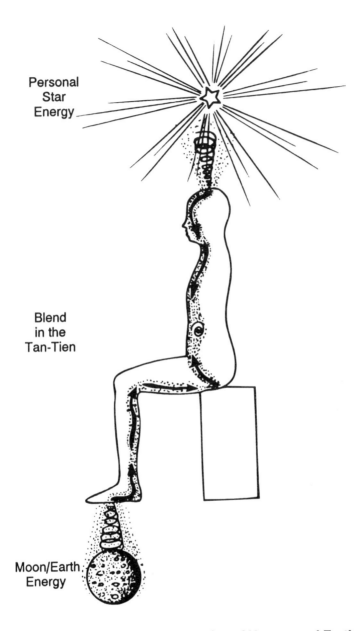

Personal
Star
Energy

Blend
in the
Tan-Tien

Moon/Earth
Energy

**Figure 2-23. Absorb the energies of Heaven and Earth.
Choose a Personal Star and picture it over your head.
Visualize the Moon and Earth Energy under your feet. Draw the
energies into your body and blend them in the Navel Center**

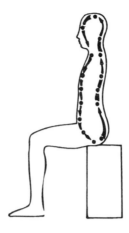

Figure 2-24. Circulate the energy in the Microcosmic Orbit

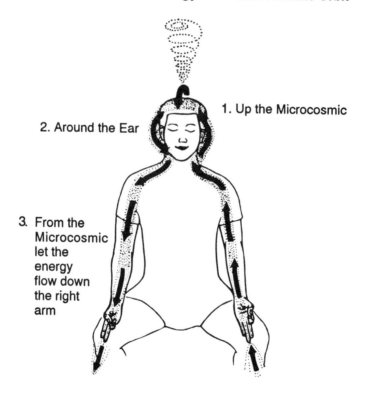

2. Around the Ear

1. Up the Microcosmic

3. From the Microcosmic let the energy flow down the right arm

Figure 2-25. Move the energy from the Microcosmic Orbit down into your right arm channel

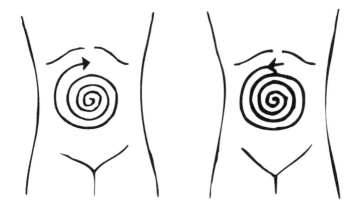

A. Men collect the energy in the navel and circle it 36 times clockwise, then 24 times counterclockwise

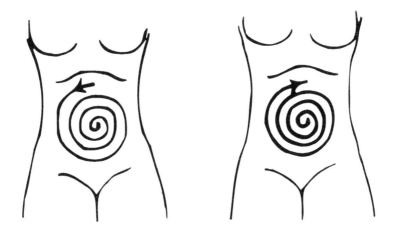

B. Women collect the energy in the navel and circle it 36 times counterclockwise, then 24 times clockwise

Figure 2-26. Finishing the Microcosmic Orbit

Learning Iron Shirt Chi Kung is very important because it is the practice that will allow you to ground yourself when working with a student. This will help you ground your energy and help send the student's sick energy into the ground. You will also learn to feel the kindness, gentleness, and openness of the Earth Force and pass the Earth Force into your student.

Giving the gift of healing energy keeps the heart channels open and both the practitioner and student benefit. Practice the Microcosmic Orbit circulation and concentrate on the point opposite of the heart and feel it connect to the Heart Center in the front. This will help to open the heart. Feel the back and the front connected like a funnel. Once the heart is open, it will be very easy to receive the energy from the Universe.

Opening the Microcosmic Orbit is very important, since this will allow the energy to circulate, balance, recycle, and transform. The meditative practices of the Healing Tao will enable you to connect with the Heavenly Force from above and the Earth Force from below. Combine them into a powerful healing force—a healing force that can be used to heal yourself and others.

G. Collecting the Cosmic Particle Force

1. Practicing Circulation of the Human Plane Energy
a. Receiving Yang Energy to Balance Yin Energy

(1) Stand or sit for this practice. Concentrate on the navel until it feels warm. If you are familiar with the Fusion I meditation, practice it, and form a pearl.

(2) When you feel the energy intensify, move the energy up to the crown. Project it out and up approximately ten feet above your head while curving it slightly forward in an arc.

(3) Be aware of the pearl and the space above the head. Feel the pearl absorb the Cosmic Particle Force.

(4) Let the projected arc continue down to a place approximately two to three feet in front of you. Absorb the Cosmic Particle Energy through the mid-eyebrow, and accumulate it like a Chi ball. Direct the energy ball down through the throat, heart, navel, and sexual center.

(5) Let the rest of the Cosmic Particle energy travel down into the Earth approximately five to ten feet. Notice that the Earth is harder to penetrate than the air.

(6) Absorb the Earth Energy through the soles of the feet. Permit this energy to penetrate and travel up the soles or backs of your feet to the perineum, coccyx, sacrum, spine, and out of the head again.

(7) Eventually you will feel this energy throughout your feet. Bring the energy up both legs to the perineum. If you practice Fusion II and your Thrusting Channels are open, let the energy pass through them and nourish all the organs and glands along the path of the Thrusting Channels. If you only are familiar with the Microcosmic Orbit, then let the energy rise to the coccyx, the spine, and to the crown. Project it out again in a forward arc.

(8) Continue this practice for nine, eighteen, or 36 rounds. (Figure 2-27) The purposes of this exercise are to balance, enhance, and purify your life-force as well as to give you practice in projecting and absorbing the force.

With continued practice absorbing the Cosmic Particle Chi and the Earth Force, you will feel the Chi thickening. You also may feel the energy around you becoming very sticky, like honey. When you project the energy outward, you may see a light. When you absorb the Chi inward, you may see the light come into you. Store the light in your Navel Center.

b. Increasing Yin Energy to Balance Yang Energy

To increase your Yin energy, you can reverse the process. Shoot the energy or the pearl down into the ground approximately five to ten feet, absorb the Earth Force, and bring it up to the space two to three feet in front of you. Absorb the Cosmic Particle Force and bring the energy upward in an arc to about ten feet above your head. Bring the energy in through your crown, down the spine, and so on. (Figure 2-28) With practice you can absorb more Cosmic Particle Chi which will enable you to help others to heal faster.

c. Practicing with a Partner

When you become proficient in directing the Chi force, you will find that you can stand about two to three feet in front of another person and perform the same Chi practice feeling the additional Chi flowing back and forth between you. If your practice partner is weaker than you, you will feel less because his or her body will absorb some Chi that you sent out and will not have as much to send back.

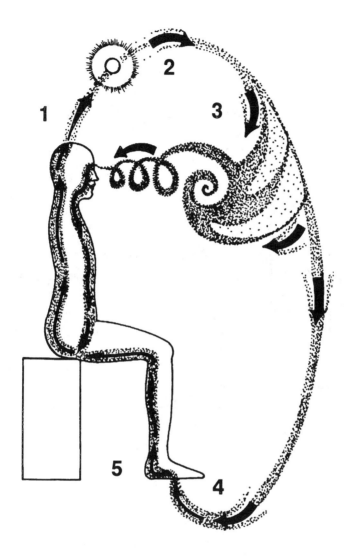

1. Send the energy out of the crown ten feet above
2. Circulate it down in front
3. Absorb the Cosmic Energy
4. Send it five feet into the Earth
5. Absorb Earth Energy through the soles up
   into the Microcosmic Orbit
6. Do this eighteen to 36 times using the pearl

Figure 2-27. Absorbing Yang Energy to Balance Yin Energy

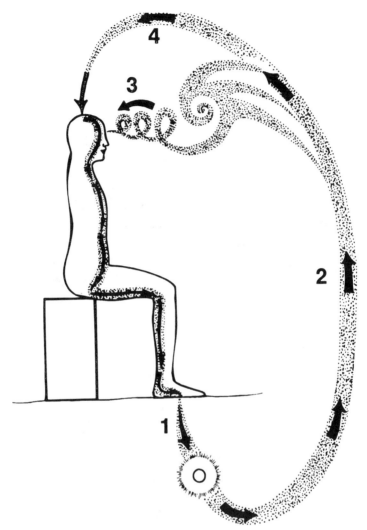

1. Send the energy out through the soles five feet into the ground
2. Bring it up the front
3. Absorb energy through the mid-eyebrow
4. Absorb energy through the crown
5. Do this 18-36 times using the pearl

Figure 2-28. Absorb Yin Energy to Balance Yang Energy. Reverse the procedure in Figure 2-27

H. Collecting Tree Energy

1. The Healing Abilities of Trees

Taoist Masters observed that trees are tremendously powerful plants. Not only can they absorb carbon dioxide and transform it into oxygen, but they can also absorb negative forces and transform them into good energy. Trees strongly root with the Earth, and the more rooted the tree, the higher it can extend to Heaven. Trees stand very still, absorbing the Earth's Energy and the Universal Force from the Heavens.

Trees and all plants have the ability to absorb the light of the energies and transform it into food; in fact, they depend on light for most of their nourishment, while water and earth minerals make up about 30% of their nutritional intake. Trees are able to live very long lives.

a. The Tree as Healer and Friend

Trees are the largest and most spiritually advanced plants on earth. They are constantly in meditation, and subtle energy is their natural language. As your understanding of this language grows, you can begin to develop a relationship with them. They can help you open your energy channels and cultivate calm, presence, and vitality. You can reciprocate by helping them with their own blockages and devitalized areas. It is a mutually beneficial relationship that needs cultivation.

b. Choosing a Tree to Work With

Throughout history human beings have used all parts of the tree for healing and medicine. The best trees for healing are big trees, especially pines. Pine trees radiate Chi, nourish blood, strengthen nervous systems, and contribute to long lives. They also nurture souls and spirits. Pines are the "Immortal Tree." Early Chinese poetry and painting is full of admiration for pines.

Although pine trees are often the best choice, many other trees or plants can be used. The larger trees contain the most energy. Among the most powerful are trees growing near running water. Some trees feel warmer or hotter than others; some feel cooler or colder than others. Practice distinguishing the varying properties of different trees.

(1) Cypress and cedar trees reduce heat and nourish Yin energy.

(2) Willow trees help to expel sick winds, rid the body of excess dampness, reduce high blood pressure, and strengthen the urinary tract and bladder.

(3) Elm trees calm the mind and strengthen the stomach.

91

(4) Maple trees chase sick winds and help reduce pain.

(5) Locust trees help clear internal heat and help balance the weather of the heart.

(6) Banyan trees clear the heart and help to rid the body of dampness.

(7) Cinnamon trees can clear coldness from the heart and abdomen.

(8) Fir trees help clear up bruises, reduce swelling, and heal broken bones faster.

(9) Hawthorn trees help aid digestion, strengthen the intestines, and lower blood pressure.

(10) Birch trees help clear heat and dampness from the body and help to detoxify it.

(11) Plum trees nourish the spleen, stomach, and pancreas and calm the mind.

(12) Fig trees clear excess heat from the body, increase saliva, nourish the spleen, and help stop diarrhea.

(13) Ginco trees help strengthen the bladder and alleviate urinary problems in women.

You do not need to go far out into the forest to find an appropriate tree to work with. Trees that are used to having people around understand our energy and are actually more accessible and friendly than those far out in the wilderness. City parks and suburban yards are filled with powerful and accessible trees that would love to have closer relationships with the humans that dominate their environment.

There is a certain size range within which trees are most accessible to human beings. When a tree is too small, it does not have enough energy to make much of an impression on you. When the tree is too big, you have the opposite problem, so it takes more persistence to get large trees to take an interest in you. As a source of healing energy, it is best to choose a large, robust tree from within the accessible size range. For playful interaction it is best to choose a small to medium sized tree. While it is not necessary to climb the tree to develop a relationship, it does open up a whole new world. Climb gently and carefully so as not to harm the tree.

c. Establishing Communion with a Tree

There are certain methods to approaching, interacting with, retreating from, and taking leave of a tree. By following specific steps you create a ritual of silent communion that both you and the tree can understand, and so increase the potential for harmonious interaction. The steps were derived from observation of the natural course of events in subtle energy communion, and apply to communion with just about anything: tree, rock, human, or animal, although the following is concerned specifically with trees.

First of all, each tree, like each person, has a personality, desires, and a life of its own. Trees differ widely in their taste for human contact. Some are very generous and want to give you all the energy you can take. Others are weak or ill and need your comforting and healing energy. Some are just friendly souls who enjoy human company. Others are quite indifferent to you. You can learn and grow by working with all of them. Try to be open and respectful, rather than pressing the trees to serve your own purposes. In this way they will provide you with more than just another source of Chi: friendship, playful expression, and love.

Trees operate on a longer time scale than do human beings. You can help to bridge this gap by returning again and again to the same tree, so that a relationship develops. Visit regularly so that the tree knows when to expect you and can look forward to seeing you. You may have the distinct impression that the tree really misses you when you are gone for a longer time than usual.

Spiritual communion with trees resembles lovemaking more than any other human activity. As such, a quality of sensuality and tenderness should be present. You do not always have to be in control of the situation. Allow some time to just relax and melt into the communion. Let the tree lead you into the wonders of its own inner life. Working with trees in this way can help to ease sexual frustration. You may find that some of the practices presented here can be easily adapted for use in lovemaking.

2. Practicing with a Tree and the Earth's Force

a. Use the Palms to Absorb Yin Chi and Help Balance Yang Energy (Figure 2-29)

Morning to noon time is the best time to practice with a tree.

(1) *Assume a Position.* Stand or sit one or two feet in front of a tree.

(2) *Open Yourself to a Tree.* Relax and center yourself. Feel your boundaries soften. Allow yourself to become more receptive and somewhat vulnerable, ready to make contact with the tree. Feel your energy field open like a flower, neither emitting nor absorbing energy, just becoming open and available (Figure 2-30).

(3) *Offer a Welcome.* Extend your arms and face the palms of your hands toward the tree. Extend your energy toward the tree with a friendly "offering" attitude. When the tree responds by extending its energy to you, accept it, breathing it into your body with an attitude of "welcome."

Use your mind and eyes as follows. With the lower part of the eyes, concentrate on the tip of your nose. With the upper part of the eyes, look at your palms and at the tree.

Let your intuition guide you as you respond to the tree again with another "offering" gesture. Proceed with several of these exchanges. Take your time and really feel what is happening.

Use the left palm, the mind, and the upper part of the eyes to absorb the Chi.

(4) *Parallel Tracking.* Remain centered within yourself, neither approaching nor retreating, and simply observe the subtle relationship between you and the tree. Use meditative concentration to become very absorbed in your connection with the tree, without actively trying to change or analyze what is going on. Do not try to deepen the communion or lessen it. Control your own energy and watch the tree while the tree controls its own energy and watches you. This is known as *Parallel Tracking.* Such a neutral state may occur several times during a session at deep as well as shallow levels of intimacy.

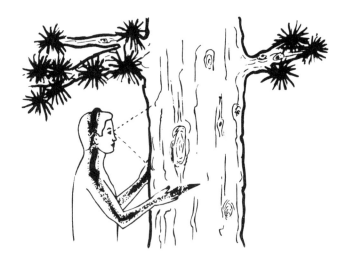

Figure 2-29. Practice with a tree to absorb Tree Energy and then return it to the tree
Yin Cycle: Use the palms and insides of the arms
Yang Cycle: Use the fingertips and outsides

(5) *Draw and Hold Close.* Allow the energy field between you and the tree to intensify, thicken, and contract to *Draw and Hold Close* the two of you together. There may or may not be physical movement involved. The sensation is that the two of you are being enfolded in a cocoon of energy while more and more of your inner cores are exposed to each other. Finally you hold each other in an embrace of deep intimacy.

Drawing and Holding Close often happens spontaneously as the offering and welcoming escalates to become circulating and sharing, or as the circulating and sharing moves to deeper and deeper levels.

(6) *Guide the Chi.* As with all Healing Tao practices, it is necessary that you train your eyes and mind to move and guide the Chi. This practice is also useful in training yourself to recognize and be aware of the quality of the tree's energy. Feel the tree's energy when it enters your body. As you send it out to the tree, combine it with Human Plane (Cosmic Particle) Energy. Notice how the energy feels when it returns to you from the tree: enhanced with a cool, healing quality. Notice also how the quality of the energy changes after nine, eighteen, 24, and 36 cycles.

Move the upper part of the eyes to guide the Chi slowly up the inside (Yin side) of the left arm, to the left shoulder, the left side of the neck, the left ear, and the crown. From the crown move the Chi down the right side to the back side of the right ear, to the right neck, the right shoulder, inside the right arm, to the right palm. Project the Chi out into the tree trunk. Absorb the Chi again in a circle (the Yin Energy Circle): 36 cycles for men and 24 cycles for women. (Figure 2-30)

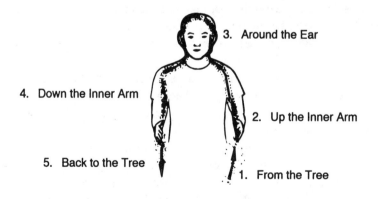

3. Around the Ear

4. Down the Inner Arm

2. Up the Inner Arm

5. Back to the Tree

1. From the Tree

Figure 2-30 Women practice 24 cycles. Men practice 36 cycles

(7) *Extend to a Deeper Level.* Now begin to exchange energy with the tree on a deeper level. To share with the tree on a deeper level means to place a particular part of your body in contact with a particular part of the tree's body, and breathing the energy back and forth between them. To circulate now means guiding the energy along a path which passes through both of your bodies and returns to its starting point. You can guide the Chi as in (6) above. Eventually you will discover many different patterns are possible.

(8) *Drawing and Holding Back to End Gracefully.* Drawing and Holding Back is very important. It prevents you from absorbing more energy from the tree than you can harmoniously utilize. It also prevents you from draining too much energy from a small or weak tree, or leaving such a tree with too much of your unprocessed negative energy. In addition, it seals off the connections you have made with the tree so that energy is not leaked into the environment after you leave. All in all, it makes for an aesthetically complete meditation and shows respect for the tree. When you have had enough and wish to begin your return to normal consciousness or just to a less deep level of communion, try to do so slowly and gradually so as not to disturb the beauty of what you have just shared. The sensation is one of gradually returning to yourself, sorting out the energy that belongs to you from the energy that belongs to the tree, and re-establishing the boundary between you.

It is important to note at this time that if, after you have done the healing, you still feel a lot of energy in your hands, close the crown point to seal it so that your healing energy will not continue to flow out.

Trees have a great liking for human contact and you will probably be ready to go long before the tree is ready to have you leave.

(a) You need to gradually withdraw your attention from the contact, and turn your attention more upon yourself.

(b) As you do this, much of the shared energy will be drawn into your body. When this happens, just "push back" at the stream of tree energy to prevent most of it from entering your body while allowing your human energy to return.

(c) Then, when your polarities reverse, allow the tree energy to flow back into the tree, but keep your own conscious energy within your body.

(d) After a couple of exchanges, the tree will get the idea and begin to cooperate with you. In a little while you will be fully back in your own body and ready for the closing.

(e) To disengage from a powerful circulation pattern, gradually focus your attention on the navel area, the place to end the meditation. As the energy collects there, allow any excess to flow into the tree.

(f) If the tree tries to feed you energy from another point, push back at this flow in the manner described above.

(g) Eventually the pattern will cease, and you will be sharing energy with the tree at the selected point. Now you can sort out what energy belongs to you and what belongs to the tree to complete the drawing back.

(h) When you are very deep into communion with a tree, you will probably have "too far to go" to draw back in one step. Instead, after a partial drawing and holding back, resume circulating and sharing, but in a less intense manner. Gradually, after several of these steps, you will come wholly back to yourself.

(9) *Closing.* Always end with a closing. The closing is a precise and somewhat abrupt gesture which breaks the connection, locks into place any healing that my have occurred, and imparts a feeling of good will, all within a second or two. The closing may be a movement, a sound, or just a change in the subtle energy field, such as the clap of the hands, or a nod of the head. A smooth movement of a fist in an upward arc, ending with a little downward punch is very effective. The sounds "Ho" or "Amen" used to end prayers are also examples of closing gestures. So is a firm handshake, or a little squeeze at the end of a hug. Follow this with a little wave of the hand, or a quick kiss on the trunk to complete your closing.

Sections (7), (8), and (9) above are used to intensify, slow down, and end the exercises below and can be used at any time to end your communication with your selected tree.

b. Use the Fingers to Absorb Yang Energy to Help Balance the Yin Energy (Figure 2-29)

(1) Stand approximately one to two feet in front of a tree. Move slowly and smoothly, gradually approaching the tree. Feel the field of energy surrounding you become thick like honey.

(2) Extend your arms out toward the tree with your palms facing the tree and your fingers extended.

(3) As you slowly adjust your position to be closer and closer to the tree, less "honey" separates you from the bright energies found at its core.

(3) Similarly, your own radiance is revealed to the tree.

(4) At the same time the honey-like energy surrounding you acts like a protective cocoon, and your awareness of the outside world fades.

97

(5) As you arrive at the tree and wrap yourself around it in a big hug, your radiant energies link up with each other and you may lose yourself for a few moments in the bliss of union.

(6) After making contact in this way, you may need to hold still for a while until the new, deeper connections between you and the tree stabilize and simplify. Soon you will find yourself in the state of parallel tracking described previously from which circulating and sharing will develop.

(7) Feel the energy of the tree first. When you feel the tree's Chi, use the mind, eyes, and lower part of the eyes to concentrate on the tip of the nose. The upper part of the eyes looks at the tips of the fingers and the tree.

(8) Use the left fingers, the mind, and the upper part of the eyes to absorb the Chi inward.

(9) Move the upper part of the eyes slowly to guide the Chi up the outside (Yang side) of the left arm, to the left shoulder, the left side of the neck, and the left ear to the crown. Move the energy down the right side beginning with the back side of the right ear, to the right neck, the right shoulder, outside the right arm, to the right palm and fingers. Project the energy out from the fingers, combine it with Cosmic Particle Energy, and guide it into the tree trunk. Absorb it again in a circle. Men repeat the cycle 36 times; women repeat the cycle 24 times. (See Figure 2-30)

(10) If you wish to end the experience at this or any point, follow the procedures of (a)(7), (8), and (9) above to intensify, slow down, and finally break your connection with the tree.

The Yang Energy Circle will help you become more sensitive to chronic and more superficial pain as well as the energy in the Yang organs (large and small intestines, gall bladder, bladder, and stomach).

c. Use the Palms to Absorb Tree Chi; the Yin Side

(1) Sit or stand approximately one to two feet in front of a tree.

(2) Extend your arms out toward the tree with your palms facing the tree. (Figure 2-31)

(3) Feel the energy of the tree first. When you feel the Chi of the tree, use your mind, eyes, and palms to absorb the Chi through your palms. Move the Chi up the inside (the Yin sides) of both arms to both shoulders, both sides of the neck, and the left and right ears, to the crown. From the crown move the energy down the Functional Channel to the mid-eyebrow, throat, heart, solar plexus, navel, and the cauldron behind the navel.

(4) Continue to move the energy down from the cauldron to the perineum, to the soles of the feet, and then approximately ten feet into the ground.

(5) Bring the energy up to the roots of the tree, then up into the tree trunk. Feel your energy flow through the tree, then emerge from the trunk into your palm. Repeat the cycle nine, eighteen, 24, or 36 times.

(6) Practice sending your energy through the tree trunk from the right palm, through the tree, to the left palm, and from the left palm, through the tree, to the right palm. Men should practice for 36 cycles; women should practice for 24 cycles. It is most important to feel your energy penetrate the tree.

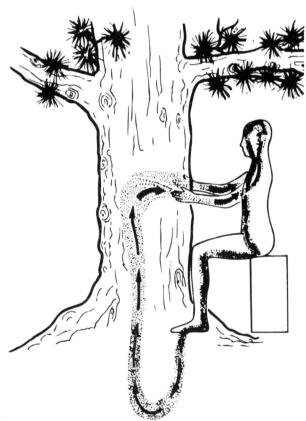

Figure 2-31. Use the palms to absorb the tree Chi and send it down into the roots about ten feet

(7) Practice distinguishing different parts of the tree. Start with the upper trunk. Send your energy into the trunk and feel it reverberate. Slowly kneel down to practice with the lower trunk. Then practice with the roots of the tree. Feel and exchange the force with the tree.

d. Absorb Tree Chi through the Crown

(1) Stand approximately two to three feet in front of a tree with your arms at your side. Feel the tree's aura. (Figure 2-32) If you do not feel it, you can move in closer.

(2) When you feel the tree's aura, use your crown to absorb the energy. The tree's balanced energy can feel very gentle and soft and have a very powerful healing effect.

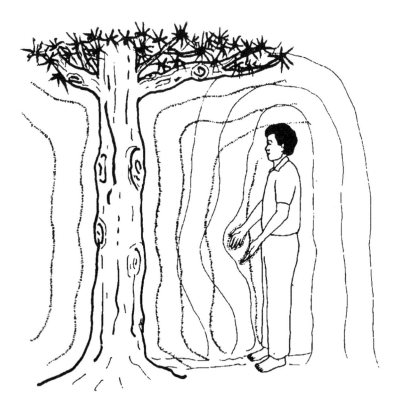

Figure 2-32 Allow the Tree's Aura to Blend with Your Own

(3) Draw the tree energy into your crown and let it flow down through the Thrusting Channels or through the Functional Channel to the perineum, then down to both feet. Move the energy out through the soles of your feet into the ground. Bring the energy from the ground to the roots of the tree, then up its trunk.

(4) Feel yourself absorb the Earth Energy and the tree energy. (Figure 2-33) Feel them purify your energy, removing negativity and sick energy. When you feel it emerge from the trunk of the tree, absorb the Human Plane (Cosmic Particle) Energy, and return the energy to your crown. You will feel the combined energies nourish your brain, glands, and organs. Repeat the process nine, eighteen, or 36 times.

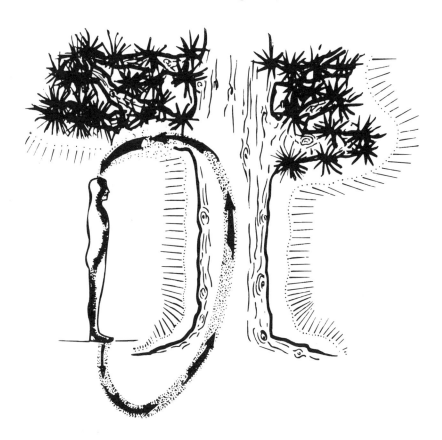

**Figure 2-33. Absorb the tree Chi
and Earth Energy through the crown**

e. Share with the Tree from the Heart

In this pattern tree energy is run through the arms and heart center. It may be used to clear a healer's arms of sick energy accumulated in work, or just to open the heart.

(1) Assume any comfortable position in which your hands can easily reach a branch.

(2) Reach one arm out to touch the tree with the palm or fingertips. Feel the vital energy just under the bark and make contact with it, allowing some time for the contact to develop.

(3) After a while you will feel the sharing begin as a gentle breathing back and forth between your hand and the tree.

(4) Gradually extend the process until you are breathing energy through the entire length of the arm, back and forth from your heart center to the tree. Let this back and forth sharing go on for some time.

(5) Next, get the other arm involved. It may rest on the same branch, near the other hand, or it may rest on an entirely different branch.

(6) Allow the tree energy to flow in along one arm, mix with your own energy in the heart center, and flow out the other arm. Every so often reverse the direction of flow in one or both arms.

(7) For a deeper experience try extending the flow from the heart down to the navel, letting it go from tree to heart, to navel, and back.

(8) Where does the energy go after it leaves your hands and enters the tree? By following it with your mind, you will begin to discover more about the subtle anatomy of the tree.

(9) You may find blocked or congested areas that you can work on by running energy out one hand and into the other. Feel the tree's response to your efforts, and let intuition guide you.

f. Absorb Earth Energy

(1) Create warmth in your navel and bring the energy up to the crown.

(2) Project the Chi out into the top of the trunk of the tree. Enter the tree and feel that you have a connection with it.

(3) During this process you can stand farther away from the tree (ten to thirty feet). As your practice continues you can project your energy easily from far away into the tree. Let the tree take in your negative or sick energy. The energy you receive back will be balanced.

(4) Let your energy flow down the trunk of the tree to its roots and into the Earth. (Figure 2-34) Let the Earth Energy purify your energy. Bring this combined energy up through the soles of your feet to the

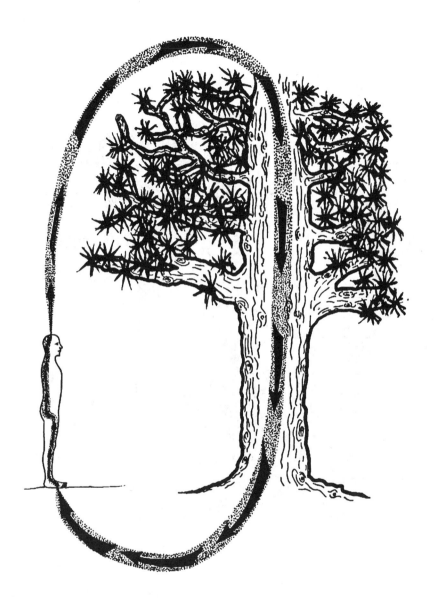

Figure 2-34. Absorb the Earth's Force. Circulate it through the tree after sending it out through the crown

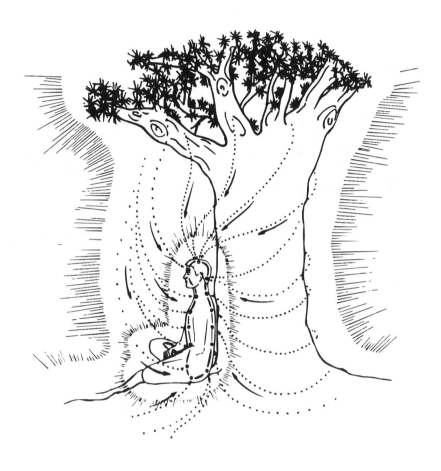

**Figure 2-35. Meditate while sitting under a tree.
Absorb the tree's energy through the stations (points)
of the Microcosmic Orbit**

perineum, then up through the Thrusting Channels, or through the Governor Channel running up the spine. Let the energy flow up to the crown and project it outward again. Repeat the process nine, eighteen, or 36 times.

The more you repeat the process, the more your energy will refine and increase. You will notice the Thrusting Channels and the Microcosmic Orbit are cleaner and brighter. Once you have established a good connection with the tree, you can send your sick energy to the tree from a far distance to refine your energy or improve your health.

g. Meditate While Sitting Under a Tree

Once you have developed the ability to feel the tree's Chi, you can sit under the tree and meditate. Draw the tree's energy into you through the stations (points) of the Microcosmic Orbit. (Figure 2-35)

I. The Six Healing Sounds

The Six Healing Sounds will help you sense the distinctive frequencies and colors generated by each organ. Practice the Healing Sounds until you can easily relate the sound to the organ and sense the qualities of that organ.

1. The Six Healing Sounds Initiate Healing

Everyone has heard stories about gifted beings who possess special healing powers. People seek out great healers. How much time can a great healer spend with you—one hour a week or one hour every day? What about the rest of the week or the rest of the day? One hour a day means one hour out of twenty-four. One hour a week means one out of 168 hours. This is why it is important for each person to learn how to clear his or her negative energy, and how to transform it into good energy. Regular practice of self-maintenance and self-healing enhances ongoing healing. The Six Healing Sounds are an easy practice to initiate healing. The Sounds are very simple, but very powerful.

When you are adept at the Six Healing Sounds and begin to practice Chi Nei Tsang, you will need to teach your students the Sounds. They can practice at home and help carry on the healing. You should teach one or two Sounds at each session and review them at each session.

2. How to do the Six Healing Sounds

a. The Lungs' Sound

Associated Organ: Large Intestine
Element: Metal
Season: Fall
Color: White
Emotions: Negative—Grief, Sadness, Depression
                Positive—Courage, Righteousness
Sound: SSSSSSS (tongue behind teeth)

(1) Position: Sit with your back straight and the backs of your hands resting on your thighs. Smile down to your lungs. Take a deep breath and raise your arms out in front of you. When the hands are at eye level, begin to rotate the palms, bringing them above your head until they are palms up, pushing outward. Point the fingers toward those of the opposite hand. Keep the elbows rounded out to the sides. Do not straighten your arms.

(2) Sound: Close the jaw so that the teeth gently meet and part the lips slightly. Inhale as you look up, eyes wide open, and push your palms upward and out as you slowly exhale through your teeth and make the sound "SSSSSSS." At first you can produce the Lungs' Sound aloud, but eventually you should practice sub-vocally (vocalizing so softly that only you can hear the sound). Picture and feel excess heat, sick energy, sadness, sorrow, depression, and grief expelled as the sacs surrounding the lungs compress. Exhale slowly and fully.

(3) Rest and Concentrate: Resting is very important because during rest you can communicate with your inner self and your internal system. When you have exhaled completely, rotate the palms down as you slowly lower the shoulders, and return your hands to your lap, palms up. Close your eyes and be aware of your lungs. Smile into them and imagine that you are still making the Lungs' Sound. Breathe normally and picture your lungs growing with a bright white color. This will strengthen your lungs and draw down the Universal Energy associated with them. With each breath, try to feel the exchange of cool, fresh energy as it replaces excessively hot energy.

Repeat six, nine, twelve, or 24 times. Practice more often to alleviate sadness, depression, colds, flu, toothaches, asthma, and emphysema.

b. The Kidneys' Sound

Associated Organ: Bladder
Element: Water
Season: Winter
Color: Black or Dark Blue
Emotions: Negative—Fear
              Positive—Gentleness
Sound: WOOOOOOO (as when blowing out a candle with the lips forming an "O")

(1) Position: Bring your legs together, ankles and knees touching. Be aware of your kidneys and smile into them. Take a deep breath, lean forward, and clasp the fingers of both hands together around your knees. Pull your arms straight from the lower back while bending the torso forward. (This allows your back to protrude in the area of the kidneys.) Simultaneously tilt your head upward as you look straight ahead and maintain the pull on your arms from the lower back. Feel your spine pull.

(2) Sound: Round the lips and slightly exhale the sound "WOOOOOOO" as if you were blowing out a candle. Simultaneously contract your abdomen, pulling it in toward your kidneys. Imagine the excess heat, fear, and wet, sick energies squeezed out from the fascia surrounding them.

(3) Rest and Concentrate: After you have fully exhaled, sit erect, separate the legs, and place your hands on your thighs, palms up. Close your eyes, breathe into the kidneys, and be aware of them. Picture the bright color blue in the kidneys. Smile into them, imagining that you are still making the Kidneys' Sound. Repeat the above steps three, six, twelve, or 24 times. Practice more often to alleviate fear, fatigue, dizziness, ringing in the ears, or back pain.

c. The Liver's Sound

Associated Organ: Gall Bladder
Element: Wood
Season: Spring
Color: Green
Emotions: Negative—Anger
              Positive—Kindness
Sound: SHHHHHHH (tongue near palate)

(1) Position: Sit comfortably and straight. Be aware of the liver and smile into it. When you feel you are in touch with the liver, extend your arms out to your sides, palms up. Take a deep breath as you slowly raise

the arms up and over the head from the sides, following this action with your eyes. Interlace the fingers and turn your joined hands over to face the ceiling, palms up. Push out at the heel of the palms and stretch the arms out from the shoulders. Bend slightly to the left, exerting a gentle pull on the liver.

(2) Sound: Open your eyes wide because they are the openings of the liver. Slowly exhale the sound "SHHHHHHH" sub-vocally. Envision expelling excess heat and anger from the liver, as the fasciae around it compress.

(3) Rest and Concentrate: When you have fully exhaled, separate the hands, turn the palms down, and slowly bring the arms down to your sides, leading with the heels of the hands. Bring the hands to rest on your thighs, palms up. Smile down into the liver. Close your eyes, breathe into it, and imagine you are still making the Liver's Sound. Repeat three, six, twelve, or 24 times. Practice more often to alleviate anger, red or watery eyes, to remove a sour or bitter taste, and to detoxify the liver.

d. The Heart's Sound

Associated Organ: Small Intestine
Element: Fire
Season: Summer
Color: Red
Emotions: Negative—Impatience, Hastiness, Arrogance, Cruelty
 Positive—Joy, Honor, Sincerity
Sound: HAWWWWWW (mouth wide open)

(1) Position: Be aware of the heart and smile into it. Take a deep breath and assume the same position as for the Liver's Sound. Unlike the former exercise, however, you will lean slightly to the right to pull gently against the heart, which is just to the left of the center of your chest. Focus on your heart, and feel the tongue's connection to it.

(2) Sound: Open the mouth, round the lips, and slowly exhale the sound "HAWWWWWW" sub-vocally. Picture the sac around the heart expelling heat, impatience, hastiness, arrogance, and cruelty.

(3) Rest and Concentrate: After having exhaled, smile into the heart, and picture a bright red color. Repeat the steps above three to 24 times. Practice more often to relieve sore throats, cold sores, swollen gums or tongue, jumpiness, moodiness, and heart disease.

e. The Spleen's Sound

Associated Organs: Pancreas, Stomach
Element: Earth
Season: Indian Summer
Color: Yellow
Emotions: Negative—Worry
          Positive—Fairness
Sound: WHOOOOOO (from the throat, guttural)

(1) Position: Be aware of the spleen and smile into it. Take a deep breath as you place the fingers of both hands just beneath the sternum on the left side. You will press in with the fingers as you push your middle back outward.

(2) Sound: Look up, and gently push your fingertips into the left of the solar plexus area, as you sub-vocally exhale the sound "WHOOOOOO." This is more guttural, or "throaty" than the Kidneys' Sound. Unlike blowing out a candle, this sound originates from the depths of the throat rather than from the mouth. Feel the Spleen's Sound vibrate the vocal cords. Feel any worries being transformed as the virtues of fairness and honesty arise.

(3) Rest and Concentrate: Once you have fully exhaled, close the eyes, place the hands on the thighs, palms up, and concentrate smiling energy on the spleen, pancreas, and stomach. Breathe into these organs as you picture a bright yellow light shining in the organs. Repeat the steps above three to 24 times. Practice more often to eliminate indigestion, nausea, and diarrhea.

f. The Triple Warmer's Sound

The Triple Warmer refers to the three energy centers of the body: The upper section (brain, heart, and lungs) is hot; the middle section (liver, kidneys, stomach, pancreas, and spleen) is warm; and the lower section (large and small intestines, bladder, and sexual organs) is cool. The sound "HEEEEEEE" balances the temperature of the three levels by bringing hot energy down to the lower center and cold energy up to the higher centers. Specifically, hot energy from the area of the heart moves to the colder sexual region, and cold energy from the lower abdomen is moved up to the heart's region.

(1) Position: Lie on your back with your arms resting palms up at your sides, and keep your eyes closed. Inhale fully into all three cavities: chest, solar plexus, and lower abdomen.

(2) Sound: Exhale the sound "HEEEEEEE" sub-vocally, first flattening your chest, then your solar plexus, and finally your lower abdomen. Imagine a large roller pressing out your breath as it moves from your head down to your sexual center.

(3) Rest and Concentrate: When you have fully exhaled, concentrate on the entire body. Repeat the above steps from three to six times. Practice more often to relieve insomnia and stress.

3. Daily Practice Before Bedtime

Practice the Six Healing Sounds before going to bed at night. This will help decelerate the body, promote good sleep, and cool down any overheated organs. Before you go to sleep, clear the negative emotions so that the positive emotions can grow. Clearing out the negative emotions will chase away bad dreams and nightmares. You can sleep well and connect to the Universal Mind to recharge your energy.

If you have problems, difficulties, or feel ill, attain the sensation of emptiness and send these disturbances up into the Universal Mind. Trust that this force will help you. In the morning smile inwardly and see if you can find answers to your disturbances. Often the answer will be there for you when you awake.

The Six Healing Sounds and Inner Smile practices are more fully explained and illustrated in the Healing Tao book, *Taoist Ways to Transform Stress into Vitality.*

J. Fanning and Venting Sick Energy

These exercises are particularly good for the CNT practitioner to practice daily to get rid of sick energy and negative emotions so that positive emotions can grow and circulate. They can also drain the excess heat from a student, but the student must practice regularly at home to receive their full benefit.

1. Fanning

Since tension causes a lot of sick, negative emotional energy to condense in the chest, the heart can easily become *jammed.* Some believe long term negative emotions such as hatred, impatience, and arrogance directly affect heart conditions or are a major cause of heart attacks. To protect yourself you can activate the heart. This process will draw the

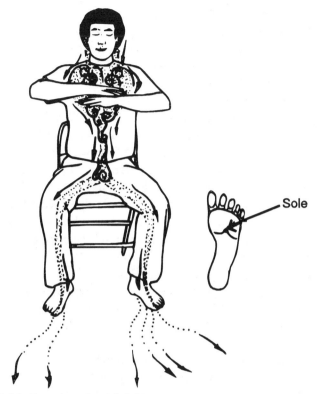

Figure 2-36. Fanning the Sick Energy and Negative Emotions from the Heart to the Soles of the Feet

negative feelings and sick energy to the heart, and you will need to *fan* this energy out of the heart and body.

a. The Purpose of Fanning

Taoists regard the soles of the feet and centers of the palms as having a connection with the heart. Therefore, Fanning sick energy involves moving the energy from the heart down to the soles of the feet. (Figure 2-36) The theory is that when the sick energy is fanned down to the soles of the feet and further down to the Earth, the soles connect with Mother Earth who can accept the sick and negative energy to utilize and transform it into useful energy. This means that if the negative energy is expressed as emotions and "dumped" from the higher place of the heart, it will not be received by Mother Earth who can put it to good use. Instead, these emotions will be received by other people involved in the person's life, a situation that can cause sickness for them as well.

111

b. Position and Practice

Fanning is an activity originating in the upper diaphragm and in the mind. With the palm facing downward, raise the left hand to the chest at the level of the Heart Center, about one and one half inches from the top of the sternum. Place the right hand parallel and above it, aligning its palm with pericardium 8.

(1) Practice the Heart's Sound (HAWWWWWW) and feel the heat from the heart start to burn, drawing in any negative feelings.

(2) Exhale this energy (using the Heart's Sound) as simultaneoulsy you lower both hands. Feel the negative energies burn out. Continue to exhale the energy down to the perineum, to the back of both feet, to the soles, and then perceive Mother Earth absorbing it. Rest the palms on the knees. Look down to the soles of the feet and feel a cloudy, grey, and cold or chilly energy go out. Rest again. Be sure to take a long time to rest since your resting time is very important.

(3) Start over again by returning both hands to the heart level. Practice eighteen to 36 times for a total of five to ten minutes. As you clear yourself of the dirty, sick energy, you will feel empty, but in a good mood. Feel the Heavenly Energy as a golden light coming down through the head and filling the body.

(5) Rest for a while. You also will feel Mother Earth's Energy, a blue color, coming up through the soles of your feet.

2. Venting

a. The Purpose of Venting

When negative emotions are causing sickness in the organs, venting is another practice to remove the undesirable energy. For example, fear in the kidneys can be vented to change the color of their energy from a cloudy, blue energy to a bright blue. Anger produces cloudiness in the liver's color which can be changed from a cloudy green back to a bright, clear green.

b. Position and Practice

After you finish Fanning as above, remain in the same sitting position to begin the Venting exercise. Venting is practiced to get rid of emotions from all of the other organs. Since fingers and toes are connected with all the organs and glands (Figure 2-37), sick energy tends to stagnate there making them feel numb.

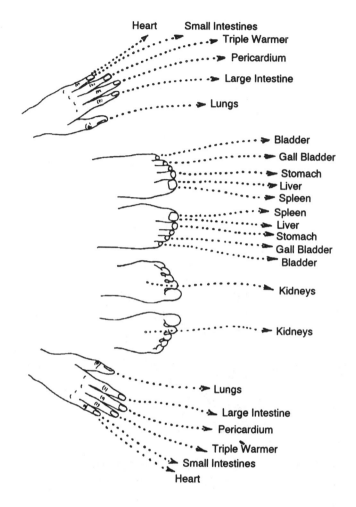

Heart   Small Intestines
Triple Warmer
Pericardium
Large Intestine
Lungs

Bladder
Gall Bladder
Stomach
Liver
Spleen
Spleen
Liver
Stomach
Gall Bladder
Bladder

Kidneys

Kidneys

Lungs
Large Intestine
Pericardium
Triple Warmer
Small Intestines
Heart

Figure 2-37. The toes and fingers correspond to the organs

(1) Sit and place your hands on your knees. Keep your fingers slightly spread apart and pointed toward the toes.

(2) Place your feet parallel to each other and point the toes up. Be aware of the area two or three inches up and directly between the big toes. Be aware of the tips of the big toes and then all of the toes.

(3) If you have sick energy affecting an organ, look at Figure 2-37 to determine the toes or fingers that correspond to that organ. During Venting you can emphasize the fingers or toes corresponding to the organ

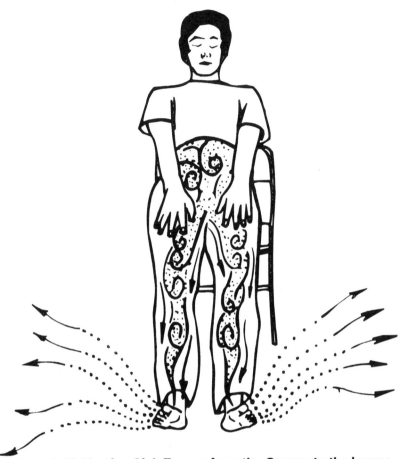

Figure 2-38. Venting Sick Energy from the Organs to the Lower Abdomen and the Toes

in which you have the sick energy to send more of the energy out of the body. For example, if you have a heart problem, you can concentrate on the pinky fingers. Feel the cloudy, grey energy exiting through those fingers.

(4) Practice the Triple Warmer's Sound (HEEEEEEE) down to the navel, perineum, and toes. (Figures 2-38 and 2-39) With the (HEEEEEEE) Sound, feel the vibration of the Sound at and moving out of the tips of the fingers and toes.

(5) Gradually feel a steaming, dark, cloudy, cold or chilly, sick emotional energy emerging from the toes and fingers.

114

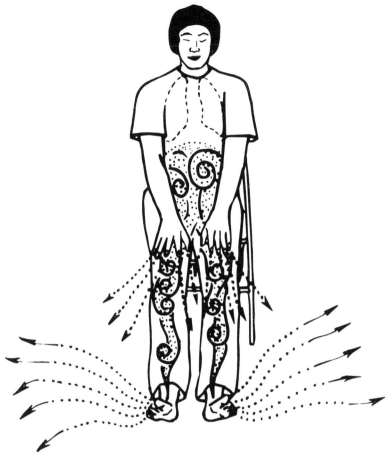

Figure 2-39. Venting Sick Energy from the Diaphragm to the Lower Abdomen

(6) Picture it becoming brighter and brighter. Continue to look at the point between the big toes to see more sick energy and negative feelings emerge.

(7) Be aware of the liver and see it become a bright green.

(8) Be aware of the spleen and the pancreas, and see them glow with a bright yellow color.

(9) Be aware of the lungs and see them glow with a white light.

(10) Be aware of the heart and see it open with a bright red.

(11) Be aware of the kidneys; see them glow with a bright blue light.

Chi Nei Tsang

CHAPTER 3

OBSERVING THE BODY: LOOKING, FEELING, AND ASKING

The techniques of observing the student's body and spirit were developed over thousands of years. You can learn procedures for looking, feeling, and asking that will indicate which organs and areas of the abdomen need attention and massage. Some of the techniques, such as pulse and tongue reading, take time to master. It is not necessary to know all of them to do the massage techniques. You can start using the easier techniques right away and practice with the more difficult ones later.

Start by observing the shape of the navel and by feeling the abdomen. When you discover soreness, tightness, congestion, distension, and toxicity, you will learn that you can help many people by using a gentle, spiraling massage around the navel area. You will learn to let your fingers educate and guide you.

A. The Abdomen

1. The Physical Structure of the Abdominal Cavity within the Peritoneum

The physical structure of the abdominal cavity contains the large intestine, small intestine, liver, gall bladder, stomach, spleen, pancreas, bladder, sex organs, aorta and vena cava, many lymph nodes, nervous system, abdominal muscles, and fasciae. They are contained in the peritoneum, a membrane lining the abdominopelvic walls. The kidneys and the adrenal glands are located toward the back, between the peritoneum and ribs. The back of the cavity is protected by the ribs, spine and

117

pelvis, and muscles. The internal organs and some blood vessels, lymph vessels, and nerves can be reached from the front of the body.

a. Feeling the Skin and Muscles of the Abdomen

The skin that covers the abdomen can help you decide the health of the organs that lie underneath it. Place your hand gently and without pressure on the abdomen. Move it in a circular motion to discern the condition of the skin. Unhealthy tissues can be too tight, too loose, or without elasticity (atonic). The better the elasticity, the healthier the organs. Healthy tissue has a normal elasticity because the nerves that influence the elasticity are not damaged by toxins. The texture and tone of the skin is normal, even, and elastic to the touch without any irregularity. Healthy skin covers the body like a well-fitting body suit. Unhealthy skin can be detoxified, and elasticity can be gradually restored.

The abdomen has many large sheets of muscles. Healthy muscles also help to create a healthy abdomen. Practice the same technique as when palpating the skin, but this time try a little more pressure. Feel the muscles under the skin and distinguish between a normal resistance of the muscle and a hard and tight resistance. If there is any inflammation in the abdominal cavity, the body will tighten up its abdominal muscles to protect the irritated area. Sometimes the abdomen feels very tough and hard. This is a good indication of an inflammation. A healthy abdomen feels soft and bouncy (like a baby's) with sufficient muscle tone to hold the organs in place. It should be without any tension or resistance, and show a clear outline of what is underneath. An overdeveloped, rock-like abdomen packs the organs too tightly and does not allow much room to expand. Such a muscle-bound abdomen also limits the range of movement of the spine, shoulders, and rib cage.

b. Breathing Properly from the Abdomen

Breathing patterns can reveal the health of the abdomen. The lungs occupy a large part of the upper chest. Under stress or emotional turmoil, a person will breathe tensely, using the chest. This causes shortness of breath and congestion in the chest. The normal breathing pattern of a healthy person is abdominal breathing. Only in this way can the lungs do their work most efficiently (oxygen exchange, activating peristaltic movements, processing Chi). Proper abdominal breathing will remove congestion and exercise all the organs.

During abdominal breathing the diaphragm moves up and down, creating a pumping and sucking massage of the intestines.

If there is a disorder or inflammation in the abdomen, or if the digestive system is unhealthy, the body provides a signal that there is a problem. To protect the irritated area, a reflex action will stop abdominal breathing and initiate chest breathing, thereby neutralizing any movement in the abdomen.

B. The Body Structure and the Abdomen

In the last twenty years, the public has become more aware of the body's needs for healthy and nutritious food. However, even if the healthiest foods are consumed, the body cannot properly use the nourishment if the digestive system isn't healthy. The result is an increasingly unhealthy state. Since the abdomen is flexible, formed by muscles and tendons, and without a stiff form, it is possible to determine any changes in the normal appearance of the abdomen.

1. Unhealthy Intestines Distort the Shape

When gas accumulates in the corners of the large intestines, the rib cage is pressed upward and outward. This can be on one side of the rib cage only, or on both sides. The intensity of the deformation depends upon how much gas accumulation there is. If this state is chronic, the ribs deform themselves. Because the ribs are attached to the spine, the vertebrae also will start changing their positions.

If there is a gas accumulation only on one side, the spine will start twisting. If there is any traction in the normal structure, the body will naturally react with a movement to adjust to this position. Thus, the body intensifies the problem. For example, suppose there is a strong chronic gas accumulation on the left side of the large intestine. The rib cage will be lifted up on the left side, and the vertebrae will move and shift to the right. The body tries to adjust to this change in structure by contracting the muscles on the left side of the spine. This will not have any affect on the vertebrae that are moved by the ribs, but it will pull the vertebrae above and below that area to the other side. Through this counter-movement of the body, the structural problem grows larger. (Figure 3-1)

2. Expansion of the Lower Back

People with weak muscles, who straighten out the natural curve of the lower back (the lumbar vertebrae), can create more room for their

119

unhealthy intestines. Because of this straightening, the head moves forward and the natural curve of the cervical spine is straightened as well.

3. Excessive Bending of the Lower Back

People with strong muscles who have problems in the upper abdomen tend to create more room for the intestines by tilting the hip down and bending the lower back excessively. Because the natural curve of the thorax straightens, the chest comes out, the neck is held tightly backward, and the scapulae close in on each other. This structure causes lower back pain and can be the reason for shortened breath.

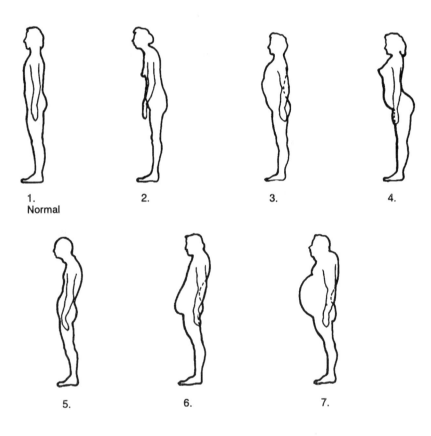

1.
Normal

2.

3.

4.

5.

6.

7.

**Figure 3-1. Distortion of the Structure Due to
an Unhealthy Abdomen**
Based on a drawing in *Diagnostik nach F.X. Mayer* by Erich Rauch

4. Excessive Bending Combined with Extension—the Duck Position

People, especially women, with strong muscles and unhealthy intestines show a structure that is a combination of an extension of the lumbar region and an excessive bending of the junction of the lumbar vertebrae. The lower back is bent, and the buttocks stick out. The upper body is held backward, but the chest is pushed out. In this structure the weight of the intestines causes them to hang down toward the back, so they are no longer pressing on the female organs. This also makes room for intestines that are full of gas.

5. Excessive Bending of the Lumbar Region and Excessive Curving of the Thoracic Spine

Those with intestinal disorders, weak muscles, and fatigue try to create more room for their intestines by excessively bending the natural curve of the lower back and rounding the thoracic curve. As a result, the abdomen protrudes and the neck is stiffly held straight and forward. The scapulae are wide apart from each other, and the chest is flat or concave.

6. Hanging Intestines

This structure of the person with hanging intestines is similar to that described in 5 above. The lower back is curved inward, the buttocks move outward, and the thorax is held back to compensate for a weak and hanging belly.

The loose small intestinal bulge often hangs over and covers the genitals, creating a fold at the height of the pubic bone. This crease easily becomes inflamed.

7. Big Belly

This body posture is the result of a big, heavy tummy. The chest and diaphram are pushed upward and become wider. The neck is almost invisible, disappearing between the shoulders and a hump at the back of the neck.

C. The Shape of the Navel

The Taoists learned by observing the most obvious things. They learned that it is possible to know a great deal about the condition of the abdominal area and organs just from examining the shape of the navel.

1. Examination of the Navel

Always note the shape and position of the navel before beginning a session. The navel is similar to a funnel, and it divides into three parts: the rim, the sidewall, and the bottom. The navel should be round, centered, and symmetrical. It should be firm and springy, not hard and tight, or soft and weak. The sidewalls should be symmetrical. The floor or bottom should be in the center of a circular rim.

The rim can be misshapen and off-center. The sidewall, and sometimes the rim, can be puffy, curved, high angled, or pulled in one or more directions. The floor of the navel can be puffy and congested, or it may be very deep. It may be twisted or pulled, and may or may not include the sidewall and rim.

The navel may be pulled in one or more directions. It may be vertical, horizontal, diagonal, teardropped, collapsed, blown out, or turned clockwise or counterclockwise.

With some practice, you will find that by reading the three parts of the navel, you can determine which way or ways it is being pulled. Distortion of the navel indicates the direction and location of tight, congested areas and blockages. Sometimes this will show which organs or systems are involved and at what depth.

2. Different Navel Pulls and their Effects

Imagine a pie six inches in diameter placed on the navel. Now divide that pie into eight sections. (Figure 3-2) Note where the navel is pushing or pulling according to the eight directions. (Figure 3-3) Notice if the navel is pulling in one or more directions simultaneously. When you learn which organs are in each pie piece and can associate them with the distortion of the navel, you will have a very good means of determining what imbalances are present in the body.

The pulling may only affect the superficial tissues or a specific organ or system. Usually the pulling affects the body's center, both superficial and deep, and involves more than one organ or system. Remember that any pulling distorts the body's center and the first system to be influenced is the Navel Center Chi system. When the Chi system is off-center, the physical body is also off-center, creating an imbalance in the emotions, systems, and organs.

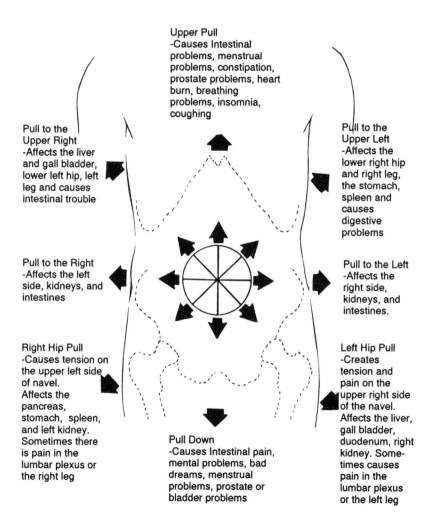

Upper Pull
-Causes Intestinal problems, menstrual problems, constipation, prostate problems, heart burn, breathing problems, insomnia, coughing

Pull to the Upper Right
-Affects the liver and gall bladder, lower left hip, left leg and causes intestinal trouble

Pull to the Upper Left
-Affects the lower right hip and right leg, the stomach, spleen and causes digestive problems

Pull to the Right
-Affects the left side, kidneys, and intestines

Pull to the Left
-Affects the right side, kidneys, and intestines.

Right Hip Pull
-Causes tension on the upper left side of navel. Affects the pancreas, stomach, spleen, and left kidney. Sometimes there is pain in the lumbar plexus or the right leg

Left Hip Pull
-Creates tension and pain on the upper right side of the navel. Affects the liver, gall bladder, duodenum, right kidney. Sometimes causes pain in the lumbar plexus or the left leg

Pull Down
-Causes Intestinal pain, mental problems, bad dreams, menstrual problems, prostate or bladder problems

Figure 3-2. Chart for Reading Navel Pulls

123

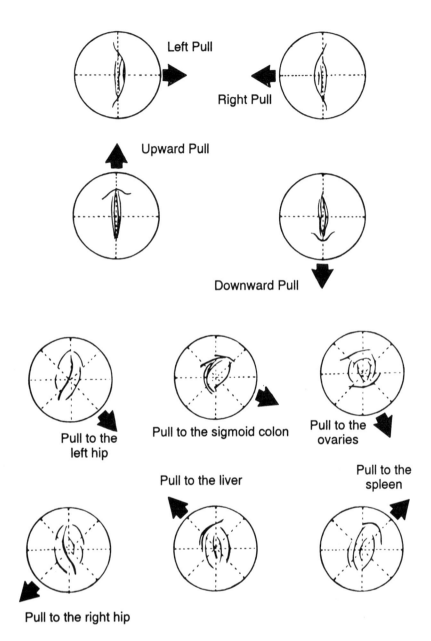

Figure 3-3. Navel Pulls

a. Pulls to the Left Hip

(1) A navel that pulls toward the lower left side can be related to tension in the upper right side. This can affect the liver, gall bladder, duodenum, and right kidney and may cause pain in the lumbar plexus or the left leg.

(2) If the left ovary is pulled off its center, it can cause menstrual problems. Gently probe to the left side of the ovary and uterus and look for tension. There may be a knot near the ovary, or between the ovary and uterus.

b. Pulls Down

(1) When the navel pulls downward toward the center of the groin, there may be tension in the solar plexus and upper chest. The navel pulse may be pulled down as well.

(2) This can cause dyspepsia and chronic pain. It also could cause pressure against the intestines, possibly bringing on mental problems and bad dreams. The small intestines are the paired organs of the heart, so any digestive problems can cause the heart to overheat.

(3) The pull can affect the upper and lower side, so there could be pain in the lower side. Tension can cause the intestines to lock together.

(4) Women can experience menstrual and fertility problems if the cervix pulls off-center.

(5) In a man you might find a knot near the pubic bone, or below the bladder, near the prostate gland, which may be causing prostate or bladder problems.

c. Pulls to the Right Hip

(1) If the navel pulls toward the lower right part of the pelvis and is tense toward the upper left side, the student can be off-center. This can affect the pancreas, stomach, spleen, and left kidney, and could pull the lumbar plexus off-center causing pain in the right leg.

(2) In women, a right ovary that pulls to one side can be the cause of menstrual problems. Gently probing the right side of the ovary and uterus can reveal a knot near the ovary or between the ovary and uterus.

d. Pulls to the Right Side

(1) If the navel pulls toward the upper right side of the pelvis, the left side of the small intestine can feel tight and painful. Problems along that line can occur at both a superficial and a deep level. This can affect the function of the intestines and the right and left kidneys.

(2) A right side pull can cause tightness in the upper right side and affect the liver and gall bladder. The pull could cause tightness in the left leg and hip and can affect the sigmoid colon.

e. Pulls to the Upper Left Side

(1) A navel that pulls to the upper left side can cause tightness in the lower right side, pull the lumbar plexus off-center, and cause pain in the right. There is the possibility of problems in the pancreas, stomach, spleen, and left kidney.

(2) In women, menstrual problems can occur.

(3) This pull suggests problems in the ileocecal valve and the digestive process.

f. Pulls to the Left Side

(1) If the navel pulls to the left side of the pelvis, the right side of the intestine can feel tight and painful. This can cause a problem on the centerline, both deeply and superficially, and the kidneys may be affected.

g. Pulls to the Upper Right Side

(1) A navel that pulls to the upper right side can cause tightness in the lower left side, pull the lumbar plexus off-center, and cause left leg pain. There could be problems in the liver, gall bladder, and right kidney.

(2) In women, menstrual problems can occur.

(3) This pull suggests problems with the sigmoid colon and the digestive process.

h. Pulls Up

(1) A navel that pulls up can pull the navel pulse above the umbilicus when it should be below. This can cause bad digestion, constipation, acidity, diseases of the heart, and an irritating personality.

(2) In women, this can pull the cervix off-center and cause menstrual problems.

D. Hand Scanning the Internal Organs

1. Each Organ Emits a Different Aura

Each organ emits a different kind of force or aura through the skin. By passing a hand one to two inches above the skin, you can feel different sensations that reflect the condition or state of the internal organs. You need to develop the sensitivity to receive the vibration or frequency of each organ.

Practicing the Aura, Tree, and Healing Hand Meditations (see Chapter 2) will help develop such sensitivity.

a. Liver and Gall Bladder Scanning

(1) Healthy liver and gall bladder energy feels warm.

(2) Negative Emotions: When you pass your hand over the liver, under the right side of the rib cage, you will feel a charged energy come up to your hand. (Figure 3-4) This is a sign of anger in the liver.

(3) Overactivity: When you pass your hand over the liver and feel a rush of hot energy, this indicates that the liver is overheating because of toxins or emotional stress.

(4) Underactivity: When you pass your hand over the liver and you feel a dense and hot energy, the liver is weak, congested, and sick.

b. Lungs Scanning

(1) Healthy lung energy feels cool and dry.

(2) Negative Emotions: Pass your hand over the lungs. Do the Lungs' Sound and listen to the echo of the sound as it rebounds from the lungs. Sadness will feel like a deflating ball pressed between your hands.

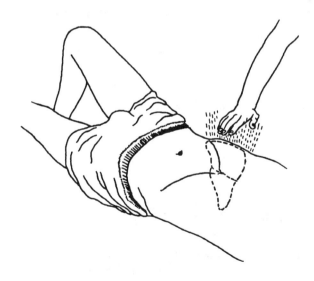

Figure 3-4. Scanning the Liver

127

(3) Overactivity: Energy that feels dry and hot indicates an overworked organ.

(4) Underactivity: Energy that feels damp and cool under the scanning hand indicates underactive or congested lungs that can lead to respiratory problems.

c. Heart Scanning

(1) Healthy heart energy feels warm and energetic.

(2) Negative Emotions: Hot and charged energy indicates impatience, hastiness, and arrogance in the heart.

(3) Overactivity: If your hand detects hot, charging, and a more expansive energy, this indicates that the heart and blood may be overheating.

(4) Underactivity: Energy that feels cool and less expansive indicates an underactive or congested heart.

d. Spleen Scanning

(1) Healthy spleen energy feels lukewarm.

(2) Negative emotions: Energy that feels damp and sinking indicates excessive worry.

(3) Overactivity: The energy feels hot and damp when the spleen is overactive.

(4) Underactivity: The energy feels cool and damp.

e. Kidneys Scanning

(1) Healthy kidney energy feels cold, but not too cold.

(2) Negative emotions: Energy that feels cold and chilly indicates fear.

(3) Overactivity: When the kidneys are overworked or over-stimulated by excessive exercise or are affected by improper diet and liquid intake, the energy can feel damp, sticky, and hot.

(4) Underactivity: When toxins are blocking the organs, the energy can feel damp and cold.

E. Traditional Face Reading

Although the most important indication of the state of the organs is the shape of the navel, there are other traditional methods of Chinese medicine that check the state of health of the body such as *Face Reading*.

Since facial features have a direct correlation to the five major organs (see Figure 1-26), as well as to the circulatory, nervous, and other systems of the body, observing the face can be helpful in diagnosing problems. (Figure 3-5)

Generally speaking, the health of a person will be reflected in an apparently balanced face. Signs of imbalances could be discoloration, deep lines, and enlarged or protruding features, such as eyes or lips. Since Face Reading is an entire study in itself, the following is only a sampling of some of the indications to look for.

1. Color of the Face

A red face indicates a problem in the cardiovascular system, especially if it is around the tip of the nose. Darkness in the face, especially around the eyes, points to kidney problems. A white, pale face suggests lung problems. A yellow-green face shows a liver problem; a yellow-orange color indicates a spleen problem.

2. Lines on the Face

The depth of the lines is an indication of the seriousness of the problem. Horizontal lines between the eyes on the bridge of the nose

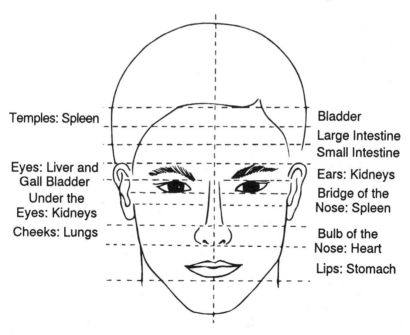

Figure 3-5. Face Reading

show congestion of the intestines and, possibly, menstrual problems for women. Horizontal lines on the forehead and under the eyes, which are caused by excess liquid in the system, can indicate a kidney problem. A deep, long vertical line above the nose and between the eyebrows indicates a liver problem.

3. Eyes

The eyes reflect the condition of every organ in the body, but perhaps most directly they reflect the liver's condition and thereby the related condition of the digestive system, and also that of the nervous system. In reflecting the liver's condition, a healthy liver is indicated by an iris with a soft, translucent quality. The pupil should be transparent; a deep black color indicates kidney trouble. Discoloration of the edges of the eyelids show an unhealthy spleen. The white of the eyes shows the condition of the lungs and, again, discoloration indicates a problem. Any bloodshot lines in the white of the eyes could indicate some imbalance in the body's condition, although four lines commonly do show in most people. Both corners of the eyes indicate the state of the heart.

4. Skin

The color of the skin can be an indication of the condition of the lungs. Observe the color of the cheeks to check for excessive whiteness. The skin of the nostrils is another indicator of the lungs' condition. Healthy skin contains a balanced moisture, so check for overly dry or overly moist skin in the nostrils.

5. Lips and Mouth

Different parts of the lips show the condition of different parts of the digestive system. The upper part of the upper lip corresponds to the upper stomach, the middle section of the upper lip corresponds to the middle of the stomach, and the lower part of the upper lip corresponds to the duodenum (the exit of the stomach, connected to the liver, gall bladder, and pancreas). The lower lip shows the condition of the intestines. If lips are swollen, the digestive tract is expanded. An outward swelling of the lower lip shows a tendency to constipation. Spots and sores on the lips show ulceration and stagnation of blood in the digestive system. Lips that are whitish in color show that the blood in the intestinal region is weak, and absorption is poor. Extreme tightness in the mouth shows that the intestines are tight, meaning absorption is poor. A healthy mouth, however, should appear fairly tight.

6. Appearance and Condition of the Tongue

Reading information from the tongue is a significant way to determine the condition of the body and spirit.

a. Areas

Various areas of the tongue reflect the state of the internal organs. The root of the tongue is related to the kidneys. The center of the tongue reflects the condition of the stomach and spleen. The tip of the tongue represents the state of heart. The area between the tip and the center shows the condition of the lungs. The right side of the tongue indicates the gall bladder. The left side of the tongue reflects the liver. (Figure 3-6)

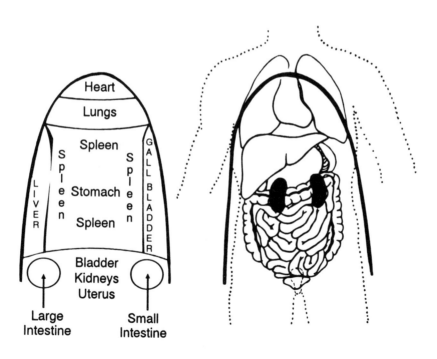

Figure 3-6. Areas of the tongue reflect areas of the body

131

b. Color

The color of the tongue indicates the state of the blood, nutritious Chi, and the Yin organs. The normal color of the tongue should be pale red. A very pale color indicates a deficiency of Yang or blood. When the sides of the tongue are pale, this indicates deficient blood in the liver.

If the tip of the tongue is crimson, it signifies too much heat in the heart. Crimson sides indicate too much heat in the liver or gall bladder, and, in severe cases, the sides may be swollen and display crimson spots. A crimson center indicates too much heat in the stomach.

An indigo tongue indicates stagnant blood. The flow of the blood and Chi has congealed. Deep purple indicates severe blood stasis, this may indicate serious liver or heart problems.

c. Shape

The shape of the tongue also indicates the state of the blood and nutritious Chi. A thin tongue indicates a blood deficiency if it is also pale, or a Yin deficiency if it is red and peeled. A swollen, pale tongue indicates dampness and Yang deficiency. A stiff tongue indicates wind problems. A flaccid tongue means not enough fluids. A long tongue means heat in the heart. A short, squat tongue indicates interior cold if pale and wet, or extreme Yin deficiency if red and peeled.

Short horizontal cracks indicate stomach Yin deficiency. A long, deep midline crack indicates heart problems. A shallow-wide crack in the midline that doesn't reach the tip indicates deficient Yin in the stomach. Short, transversal cracks on the sides and/or in the middle of the tongue indicate chronic Chi deficiency in the spleen. A quivering tongue also indicates deficient Chi in the spleen.

d. Coating

A normal tongue coating or tongue fur is thin, white, and moist. This indicates that the stomach is digesting food properly. A thick white coating indicates cold problems. A yellow fur means heat problems.

e. Moisture

A normal tongue should be very slightly moist. Too much moisture indicates that the fluids are not moving well. If it is too dry, there is too much heat in the body.

7. Tone of the Voice

A loud voice shows overactivity of the liver. If it is joyful and laughing (overexcited), there is an overactivity of the heart. If the voice is singing, there is an overactivity of the spleen. Overactivity or irritation in the lungs is indicated by a weeping sound. A weak or trembling voice shows weakness in the kidneys.

F. The Wrist Pulses

The reading of the wrist pulses developed into a complex art. An experienced therapist can feel 28 pulses and tell a great deal about the body. Such an art takes a lifetime to master. However, a novice can learn valuable information about the organs. In CNT you only need to know a few simple pulse readings, for there are many other ways of determining the state of the organs.

1. Reading the Pulse

a. The purpose of pulse reading is to detect what is going on with the individual spiritually, emotionally, and physically. Feel the spirit of the pulse. See if the student is alert. Look at the big picture first, not the small details. If you grasp the big picture, the small details will fall into place. Feel for clearness; if the pulse is turbid, the energy is not positive. Feel for consistency; note how pure, mixed, or unified the pulses are. People can change their pulses over a period of time. One can change their mind and make the pulse change.

The Taoists discovered that the pulse is the sound of the blood leaving an organ. If there is something in the organ to obstruct the blood, there will be a delay or distortion in the pulse. Each organ has a different sound or echo. If the person is healthy, there are probably no obstructions. Some blockages can't be changed, but many can be removed by working directly on the organ. This will cause a new and different pulse.

b. It is important to realize that where the Chi goes, the blood follows. Therefore, it is possible to find out the flow of a person's Chi by observing the blood flow. You can externally determine what someone's internal conditions are.

2. Locating the Wrist Pulses

When taking your own pulse, hold one hand palm upward and use the fingers of your other hand to locate the radial artery passing through the top of your wrist. Feel for a prominent bone (called the styloid process of the radial) that is about one inch below the outside of the wrist. Place the middle finger on this point. That is the center of the pulse area. There are two other pulse positions, one on either side of this bone, where you can feel the artery pulsate. You can easily locate the other two pulse positions by placing your index and ring (or fourth) fingers on the artery. Your index finger will lie closest to the thumb, while your ring finger will lie farthest from the crease formed at the connection of the hand and wrist. (Figure 3-7)

This pulse is located along the Lungs' Channel which starts in the shoulder area near the clavicle and runs down the arm around the biceps, passes the elbow crease, runs along the top of the wrist, and ends near the tip of the thumb. You can ascertain the condition of the whole body by feeling the pulses at the wrists along the Lungs' Channel.

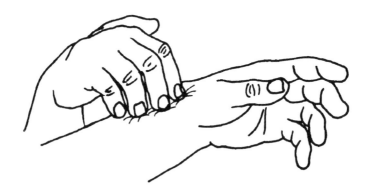

Figure 3-7. Locating the pulses on the left wrist

3. Feeling the Pulse

a. Feel what is called the *area of the pulse*. The pulse may extend in either direction, or the area may only feel like the head of a pin.

b. You may not feel the pulse unless you press hard; or, again, it might not even have to be pressed because it is plainly visible. This is called the *depth of the pulse*.

c. Also feel for the *quality of the pulse*. There may be an *urgent or fighting pulse* that feels like it is banging against your fingers. Its opposite is the *weak* pulse, for it seems to disappear as you feel for it, like a ball of cotton.

4. Noting Some Common Pulse Qualities

a. *Healthy Pulse:* A healthy pulse feels moderate. It is not too fast or slow, too big or small, too strong or weak, too superficial or deep, and not too rough or hard. A healthy pulse is gentle, steady, clear, smooth, calm, balanced, and soft (but not too soft). It beats four beats per respiratory cycle. Visualize this healthy pulse when you start to take someone's pulse.

b. *Empty Pulse:* When you palpate this pulse, it feels as though you are pushing down on a cotton ball. There is very little resistance. The body is weak and has low resistance.

c. *Fast, Inflamed Pulse:* A fast pulse is very Yang and beats more than five times per respiration. This pulse is so forceful that it feels as though it were trying to push your finger away. You can see it pounding. The heart may be beating quickly, which would indicate that there is excess energy in the heart, and, thus, not enough energy elsewhere.

An increased pulse rate can suggest an inflammation.

d. *Full pulse:* This pulse is full and long, hard and forceful. It feels like the tight cords of a musical instrument. It is commonly associated with liver problems.

e. *Slippery Pulse:* A slippery pulse feels smooth and rounded like slippery pearls rolling around. It means that there is a mucous problem or stagnant Chi in the organ, perhaps due to digestion problems.

f. *Choppy or Rough Pulse:* It feels rough, uneven. This indicates that the blood is deficient in Chi, because of a decreased organ function.

5. Observing the Body Type

Body type makes a difference. For a bigger person, expect a wider pulse; whereas someone thin will have a thinner pulse. Look at the trunk of the body; if it is thin, then a thin pulse is proper. Consistency of pulses and body type must exist. This means the consistency of the speed, depth, strength, shape, and length of the pulse must also be consistent with the body type. So, if the person is big and the pulses are small, then there is a serious imbalance.

6. Feeling the Lungs' Channel and the Pulse

The Lungs' Channel and lungs' energy are extremely important to the healthy functioning of the body. The heart and lungs both work closely together rhythmically circulating blood and Chi. The Lungs' energy carries the Chi and the Chi causes the blood to flow. This is how

135

the energy of the lungs enters the blood. The Lungs' energy is also directly connected to the Triple Warmer. You can see the position of the pulses in relation to the Triple Warmer.

Rest the back of your left hand in the palm of your right and wrap the index finger, middle finger, and ring finger of your right hand around the thumb side of your left wrist. Now gently push with those three fingers, one at a time, until you find the strongest beating at each of those locations. With all three fingers depressed, connect your index finger to your chest. Connect your middle finger, resting on the styloid process with your digestive organs, spleen, liver, gall bladder, and pancreas. The lower position, farthest from the crease of the wrist, is the urogenital area, the place of Original Chi found between the kidneys.

7. Taking a Student's Pulse

When taking a student's pulse, it is best to work on the student from the side. Don't put your arm across the body. It is easiest to use your left hand on his or her right wrist. Place the tips (not pads) of your fingers on the wrist at a 90 degree angle. Line up your fingers as in Figure 3-7.

Feel with sensitivity and receptiveness. Don't feel as though you were touching something; feel as though something was trying to touch you, to impress itself upon you. Relax, as if in meditation. A healthy pulse feels firm, not too strong or aggressive, and does not feel like it is hiding, weak, or vulnerable. Look for moderate resistance and moderate strength when treating someone.

Is the pulse weak in one of those three positions? Or is it weak in all of them? Perhaps it grows weak and strong, reflecting the student's energy level in response to a disease factor. The student may have an excessive pulse which feels tense. It may be tense in some places and weak in others. This is something to watch for. See if it relaxes and if some of the weak places fill up so that the pulsations even out.

It may feel as though you were pressing on the steel or fiberglass string of a musical instrument. The steel string feeling that really hits your fingers would be described as a wiry pulse. When it is a little softer, it is called a cord pulse. Both of these primarily reflect emotions. The wiry pulse is associated with disharmony in the liver and gall bladder.

Other qualities to look for are superficial and deep. Ideally, there should be a balance between the two with a presence of fullness. Some people may have a really faint pulse that is just superficial or deep. If you have to press very hard to sense anything then you would say that the

136

energy is deep, and that there is not much energy on the surface of the body to defend itself. This could lead to catching cold easily. If the energy is superficial it is called a floating pulse. You hardly touch the wrist, and you already feel the pulse to be quite strong. With such a pulse you might have to strengthen the kidneys, spleen, or Yin energy.

If you have a problem in the lungs or large intestine, you may have a superficial pulse that shows the body's skin surface is struggling with sick energy and is in conflict with the rest of the body. You can feel that conflict when it is in the superficial part of the body as a floating pulse. The person might have a cold because the lungs and intestines are conceived of as a continuation of the skin.

The main pulses to work with when you are starting out are the excess and deficient, the full and strong, and the weak, thin, and empty. When you are feeling a blood vessel and it is thin, it indicates a lack of blood. Blood is something to which all the organs contribute. It is involved with supplying the entire body with food and oxygen, and with getting rid of waste and excess water. A weak, thin pulse is a sign of weakness while a full pulse that has a slippery quality shows that the blood is full of energy.

8. Working with Specific Pulses

You may also feel each organ individually along the wrist pulses. Feel for the different qualities listed above.

a. The Pulses on the Left Wrist

On the left wrist (Figure 3-8) the position of the index finger, nearest the crease of the wrist, reveals the condition of two organs. The small intestine is the surface position. When you press down with your finger, you can read the condition of the heart.

Your middle finger reads the condition of the gall bladder superficially. Pressing down will reveal the state of the liver.

Your ring finger, farthest from the crease of the wrist, reads the bladder in the superficial position, and when you press down you can read the kidneys.

b. The Pulses on the Right Wrist

When feeling the student's right hand pulses (Figure 3-9), your index finger, placed closest to the crease of the wrist, feels the large intestine superficially and the lung at the deeper position.

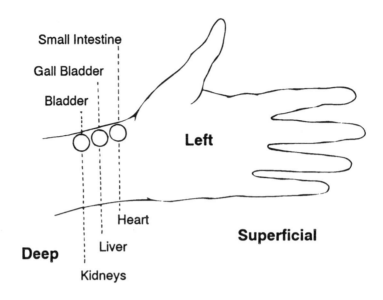

Figure 3-8. Pulses of the Left Wrist

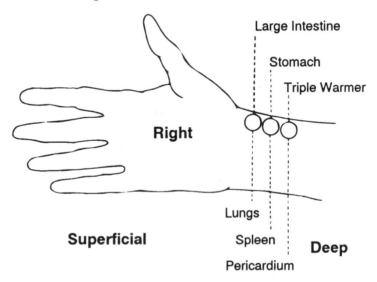

Figure 3-9. Pulses of the Right Wrist

Your middle finger reads the condition of the stomach at the surface position, and feels the spleen at the deeper position.

Your ring finger can feel the condition of the Triple Warmer at the superficial position, and it feels the condition of the pericardium or heart controller in the deep position.

G. The Tendons and Muscles

1. Emotions, Weather, and Toxins Can Harden the Tendons and Fasciae

An important factor affecting the smooth operation of the body is the condition of the tendons. The tendons have to be elastic and in their proper place at the proper time. Anger and very hot weather heat and expand the tendons. Negative emotions, such as fear, and very cold weather can cause contraction of the body's vital systems and the tendons which creates problems. As the tendons expand or contract, they do not always return to their original size, shape, and position. This can cause muscles and organs to be pulled out of shape and position. Knots and tangles start to form. As the knot lengthens and becomes larger, it becomes tighter. It then pulls the tendons, nerves, blood vessels, and lymph vessels tighter together.

Since the internal organs are also related to colors, temperatures, seasons, etc., when there is a change in the emotions, weather, or color of clothes you are wearing, there is also a change in the structure of the body, particularly of the tendons. The fasciae and tendons of the body are an integral part of the five major systems and the internal organs. Smooth operation of the tendons and fasciae is vital to good health.

2. Muscles: the "Backup Tanks" of the Organs

Muscles are like backup tanks. When the organs become overloaded with negative emotions or toxins, they will unload their energies into the muscles. When you have problems in the organs, you will feel aches and pains in your muscles. The main causes of the problems are the organs, not the muscles. The organs are deep inside making their problems difficult to feel. Unless a problem is truly serious, it will usually first show up within a muscle.

In studying Chi Nei Tsang, the root of the problem is determined (usually in one or several of the organs) by feeling the abdominal conditions of the lymphatic system, the nervous system, the circulation system, and the Chi channel system (energy system). Once the major cause of the problem is corrected, the muscular system can be worked on. The muscles then gradually release their tensions, aches, and pains.

H. Questionnaire

Use this questionnaire to interview a new student before you start working on him or her. You can begin to get an accurate picture of what is going on with and within the student. Some conditions, explained in this book, should not be worked on with Chi Nei Tsang techniques. Type this list of observations and questions and make copies to distribute to your students.

Date: _____Referred by: _____

Name: _____

Address: _____

Tel:_____Emergency # _____

Birth Date: _____

Marital Status: _____Children: _____

Job: _____

Complaint: _____

1. ASK QUESTIONS

Ask about the following conditions, systems, and situations:

a. Problems with liver, heart, lungs, kidneys, spleen, pancreas, intestines, stomach, bladder, gall bladder

b. Urogenital or gynecological problems

c. Surgeries, hospitalization

d. Accidents

e. Under care of psychologist, psychotherapist, psychiatrist

f. Medications now being taken

g. Coffee, cigarettes, alcohol, drugs

h. Appetite, digestion

i. Dominant emotion, nerves

j. Sleeping trends

k. Sexual energy

l. Immune problems

m. Diabetes

n. Hernias, ulcers

o. Infectious diseases, inflammations, skin infections

p. Cancers

q. High blood pressure (Can the student exercise, run, walk up stairs?)

r. Stroke

s. Pacemaker for stimulating the heart, artificial hip joint, or other artificial parts of the body

t. I.U.D. birth control device

u. Aneurism (a sac formed by the dilatation of the wall of a blood vessel)

v. Thrombosis (blood clots)

w. Phlebitis (inflammation of a vein)

x. Melanoma (a tumor made up of dark pigmented cells, usually visible)

y. Lymphoma (disorder of the lymph nodes)

2. OBSERVE

a. Face color, hues, lines

b. Breathing

c. Tone of voice

d. Gestures

e. Tics

f. Posture, build

g. Symmetries (shoulders, legs, eyes, mouth, muscle tension)

h. Skin texture, vascular spiders, pigmentation

i. Varicose veins

j. Shape of the navel

k. Moles in or very near the navel

l. Tongue analysis

m. Mannerisms

3. FEEL

Many CNT practitioners have made a copy of the CNT chart in Chapter 6 (Figure 6-13) so that they can mark the problem areas.

a. Muscle and skin tone of the navel and abdomen

b. Knots, tangles, tensions in abdomen

c. Results of organ scanning

d. Pulses

Chi Nei Tsang

CHAPTER 4

OPENING THE GATES
AND CHASING THE WINDS

If you are unfamiliar with Taoist concepts about the body, mind, and spirit, then in the first three chapters you have been introduced to more than a few novel and strange ideas: an invisible energy called Chi that powers the body; changes in the organs that generate varying emotions; and pulses in the wrist that reveal the condition of the organs. It is not important that you believe in these concepts to begin the practice of CNT. However, you need to be aware of the ideas and have an experimental attitude. One day they will become very real and evident to you.

This chapter discusses a similarly strange observation: there are winds circulating inside your body, affecting your health and emotional life. These winds are created inside and outside of the body. The idea of outside winds affecting us is not as foreign as you may think. The people of southern California and Los Angeles dread the late summer arrival of the "Santa Ana winds," which arise in the desert and are felt to be the cause of accidents and psychological problems. The serenity of people living in many valleys in Switzerland is often disturbed by the annual arrival of strange winds that descend on peaceful valleys. People who have lived long lives or live close to nature have learned to recognize that some winds and weather are more than what they seem.

Wind is Chi that can enter from the exterior of the body or can arise in the interior of the body. Winds enter and exit through the navel, back of the head, forearms, and lower legs. Good wind is Chi that is healthy and good for you. The ancient Taoists identified unhealthy, abnormal, and foul winds as winds that are pathological and perverse and called them *evil winds*. Evil winds become trapped as toxins, blockages, and energy that can't move. Chi composes these winds, and when they are expelled from the body, the Chi becomes healthy again. The Chi itself is

143

good, but it is in a bad situation. It is like having a room in your home that normally is full of good air, but if there is a dead fish or dead mouse in that room, then the air becomes unbearable and foul. Remove the offending cause, open the windows, and the air will be pleasant again.

Nature's winds arise from a difference in atmospheric pressure that moves the air from low pressure regions to high pressure regions, and by differences in temperature which move the wind from cold to hot regions. Who knows where the winds come from? Who can control them? They arise and come on quickly and easily shift directions.

Within the body there are different pressures as well. They arise at places of congestion, hyperactivity, obstructions, and movements. Different temperatures arise in hyper (high) and hypo (low) activity areas. Remember that the five organs' functions happen at different temperatures and levels of moisture or dryness. When the body is balanced, the heart is hot, the kidneys are cold, the lungs are cool and dry, the liver is warm and moist, and the spleen is damp and warm. The mixture of the "weather" in the body is pleasant. The organs maintain a homeostasis in the body by balancing each other automatically. The conditions of the organs are rarely ideal, and the organs are always going through different temperature changes. Such changes affect the body's "weather" and could cause winds or breezes to develop internally.

Winds carry toxicity out of the body. When winds exit the body they often exit as flatulence, a burp, a yawn, or a pop in a joint. Sometimes, the winds get trapped in the body and cause hiccups, wandering pain, itching, fevers, pain in the joints, heaviness, sluggishness, cramps, headaches, vertigo, and in extreme cases, gout, paralysis, and arthritis. Winds can cause the hands and limbs to feel heavy and numb. Cramps are winds that are trapped around nerves, pulling on them and causing pain. Winds also cause migraines, eye pains, kidney pains, muscle pains, and poorly functioning organs.

Skin rashes are the clearest sign of wind problems. Look for rashes in the crease of the elbow, around the neck, and at the back of the knees. This is a good sign, since it indicates that the winds are leaving the body. However, they are having a difficult time exiting, and you need to do more detoxification work.

A. Sick Winds (Trapped Gases)

Gases can be formed by certain kinds of food you eat, extremes in the weather, changes in seasons, toxic substances in the environment, negative emotions, and other factors. These gases can become trapped in knots, tangles, and blockages within the body's systems, vital organs, and spaces between, gradually to become sick or evil winds.

Opening the wind gates is the first procedure in Chi Nei Tsang massage. With the application of the CNT technique of applying pressure at appropriate points, the wind can be released and passed from the body.

Again, not all winds are sick. Wind is air or gas. The process of breathing, of moving air in and out of the body, involves wind. Each organ has an intrinsic wind. The wind becomes sick only when it is inappropriate to the part of the body in which it is found, or when it has been trapped and becomes stagnant. The trapped energy, taking the form of blockages or knots, needs to be released, so that the life-force wind can flow freely throughout the body. Good energy flow prevents more sick winds from arising.

1. Sick Winds Can Run and Hide

The Chi Nei Tsang techniques are excellent for wind maintenance. Sick winds (bad gas) can be eliminated before they can cause any problems. Stiffness, tightness, and numbness from trapped energy (winds) can be alleviated. Although massage will sometimes give temporary relief to these problems, the sick winds can simply run away and hide in another place. The Chi Nei Tsang practitioner has to know how to chase the sick wind out of the body, since any trapped energy in the body prevents healing energy from circulating freely through the main channels and meridians.

Most people have blockages and trapped winds. Blockages affect circulation of the system directly involved and the circulation of other systems since they are all interconnected. Thus, it is vitally important to clear the abdominal area of blockages and trapped winds so that the Chi can flow freely through its various channels, and the body can function more efficiently.

145

2. Sick Winds Can Cause Illness

Traditionally in the Chinese system, sick winds cause illness. When there is sick Chi, toxins accumulate in the body. The body attempts to eliminate them through the lymphatic system. When a chronic state of sick Chi is present, the lymph nodes at the navel, neck, and armpits become hard and enlarged. Gently massaging these areas releases the toxins there and enables the lymph nodes to function more freely. Occasionally sick Chi gets trapped in the blood and travels in a bubble.

Each organ has a particular kind of wind or energy associated with it when it is unhealthy. Through CNT and the meditation practices of the Healing Tao System, sick energy can be cleared from the body.

3. What Sick Energy Feels Like

Some people see sick wind, but others sense the energy in different ways. You will be taught five of the sick energies found in the body's organs along with the sensation each produces.

a. The lungs can produce a crawling, itchy, and sick energy that can accumulate on the skin of the practitioner and will eventually penetrate into the body. On the student's skin it may appear as a rash which can easily be transferred to the practitioner. Though this energy may not be felt immediately, it can eventually produce a terrible urge to itch.

b. The kidneys, bladder, and other Yin organs produce a cold, chilly energy when they are not well. This chill can go into the bones and is very difficult to remove.

c. The liver makes a biting, sick energy, somewhat similar to itchy, sick energy but with more of a stinging quality. It feels like ants are pinching the skin.

d. The heart produces a hot, burning form of sick energy that surfaces as a red rash.

e. The spleen, stomach, and pancreas produce a damp energy. When it penetrates into the hand, it can feel wet and sticky.

4. Combinations of Itchy, Biting, Hot, and Cold Energies

As previously mentioned, the combination of cold and biting energy is, by far, the worst to experience. It is important for you, as a practitioner, not to allow this energy to penetrate into your body and rest inside one of your internal organs.

A practitioner may find that the skin is warm or hot to the touch because of the laws of convection currents that cause heat to rise. You will notice that this heat, generated in the internal organs and other tissues and spaces in the body, will rise to the upper torso, head, neck, and upper organs. This creates a thermal layer within the body. The cold, sick energy gets trapped beneath a layer of hot energy that has risen. This is why people who have itchy, sick, and biting energies tend to develop rashes in the upper portions of the body.

You also may find that there are multiple layers of cold and hot energies within the body. Because of these layers of trapped energy, the resultant rashes also encourage rashes to develop in other portions of the body, such as behind the knees and in the creases of the elbows. It is important to remove these layers one at a time until you can reach the source of these problems.

The organs generate the different energies because of accumulated toxins. These toxins get trapped in the liver or the heart and often in the blood. When there are excess toxins in these systems, there is also excess heat produced.

5. A Closer Look at Cold, Sick Energy

a. Cold, Sick Energy Chills the Bones

People who have cold, sick energy will exude a cold chill into your hands when touched. This condition is caused by a cold wind that has been trapped in an organ or somewhere else in the body. A kidney or bladder disorder also causes this problem. This chill can travel into the bones and become very difficult to remove. Cold, sick energy is also slow to move, but will try to hide in a new location in the body.

b. Cold, Sick Energy Feels Heavy

Cold, sick energy has a cold, wet nature, and is also heavy. It seeks out the depths of the body, and, in particular, the lower limbs and the lower internal organs because of gravitational force and convection currents. This cold, sick, heavy energy mixes with the accumulated toxins also trapped by gravity in the lower tissues of the body and the internal organs making it more difficult to remove.

c. Identifying Cold, Sick Energy

When looking at a person, you can easily identify cold, sick energy. You will notice a pale blue or gray color in the skin, especially in the face, around the cheeks, under the eyes, beside the nose, in the ears, the lips, the gums, and the tongue. The fingernails and toenails may be blue or pale, and the fingers and toes will be cold. The pulse will be slow, tight, weak, and feel cold, especially when taken at the aorta, vena cava, and other major vessels. You also will find varicose veins and sometimes skin mottling. After having practiced the Taoist meditations and Chi Nei Tsang for some time, you will become sensitive to cold, sick energy.

B. Opening the Wind Gates

It is important to master and clear out the winds at the beginning of every session. This will help to activate the abdominal energy and loosen the tightness and tension in that area. Some persons will have abdomens that are too painful to bear the pressure of this procedure. In such cases, first do gentle skin detoxification.

C. Techniques for Opening the Wind Gates

Sick winds can leave through the navel if they have a way to get out. By opening points around the navel, you can draw these winds from organs and different parts of the body. Numbers one through eight on the illustration of the Navel's Pressure Points (Figure 4-1) list the sequence to follow; they also indicate which organs you will affect. The Wind Gate Chart (Figure 4-2) is more detailed than Figure 4-1 and serves as a daily guide to working on the Wind Gates.

1. The Wind Gate Chart
a. Open the winds gates in the order listed. (Figure 4-2) Visualize the Tai Chi symbol as the navel.

b. Follow the navel center guides I-VIII and use the thumb or elbow to press at the point indicated. (Figures 4-3 and 4-4) For example, after you do the groin gates and the Gate to the Sea of Winds (Tan Tien), go to point I and notice that on Monday the pulse is held for eight beats of the pulse. If it were Tuesday, you would hold the pulse for seventeen counts, on Wednesday nineteen counts, on Thursday 21 counts, and so on, through the end of the week.

c. Then go to point II. The point in that area would be held for seventeen counts Monday, nineteen counts Tuesday, and so on.

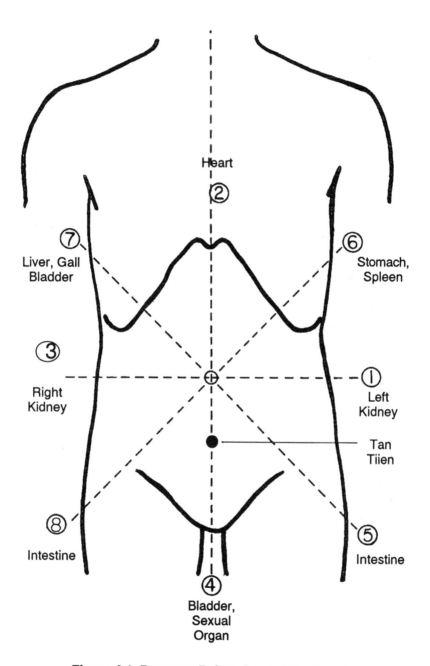

Figure 4-1. Pressure Points Around the Navel
Numbers one through eight list the sequence to follow
and indicate the organs you will affect

Chart of the Wind Gates

Point No. Day	Tan Tien Point below Navel	1	2	3	4	5	6	7	8
Monday	15	8	17	19	21	10	12	6	15
Tuesday	8	17	19	21	10	12	6	15	8
Wednesday	17	19	21	10	12	6	15	8	17
Thursday	19	21	10	12	6	15	8	17	19
Friday	21	10	12	6	15	8	17	19	21
Saturday	10	12	6	15	8	17	19	21	10
Sunday	6	15	8	17	19	21	10	12	6

Working on a Student: Monday Sample

a. Press both groin areas with the knife edge of your hands for 36 to 72 pulses or count your own pulse.

b. Press your thumb or elbow on the Tan Tien (3 inches below the navel) for the indicated count (15 times). You won't feel the pulse.

c. Press the Navel Center points 1-8 for the indicated count.

On the left side is the aorta at which you can feel the pulse; on the right side is the vena cava at which you can feel the pulse strongly.

1. Left Kidney; 8 times or pulses.
2. Heart: 17 times or pulses.
3. Right Kidney: 19 times. You will not feel the pulses because of the vena cava.
4. Bladder and sexual organ: 21 times or pulses.
5. Large and small intestine: 10 times or pulses.
6. Spleen, right lung, stomach: 12 times or pulses.
7. Liver, left lung: 6 times or pulses.
8. Large and small intestine, right ovary: 15 times or pulses

Figure 4-2. Chart of the Wind Gates

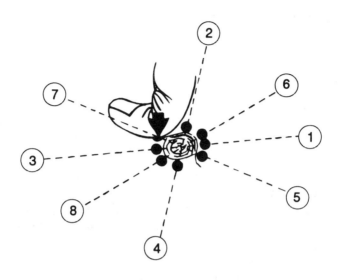

**Figure 4-3. The Wind Gate points
are on the sides of the navel and not in the navel**

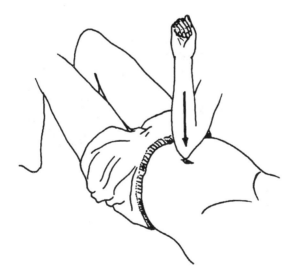

**Figure 4-4. If you are working on someone who is very heavy
or muscular, you may need to use your elbow**

d. You will travel all round the navel opening the gates. After each point pause to let the effect take place and the energy settle. The daily number guide is traditional the Taoist numerology practice for opening the Wind Gates.

2. Flushing the Blood at the Groin

a. Stand or kneel beside the student (unless the person is very large, in which case it is best to kneel between his or her legs.) Press the edge of each palm into the femoral artery pulse at the crease of each leg in the groin area. (Figure 4-5)

b. One pulse will probably feel stronger than the other. In that case, press down on the pulse that is strongest. This will help bring more blood and Chi to the weaker pulse. You should feel them equalize.

d. Hold the pulse for 36 or 72 counts to stimulate the circulation in the lower abdomen and legs and break up obstructions. Some winds will exit through the legs. This procedure will open the passageways.

NOTE: Do not practice this technique on someone in danger of, or afflicted with, thrombosis or a severe case of vericose veins.

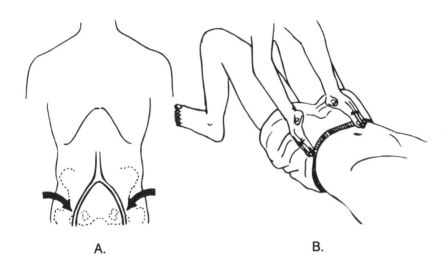

A.   B.

Figure 4-5.   A. Pressure Points for Opening the Groin
B. Opening the Wind Gates of the Groin

3. Opening the Gate to the Sea of Winds

You may remain between the student's legs, or move to the side of the body.

a. Locate the Tan Tien pulse (the Gate to the Sea of Winds) in a depression approximately one and a half inches below the navel at six o'clock. (Figure 4-6).

The first pulse you will feel is the aorta pulse which may feel more like an energy sensation. You may have to practice this procedure for some months before you can distinguish it. At all the other positions, just feel for the aorta pulse.

b. Press down until you feel the pulse. Usually a thumb is used; if you are working on someone who is very fat or very muscular, you may have to use your elbow to find a pulse. (Figure 4-4) Whether you use your finger or elbow, be gentle and don't slip. Sometimes you cannot find a pulse; in that case, all you can do is slowly count out the number for that day (one thousand, two thousand, three thousand, and so on.)

c. Figure out the number of pulse counts you will hold for that day. Consult the chart under "Tan Tien." On a Monday you would hold for fifteen counts, Tuesday eight counts, Wednesday seventeen counts, and so on.

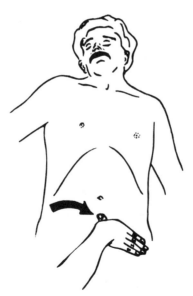

Figure 4-6. Opening the Gate to the Sea of Winds

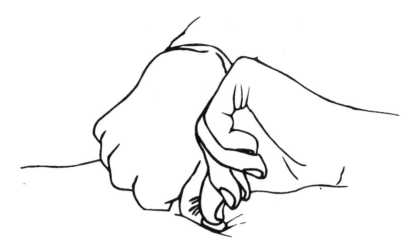

Figure 4-7. Working on yourself—Pressing the Navel Points

d. Release the pressure after the required number of counts has expired. The student should feel energy flowing down to the lower part of the body.

e. To gain experience you should do all the points or gates on yourself as well. (Figure 4-7)

4. Opening the Wind Gate to the Left Kidney— the Western Gate

a. Check point 1 on the chart to note the daily count.

b. Press the point just to the left of the navel at three o'clock until you feel the pulse. (Figure 4-8)

c. Hold for the count.

d. Just before you release, direct the energy to the left kidney by using your mind and intention. The student may feel warmth and comfort spread to that area.

5. Opening the Wind Gate to the Heart— the Southern Gate

a. Check the chart for point 2 and note the daily count.

b. Press the point above the navel at twelve o'clock. (Figure 4-9)

c. Hold the count with moderate pressure.

d. Before you release, direct the energy toward the sternum. The student may feel warmth and comfort spread to the chest and heart area.

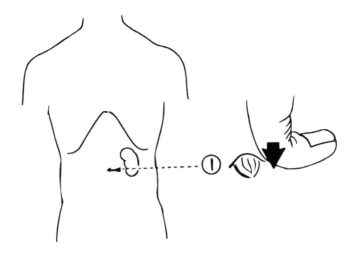

Figure 4-8. Opening the Gate to the Left Kidney

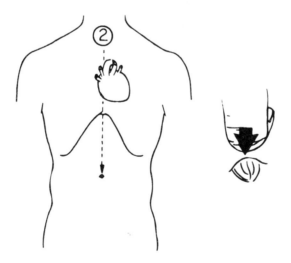

Figure 4-9. Opening the Gate to the Heart

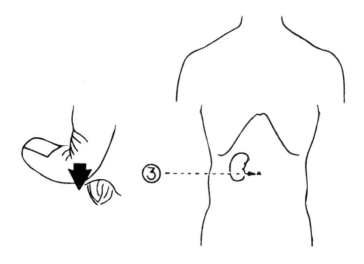

Figure 4-10. Opening the Gate to the Right Kidney

6. Opening the Wind Gate to the Right Kidney— the Eastern Gate

a. Get the daily pulse count from the chart for point 3 and press at nine o'clock. (Figure 4-10)

b. Send the energy to the right kidney just before releasing.

7. Opening the Wind Gate to the Sexual Organs and Bladder—the Northern Gate

a. You should now be at point 4. Check the pulse count for that day.

b. Hold at six o'clock just below the navel. (Figure 4-11)

c. Send the energy to the sexual center and bladder before releasing.

8. Opening the Wind Gate to the Small and Large Intestines and the Left Ovary— the Northwestern Gate

a. See what the daily pulse count is for point 5.

b. Note that the point you will press is between four and five o'clock. (Figure 4-12)

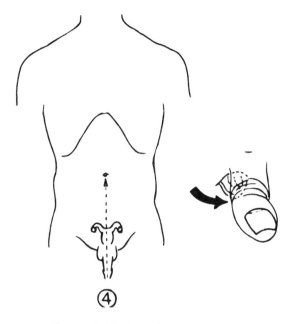

**Figure 4-11. Opening the Gate
to the Bladder and Sexual Organs**

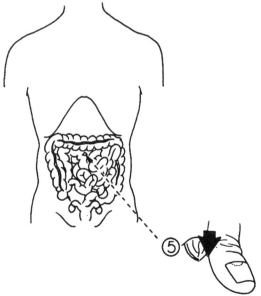

**Figure 4-12. Opening the Gate
to the Intestine and Left Ovary**

c. Press closely to the navel until you feel the pulse.

d. Direct the energy to both intestines and to the left ovary.

9. Opening the Wind Gate to the Spleen, Stomach, Pancreas, Triple Warmer, and Left Lung— the Southwestern Gate

a. Look at point 6 on the chart. Note the daily pulse count.

b. Find the pulse between one and two o'clock. (Figure 4-13)

c. Press it for the required number.

d. There are five places to direct the energy, so be prepared. The student should feel blood and Chi flow to the spleen, stomach, pancreas, Triple Warmer, and Left Lung.

10. Opening the Wind Gate to the Liver, Gall Bladder, and Right Lung—the Southeastern Gate

a. Point 7 is between ten and eleven o'clock. (Figure 4-14)

b. Press for the daily count. Be sure to feel the pulse.

c. When you are done, direct the energy into the liver, the gall bladder, and the right lung.

11. Opening the Wind Gate to the Small and Large Intestines and the Right Ovary— the Northeastern Gate

a. Check the chart for the last time. Get the count. Point 8 is between seven and eight o'clock. (Figure 4-15)

b. Hold the point with moderate pressure, as you did at all the other points. Before you release the point, send the energy to the intestines and right ovary. The student may feel warmth and comfort in those areas.

C. Baking Sick Winds

Use the baking technique to "cook" or "bake" sick winds, that are hot and expansive, or cold and contractive.

1. Baking Hot Wind

a. The best place to cook wind is in the small intestine. Place both hands over the small intestine and do the Heart's Sound together with

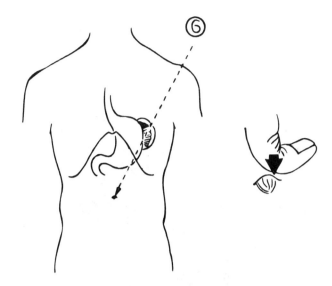

**Figure 4-13. Opening the Gate
to the Stomach and Spleen**

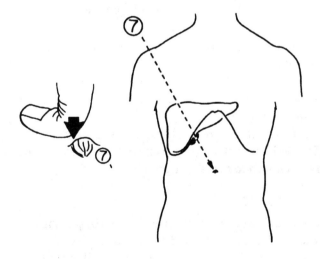

**Figure 4-14. Opening the Gate
to the Liver and Gall Bladder**

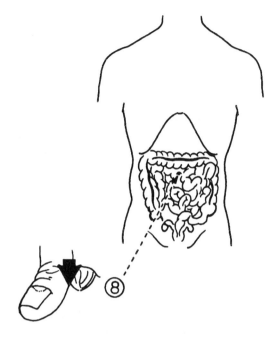

**Figure 4-15. Opening the Gate
to the Intestine and Right Ovary**

your student. This will attract the hot energy. You are calling the hot wind into the small intestine.

b. Feel the pressure and heat of the hot wind entering the small intestine. Leave the right hand on the abdomen over the areas where the winds are trapped. (Figure 4-16)

c. Place the left hand on the back, opposite the right hand.

d. Do the Heart's Sound together again to raise the temperature of the area just enough to move it or cook it.

2. Baking Cold Wind

a. Cold winds can be attracted and directed by placing the right hand on the cold wind and the left hand on the small intestine.

b. Attract the cold wind and build a cold ball in the small intestine by doing the Kidneys' Sound together with your student. (Figure 4-17)

c. After the cold wind has entered the small intestine, bake it by keeping one hand on the abdomen and placing the other hand beneath it

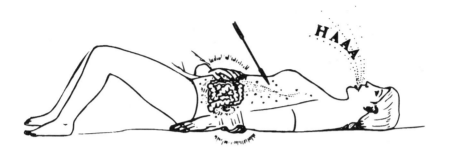

Figure 4-16. Baking the Small Intestine

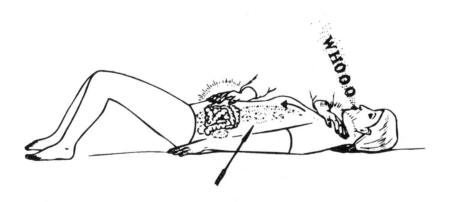

**Figure 4-17. Moving a Cold Wind
from the Chest to the Navel and Baking It**

on the back. Do the Heart's Sound together and bake the wind. Be sure to bake the cold wind thoroughly to avoid cramps in the small intestine.

d. Using a vibrating or shaking palm speeds up the process. Tapping vigorously around the navel with the fingertips in a firm manner will also help purge these winds.

e. If the cold wind will not cook off, you can use your fingernails to lightly scrape the skin over the affected area. This will create a gate through which the winds can escape.

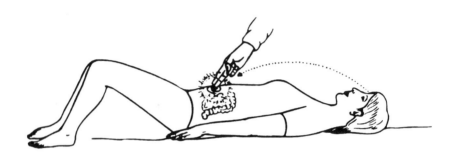

Figure 4-18. The student concentrates on the wind as it is burned out at the navel

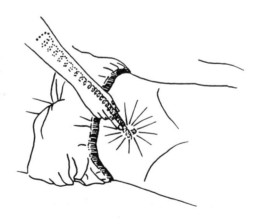

Figure 4-19. Burning a Sick Wind

3. Burning Sick Wind

a. For sick wind energy in the abdominal area, use the scooping technique to scoop the sick energy into the Tan Tien area, one and one half inches below the navel. You will gradually feel a cold or chilly energy ball form there.

b. Use your index and middle finger to press on the area, while your student concentrates on this point. (Figures 4-18 and 4-19)

c. Concentrate on the area and spiral with the fingers. Feel a "sunshine" heat in that spot as you gradually feel the warmth displacing the cold, chilly, sick wind.

Chi Nei Tsang

CHAPTER 5

DETOXIFYING THE SKIN AND THE LARGE AND SMALL INTESTINES

The skin around the navel is an area that can be worked to reach deeper levels of the body's operations. When you press around the navel point, you can bypass muscle, fat, and intestines to reach the lymphatic, circulatory, and nervous systems. These systems tend to be blocked at the navel area, so toxins and waste material accumulate there. When the lymph system clots, the body's defense system is inefficient. When the circulatory system tangles or clots with fat and sediment, the blood will not circulate well. When the nervous system tangles, nerve impulses will travel very slowly through the whole system or will jam. When Chi backs up, growths and tumors develop.

Detoxification always comes first because the skin, organs, and lymph glands will not work efficiently unless they are detoxified. The body's systems make up a great part of a human being. When their work load piles up, the work rate slows down. When the work gets to be too much, these three systems want a rest.

CNT will help the skin, lymphatic system, and organs handle the overload. You will be doing their work with your fingers. Massaging primes these systems, "jump-starts" them, and gets them moving. When there is less work to do, they get more energy and can complete the task. Once the extra toxicity is eliminated, the next toxin to enter the body will be quickly eliminated.

When the organs try to cleanse themselves and cannot get rid of their excess toxins, they push the toxins out to the muscles and skin (the body's largest organ), and store them there. Poisons can be easily removed from the skin, but the organs will benefit greatly from the application of some special techniques.

Toxins exit the body in a variety of ways. Sometimes they evaporate through the skin; at other times they exit as pimples, rashes, boils, and sweat. They also exit via the large intestine or the bladder.

It is important not to over-eliminate toxins. You have to be aware of the body's ability to eliminate waste material. You should be particularly cautious when working on the very ill, old, and young. If too many toxins are released for the body to eliminate efficiently, the student can become sick or experience a cleansing crisis. This could show up as a rash, a fever, or nausea. There are limits to the body's ability to eliminate. It is possible that some material released, and not eliminated, will find its way back to where the body has become used to having it. It will then have to be released again in the next session.

A. Skin Detoxification

In CNT we treat the skin of the abdomen, starting at the navel. This is where the umbilicus of the fetus received nutrition and eliminated toxicity. As the original center of the body, the navel is still connected with all the organs. Whatever toxins the organs cannot process, they store in the navel for later detoxification.

By massaging the skin lightly and stimulating its surface, you can draw the pressure and toxicity from deep within all parts of the body to the surface. It is easier to reach the toxins on the skin to break them down. The longer you work on the skin, the easier it will be to work deeper later. The skin is a storage space for whatever extra toxicity the organs have. When you release the toxins stored in the skin, you create an open area on the skin. The organs can now release more toxins to the new storage space just made available. Instead of clearing, sometimes the skin may swell. This is because more toxins have been released from the organs to the skin. Once cleared, the skin will recover its balance.

The toxins, tightness, and tension in the abdomen also block the flow of energy from the vital Navel Center or Tan Tien. When you clear the area, the pre-natal Chi can begin to flow through the body more forcefully.

WARNING AND CAUTION:

IF THERE ARE ANY WARTS OR MOLES VERY CLOSE TO THE RIM OF THE NAVEL, DO NOT WORK ON THE STUDENT. THIS SUGGESTS THAT THERE IS A SERIOUS VIRAL PROBLEM AND A DOCTOR SHOULD BE CONSULTED. YOU CAN, HOWEVER, TEACH THE STUDENT TO WORK ON HIMSELF OR HERSELF.

1. Spiraling Technique

The Spiraling Technique is the main technique for skin detoxification. Gently use both hands on the abdomen to loosen the tissues. Begin by massaging with the thumbs, finger, or fingers together in small, tight, clockwise circular motions around the navel. (Figure 5-1) The sequence for each point is to press in, spiral, and loosen the skin. Continue to create tight, clockwise circles outward from the previous points you have worked on. This will create a large spiral, extending from the navel to the outer edges of the abdomen. (Figure 5-2) Although this procedure mainly influences the small intestine, the clockwise direction also follows the path and motion of the large intestine, the body's "great eliminator." With this movement toxins are encouraged to pass from the body. This technique is especially powerful for breaking up a constipated large intestine.

Conversely, if your student has diarrhea problems, you should teach him or her how to spiral in a counterclockwise direction. This will encourage the watery waste to slow its exit, until it has formed into normal stool consistency.

If your student's abdomen is tense, nervous, hot, hard, and too Yang, this means there is excessive energy and you should drain some off. Spiral counterclockwise to withdraw the energy. Use your concentration. Ask the energy to leave. Direct it into the Microcosmic Orbit, where it can be circulated and stored safely in the Navel Center. You can also direct it to go into the Navel Center.

If the abdomen is cold, soft, weak, sick, and too Yin, this means that there is deficient energy. Spiral clockwise to add energy. Concentrate to direct some of your energy to pass from your fingertips into the student's abdomen, to help warm the area.

When you finish the finger spiraling technique, apply the following hand techniques. You will become very familiar with these techniques, for they are used repeatedly in CNT.

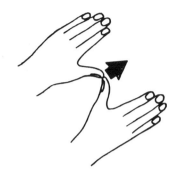

a. Use Two Thumbs

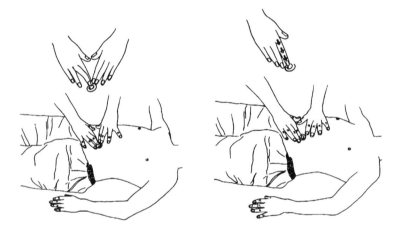

b. Use Four Fingers   **c. Use a Single Finger**

Figure 5-1. Spiraling Technique: Use the (a) thumbs, (b) fingers, or (c) finger to press in, spiral, and loosen the toxins locked in the skin

2. Scooping Technique

With your fingers together, press inwardly and scoop in, or press downward and scoop out. There are many variations to the direction and use of this technique. (Figures 5-3, 5-4, and 5-5)

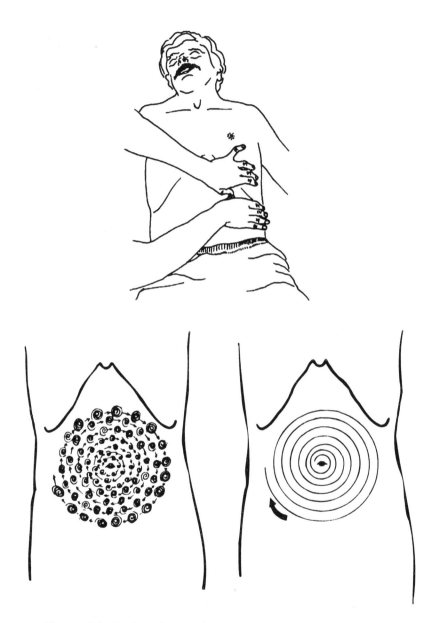

Figure 5-2. Create tight spirals. Move in clockwise circles beginning near the navel; gradually spiral out toward the perimeter of the abdomen

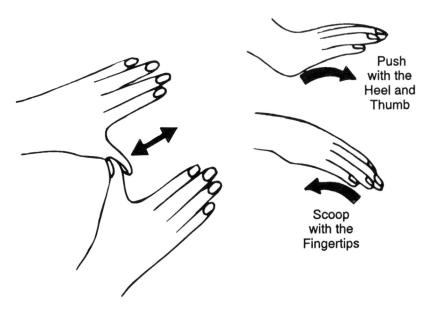

**Figure 5-3. Pushing with the Palm-Heels
and Scooping with the Fingertips**

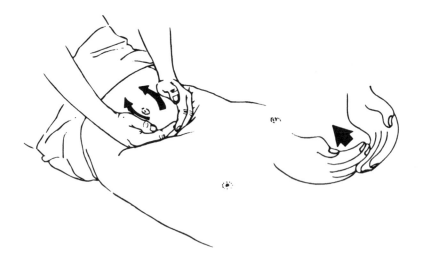

Figure 5-4. Scooping with Two Hands

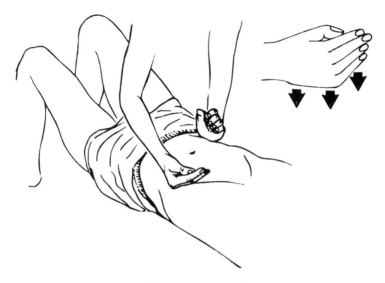

Figure 5-5. Scooping with One Hand

3. Rocking Technique

Use all the fingers to hold the abdominal muscles while rocking forward and back. Spread your fingers to cover the ascending and descending colon, or change the width and cover the small intestines. (Figure 5-6)

4. Kneading Technique

Use all the fingers of both hands to scoop the intestine into the navel and central area. Follow by pressing with the heels of the palms into the navel and the central area as though you were kneading a loaf of bread. (Figure 5-7)

5. Shaking Technique

Use either the index or middle finger to press on the knot or problem area. Move the finger quickly up and down or from side to side. Use two or three fingers to cover a larger area. (Figure 5-8)

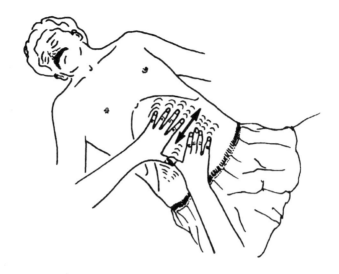

Figure 5-6. Rocking

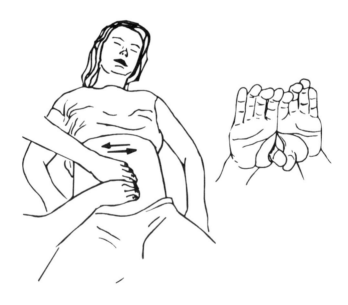

Figure 5-7. Kneading

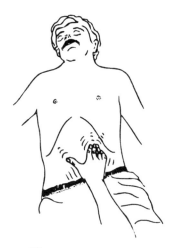

Figure 5-8. Shaking

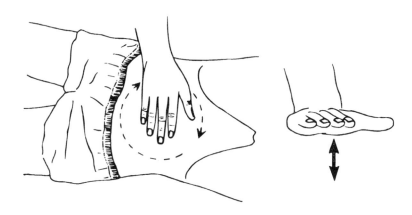

Figure 5-9. Patting

6. Patting Technique

Pat around the navel and the entire abdominal area with the fingers and with a soft, open palm. (Figure 5-9) (Patting is generally used to finish a CNT session.)

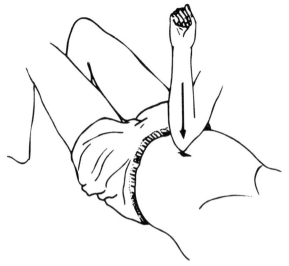

Figure 5-10. Elbow Press

7. Elbow Press

Remember, if you are working on someone who is very large or very muscular, sometimes the only way you can have an effect is to use your elbow. Press straight down or spiral with your elbow. (Figure 5-10)

B. Detoxifying the Large Intestine

1. Shape and Function of the Large Intestine

The large intestine includes the cecum, with the appendix, colon (divided into ascending, transverse, descending, and sigmoid parts), anal canal, and rectum. (Figure 5-11) It is a tube five feet long that starts in the lower right side of the abdomen at the ileocecal valve (the junction with the small intestine), and ascends toward the liver. Under the liver it makes a left turn and goes across the body toward the spleen, where it makes another bend, and goes down the left side of the abdomen. It turns at the area of the left hipbone and becomes the sigmoid colon. It then curves into the middle of the pelvic cavity and ends in the rectum and anal canal. The bends in the large intestine, especially on the left side, are tucked away deep in the corners of the abdomen, and are not easily accessible. (Figure 5-12)

Undigested food and other products pass through the colon. It absorbs whatever water, nutrients, and vitamins it can, and expels the unabsorbed products as feces. In its passage from the cecum to the rectum, the material is sloshed around and shifted by peristaltic movement. This alternating, worm-like, propelling movement is caused by the contraction of the longitudinal and circular muscles of the intestine. This action is especially noticeable during bowel movements, which are brief bursts of peristaltic movement.

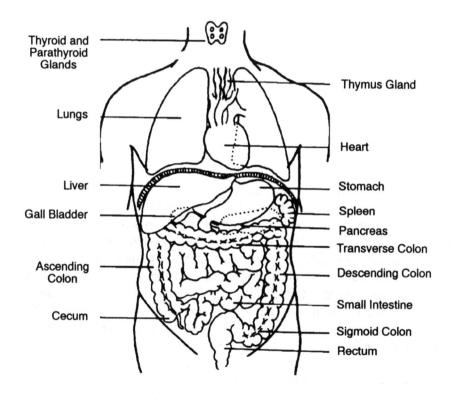

Figure 5-11. The Large Intestine and the Viscera

175

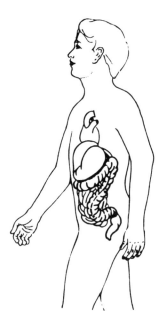

**Figure 5-12. The corners of the large intestine
are not easily accessible**

2. Constipation

The peristaltic movement does not always propel the contents toward the rectum, sometime it sends it back toward the cecum. During this process the intestine is absorbing salts and water from its contents. Constipation can result when the intestine absorbs too much water and the material is too dry to move easily. Sometimes the cause is very simple, such as not paying attention to the need to eliminate. The stool backs up and gets very dry. Constipation can also be caused by the poor functioning of the intestine's muscles; they have lost their tone and strength, or have become spastic. Laxatives poison these muscles causing the intestine to twist and twitch like a dying snake.

To the Chinese the main cause of constipation is excess heat in the stomach and intestines, causing them to evaporate too much liquid. Another cause is stagnation of liver Chi, which also creates heat.

The processing of food is not the only cause of constipation. Some people lack the ability to commit themselves and hold back from normal human involvement, perhaps through fear. They may be unaware that this behavior may be the reason they are often constipated.

If the large intestine gets constipated and enlarges, it will stop the free motion of the diaphragm. Roemheld, a German doctor, discovered a syndrome that was later named after him (the Roemheld Syndrome). He found that gas pressure building up in the intestine causes increased contraction of the rib cage and attracts stagnant toxicity all along the length of the diaphragm area. This will eventually press against the heart area under the rib cage and can create feelings of anxiety, heart pains, and breathing difficulties. This energy back up is sometimes referred to as "constipation" of the heart.

Constipation can cause an accumulation of mucus in the lungs resulting in asthmatic symptoms. It can also be the cause of psoas muscle, leg, and back pain

3. Diarrhea

Diarrhea is the abnormal frequency and liquidity of the feces. Western medicine has named over 50 varieties. It can be caused by failure of the ileum (the lower part of the small intestine) and the colon to absorb sufficient water. Sometimes worry and anxiety causes over stimulation of the nerves, which cause hyper-peristaltic movement and premature discharge. Diarrhea can be beneficial if the body needs to expel toxins or parasites.

In Chinese medicine the most common cause of diarrhea is too much Yang energy in the spleen and kidneys. This energy needs to be balanced, a technique you will be taught in Chapter 7.

4. Colonic Irrigation

It bears mentioning that while CNT probably offers the best techniques available anywhere for irrigating and clearing the large intestine, it is advisable to have at least one high colonic irrigation to have a healthy digestive and elimination system. This involves full irrigation of the colon all the way to the cecum. The colon is full of cracks, fissures, and bends. Usually its walls are caked and lined with junk material that has been collecting there since childhood. The only way to clean it properly is to give it a good hosing; this means running twenty to 30 gallons of filtered water (from a tap though a water purifier) through it. The constant water pressure will gradually eat away at the plaque and build-up. Complete irrigation on the entire large intestine is necessary to restore its function. After that, CNT and diet can help the normal process of the large intestine. Since it is very easy to rely on colonic irrigation, such reliance can interfere with the normal function of the large intestine and, therefore, is only recommended as an initial cleansing.

We agree with V.E. Irons, a man who has spent his life trying to educate the public about this important organ. One of his handouts addresses the problems with this organ. It is slightly overstated, but effective:

"To no other single cause is it possible to attribute one-tenth as many various and widely diverse disorders. It may be said that almost every chronic disease known is directly or indirectly due to the influence of bacterial poisons absorbed from the large intestine. The colon may be justly looked upon as a veritable Pandora's box, out of which comes more human misery and suffering, mental and moral, as well as physical than from any other known source.

The colon is a sewage system, but by neglect and abuse it becomes a cesspool. When it is clean and normal we are well and happy; let it stagnate, and it will distill the poisons of decay, fermentation and putrefaction into the blood, poisoning the brain and nervous system so that we become mentally depressed and irritable. It will poison the heart so that we are weak and listless; poison the lungs so that the breath is foul; poison the digestive organs so that we are distressed and bloated; and poison the blood so that the skin is sallow and unhealthy. In short, every organ of the body is poisoned, and we age prematurely, look and feel old, the joints are stiff and painful, neuritis, dull eyes and a sluggish brain overtake us; the pleasure of living is gone."

The ancient Taoists, and many country doctors early in this century, knew the importance of a healthy large intestine. In fact, Taoists would fast for *years* to make sure this organ was clean. Many modern health experts underplay the crucial role of this organ. In the United States colon cancer takes the lives of more people than any other cancer, except lung cancer: typically one out of every fifteen people. Pockets growing through the wall of the colon occur in one out of five people over the age of 45.

We would like to help reintroduce their wisdom and concern, especially since CNT makes it is so easy to care for the large intestine properly.

5. An Unhealthy Large Intestine

An intestine that is too tight is sensitive to pressure and feels like a tight string. Use two thumbs or the edge of your palm to probe the cecum

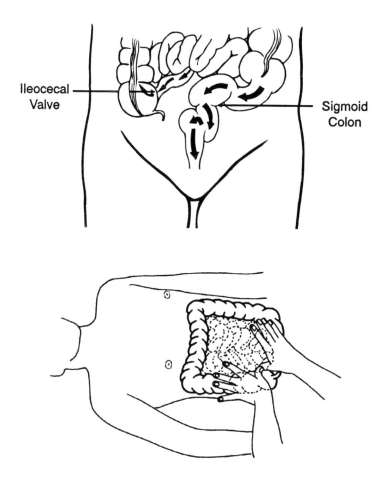

Ileocecal Valve

Sigmoid Colon

Figure 5-13. Probe the ileocecal valve and sigmoid to determine the condition of the large intestine and if there is constipation

and sigmoid colon. (Figure 5-13) Use light, medium, or heavy pressure. If you use a very light touch on the cecum or sigmoid colon and cause pain, this indicates a very serious problem and heavy constipation. If you use medium pressure and there is pain, the problem is not so serious. If you use deep pressure and there is no pain, then this is very good and you can probably release the cecum and large intestine at once.

A healthy large intestine that can be palpated with the hands without generating any pain or discomfort is rare. (Figure 5-14) Sometimes it is

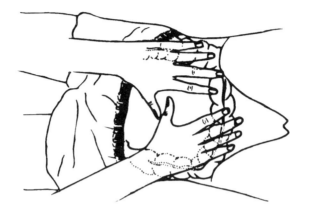

Figure 5-14. Feeling the Large Intestine

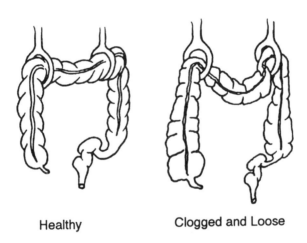

Healthy   Clogged and Loose

**Figure 5-15. A healthy intestine hangs naturally;
a clogged intestine sags and bulges**

often only a finger's width wide on the traverse section. A loose, clogged traverse colon hangs down in a big curve. (Figure 5-15) Because of the extreme bending, there will be a blockage of stool in the left curve. This becomes fertile ground in which bacteria can grow, causing inflammation and gas pain. A large intestine full of gas pockets can push on the left side of the rib cage, deforming the structure and moving it off-center. (Figure 5-16) Figure 5-17 portrays some different types of unhealthy large and small intestines.

6. Open the Large Intestine

Many of the problems with the large intestine occur at the cecum/ ileocecal valve or at the sigmoid colon. (Figure 5-18) Your palpation of

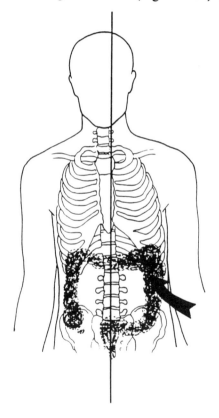

Figure 5-16. A large intestine full of gas pockets on the left side can deform the structure

181

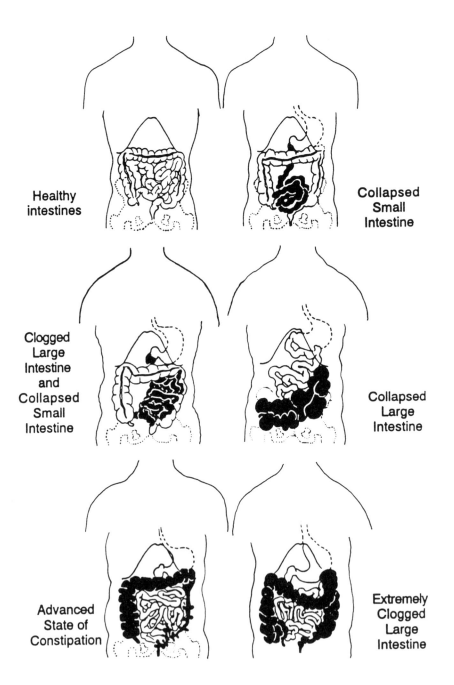

Healthy intestines

Collapsed Small Intestine

Clogged Large Intestine and Collapsed Small Intestine

Collapsed Large Intestine

Advanced State of Constipation

Extremely Clogged Large Intestine

Figure 5-17. Healthy and Unhealthy States of the Large and Small Intestines

182

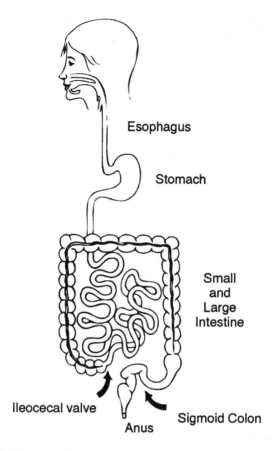

Figure 5-18. The digestive system is one continuous tube, beginning at the mouth and ending at the anus

these areas should indicate the problem. If the problem is in the sigmoid area, don't start there but work around it. Never work directly on a painful area (in the large intestine or anywhere else); prepare a place for the pain and congestion to go. To release the congestion in the large intestine, start at the left side of the rib cage at the splenic bend. This will release congestion there and make room for more congestion coming from the problem area.

a. Figure Five Technique

The Figure Five technique is a hand pattern that outlines the number "5." It can be used to open the descending colon at the splenic curve.

(Figure 5-19) Gas and matter get stuck in this area and need to be cleared out. This motion mimics the peristalsis movement and activates the intestine.

(1) Start by standing or sitting on the right side of the student's body to work on the left side of the body and colon. Reach over the body and stroke up with both palms toward the sternum. Use an overhand palm to brush on the left rib cage in the direction of the sternum. The hand action

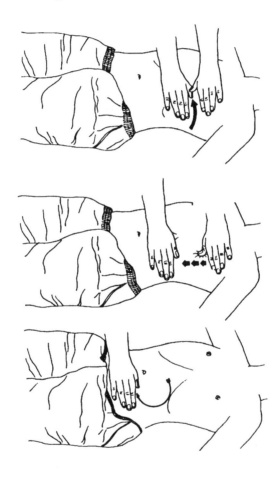

**Figure 5-19. The Figure Five Technique outlines
the Arabic numeral "5" on the body**

is a little more forceful than a brush. You want to move the rib cage as well. This will concentrate the fluids toward the center of the rib cage and release the splenic curve.

(2) Position the right thumb on top of the sinking point below the nipple between the eighth and ninth rib. Stroke down toward the abdomen, in a line parallel to the midline, to a point midway between the sternum and the navel.

(3) Then circle to the left under the left rib cage and make a wide half-circle following the descending colon, ending at the sigmoid colon.

b. Mouse Technique

Starting at the cecum, use the fingers of each hand, side by side, to nibble like a little mouse in short two inch bursts along the large intestine. This nibbling movement mimics the normal peristaltic movement of the large intestine and will help the energy to flow again.

c. Scooping Technique

Use the scooping technique to move the large intestine into its proper position.

d. Clockwise Wave Technique

Practice the Wave Technique. (Figure 5-20) Reach into the abdomen with both hands and create a relaxing, alternating, rotating movement between the two hands. By creating a wave of motion inside the bowels, you will increase the peristaltic movement of the intestines. Do this two to three times or longer. This technique is always nice and relaxing in between other techniques.

Using the edge of the left palm, press down and upward along the ascending colon toward the transverse colon. Follow by using the fingers of the right hand along the descending colon. This will end in a circular motion as you bring your elbow in toward your rib cage on the right side and press the palm of your right hand toward the sigmoid.

e. Releasing the Sigmoid Colon

The sigmoid colon is inside the left hip and is part of the large intestine. Most problems occur here or in the ileocecal valve.

(1) Sit on the left side facing the student and have him raise the left knee. Using the edge of the right hand, place it against your student's left hip bone. Place the fingertips of your left hand on top of the pubic bone as counter pressure. (Figure 5-21)

(2) With your right hand, press underneath the sigmoid. If you are on top of it, you can cause pain.

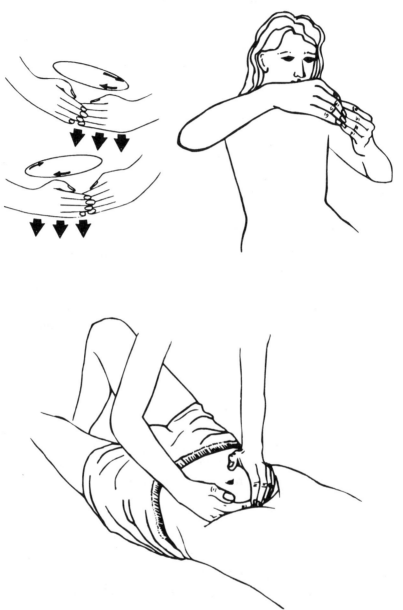

Figure 5-20. Hand Formation of the Wave Technique

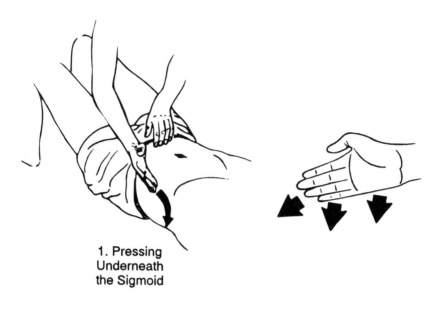

1. Pressing
Underneath
the Sigmoid

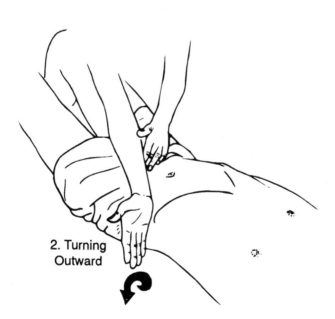

2. Turning
Outward

**Figure 5-21. Use the edge of the hand to
release the sigmoid colon**

(3) As you feel underneath the sigmoid, roll out with the back of your right hand toward the rib cage. Feel the stretch of the sigmoid, which will release any blockages or knots. Repeat this motion several times.

(4) Finish by doing the Wave Technique three to six times.

f. The Cecum (Figure 5-22)

The cecum is inside the right hip.

(1) Use your finger to press around the right hip and feel for a bulge, which can be about an inch long, just under the ileocecal valve. If this area is irritated or congested, it also will cause irritation or blockages of the appendix. This is where the large intestine starts. Sometime when you are able to release the tension and congestion in this area, you can feel an explosion of energy travel through and clear out the whole intestine.

(2) Be sure that you have first released the congestion at the splenic bend and liver bend to allow room for the congestion to move.

(3) Release by using your thumbs to inch up toward the ileocecal valve. Use a consistent and firm pressure, like squeezing a tube.

(4) Repeat two to three times until the area is clear of congestion, hardness, obstruction, or pain.

g. The Ileocecal Valve (Figure 5-22)

(1) The ileocecal valve should be about half way between the navel and the right hip bone. This valve is the connection between the large and small intestine. Blockages cause this valve to close. It is a one-way valve opening into the large intestine at the cecum. It opens when the pressure inside the cecum releases, and closes when the pressure inside the cecum builds. It is also activated by food entering the stomach, which initiates a contraction of the small intestine, expelling contents of the lower part of the small intestine into the large intestine.

This is a very important valve. If it is not working and closed, it causes constipation and headaches. If it is stuck open, it causes diarrhea. Again, to work on constipation, it is necessary to release the whole of the large intestine and the cecum. Then the ileocecal valve can open automatically. If it doesn't open automatically, do the following technique. When it opens, you will hear it make a gurgling sound and the cecum will fill.

(2) Place the edge of your right hand along the right hip bone and your left hand on the back, supporting the kidney.

(3) With the edge of your right hand, slowly apply downward pressure, then roll the palm of your hand up and out toward the rib cage

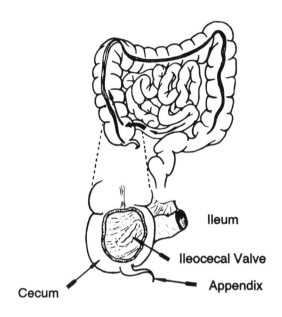

Ileum

Ileocecal Valve

Cecum

Appendix

Figure 5-22. The Cecum and Ileocecal Valve

at a diagonal. This is a small movement, used only to open this gate between the two intestines.

(4) Do not do this movement more than once or twice, since the tissue is very sensitive. You should remember to press before you make the movement.

(5) In cases of diarrhea, the large intestine is open. This causes the ileocecal valve to remain stuck wide open. Use your fingers to close it. Do a counterclockwise wave technique to re-establish its peristaltic contractions so that it may start to absorb moisture from the small intestine. Drink plenty of water to replace the lost fluid.

C. The Small Intestine

The small intestine is the digestive tract between the stomach and the cecum. It is in charge of absorption and digestion. The small intestine divides into the duodenum, jejunum, and ileum. The small intestine is about twenty feet long and fills up the central space of the abdomen. (Figure 5-23) Its main role is the absorption of food. It allows the digested

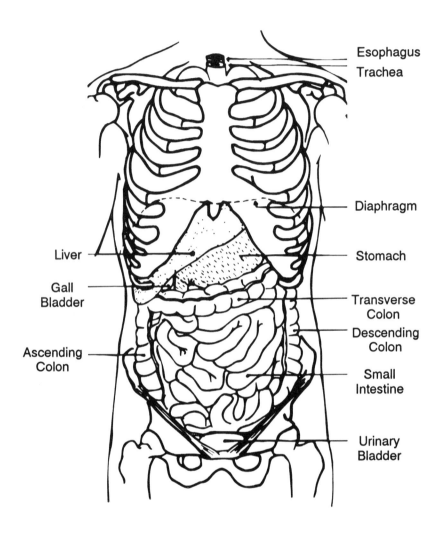

Figure 5-23. The Small Intestine and Neighbors

food to go through its lining to the liver via the portal vein system, where the food is further processed before reaching the rest of the body.

1. The Abdominal Brain

The small intestine is in charge of digesting emotions as well as food. Different contractions of this intestine correspond to undigested emotions. In Chinese medicine it is called the *abdominal brain*. All negative emotions are expressed in the small intestine by contraction and circumvolutions. Anger contracts the right side of the intestine near the liver. Worry affects the upper left side near the spleen. Impatience and anxiety affect the top. Sadness affects both lower lateral sides. Fear affects the deeper and lower abdominal areas. (Figure 5-24)

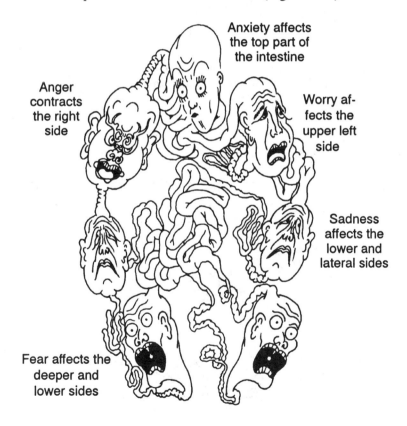

Figure 5-24. The Effect of Negative Emotions on the Small Intestine

191

2. Toxins in the Small Intestine

Toxins travelling inside the intestines are still outside the body, since they do not penetrate the membranes of the digestive system. They are on their way to being eliminated. These are toxins that have not been digested or broken down by the stomach and its digestive juices into particles small enough to go through the digestive membrane and into the blood system. When the intestines become too crowded with toxins, the speed of digestion will slow down and the absorption function of the small intestine will be impaired. The intestine will become congested and cannot perform all its physiological functions. Though you may eat well, you may be undernourished.

3. The Healthy Small Intestine

A healthy small intestine can be covered with one spread hand. (Figure 5-25) When touched, it should feel even and soft. It should move easily, painlessly, and give way to the fingers without creating any muscle reflex reaction. It will move back to its normal position after releasing the pressure. A light small intestine will be firm when touched and will often allow you to feel the pulse of the aorta very strongly. A loose and weak small intestine will be unevenly shaped and filled with bubbles of gas and fluid. Often some parts are too tight and others too loose.

4. An Unhealthy Small Intestine Damages the System

The small intestine gives the abdomen its form and size. If the small intestine is full of toxins, resulting in loss of tone and enlargement, it can

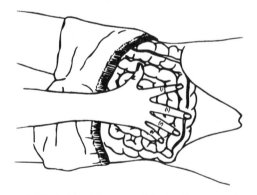

Figure 5-25. A healthy small intestine can be covered with a spread hand and should feel soft and even

press downward and disturb the blood flow in the lower abdomen. This creates pressure on the veins and encourages the growth of hemorrhoids and varicose veins. It can create hormonal and menstrual disorders for women.

The weight of an unhealthy intestine often pulls at the spine. The weight excessively bends the curve of the lower back and rounds the thoracic curve. (Figure 5-26) The weight distorts the breathing reflex, pulls the diaphragm, and overextends the rib cage opening. This causes chronic contractions of the intercostal muscles. It also promotes the formation of mucus in the lungs and weakens the lymphatic system through lack of abdominal motion. This creates a vicious cycle of toxicity and tension formation.

The buildup of toxicity in the small intestine creates a pressure that weighs on and against the nerves and communication center of the lumbar and sacral plexus. This numbs the messages that the nerves should be getting from the organs and lower abdominal area. Important infor-

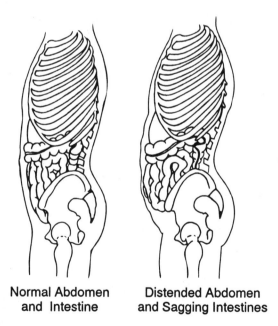

Normal Abdomen
and Intestine

Distended Abdomen
and Sagging Intestines

Figure 5-26. Normal and Abnormal Intestines

mation is not able to get to the brain. Conversely, messages from the brain cannot get to the organs.

This is how emotional tensions stored in the intestines can be turned into muscular tension in the back, legs, and psoas muscles. The pressure exerted on the plexus triggers a reaction in the back. You don't feel it, and even if you did, the muscles would be unable to relax because of the pressure blocking the nerves. It takes a while, but the contraction begins to irritate the nerves in different areas causing pain. Even then you can't alleviate the pain because of the pressure on the nerves. This is why when you are working on the small intestine, and you press a certain point, you trigger a sharp pain somewhere else in the body, such as the leg, back, shoulder, or arm.

5. Massaging the Small Intestine

The student should have an empty stomach. Sometimes the area is very painful, and extremely congested. If this is the case, ask your student to eat white rice for two to three days, chewing each mouthful 50 to 100 times, three times a day. This will cause the saliva to collect. The saliva will help to clear the area. The student may supplement the saliva with a little yogurt. This will help heal the intestine.

Now, when you do the work, it will be easier to feel the blockages and twisted parts of the intestine. By massaging the small intestine, you will be helping it to digest food and eliminate the waste material more quickly. Remember also that you are helping to eliminate the emotional trauma as well. You want to eliminate congestion or obstructions that would prevent a healthy flow inside it.

Sometimes it will not be possible for the person to follow the rice and saliva diet. In that case you can start detoxifying by using some very gentle basic techniques.

6. Small Intestine Techniques

Working on the small intestine is of primary importance to the practice of CNT. Any congestion, toxification, or stagnation, including trapped emotions, will inhibit the Navel Center from supplying the rest of the body. These are not only techniques; they involve using your personality and spirit. When you push in to massage and spiral your student's stomach, you may feel your stomach being massaged and spiraled as well. You attach the spirit of your intestine to his or her intestine and connect your healing energy as well. It will take some time before you can do this well, but start trying immediately. The small intestine work is very much like playing and should be approached with a bubbling kind of joy. If you are tight, it is transmitted to the student. Therefore, you have to be very grounded, safe, comfortable, relaxed, and spontaneous.

a. If the student's abdomen is very hard and so painful that you can hardly touch it, you will have to be softer and more patient. Your fingers can only skim over and lightly touch them with a feathery pressure. You can lay the whole surface of the palm or the heel of the palm on the skin and gently spiral it. After some time it will start to soften. The harder the abdomen, the softer your fingers should be. If you want to go in deeply, your fingers must also be soft.

b. Practice deep skin detoxification and use the Wave Technique.

c. When doing the Wave Technique, your fingers may feel one area of the intestines is tighter than another, or you may feel knots. This could be chronic contraction of the involuntary muscles within the tissues of the intestine, a diverticulum (a pouch or sac), or a hernia. As long as it is not a painful spot, massaging this area will progressively alleviate the problem.

d. The small intestine has a serpentine or S-shaped design, with one curve of it lying on top of the other. When you detoxify the intestine, use the basic spiraling techniques of the fingers, but try to feel and follow its sinuous design. When your fingers come to a "switchback," shake it until it feels loose. This will help to move the food (chyme) and activate the intestine.

e. Work with short, bubbling bursts, back and forth, counterclockwise and clockwise half spirals. You can use a left-right-left-right, one, two, three, four motion or longer sets. Always end by pulling the fingers and energy toward the cecum, which is where the contents of the small intestine flow into the large intestine. (Figure 5-27)

f. Keep working until you have stimulated the entire small intestine.

g. Cover the small intestine with your hands and have the student breathe into your hands. Both of you do the Inner Smile. Breathe with the student. Fill yourself with light and exhale through your hand into the student as he or she inhales. Teach the student deep abdominal breathing.

h. A good time to work on your own small intestine (and all other areas) is when sitting on the toilet. You can bend over, lean into your finger, and probe deeply. (Figure 5-28)

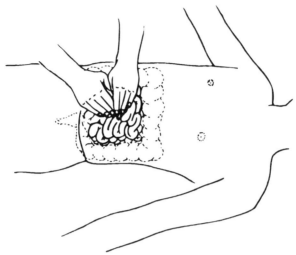

Work in clockwise and
counterclockwise half spirals.
Always end by pulling the
energy toward the cecum

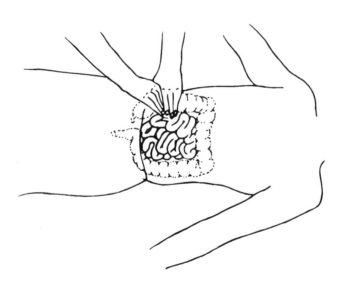

Figure 5-27. Working on the Small Intestine

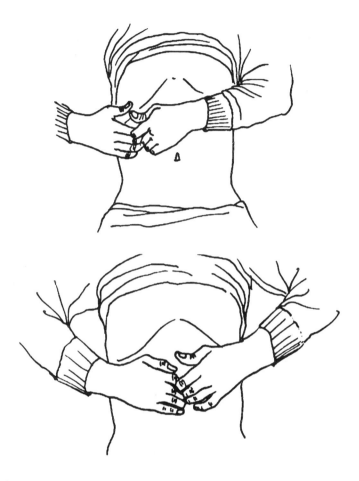

Figure 5-28. Working on Yourself

D. Knots and Tangles

1. Knots

As knots in the small intestine grow, they build pressure against the nerves coming out of the spine. Nerves don't tense up, muscles tense up. The nerves just transmit information. When you are subjected to stress, whether through anger, illness, or fear, the sympathetic nervous system is stimulated causing contraction in the muscular system. As a result, the

197

muscles, nerves, lymph, and blood vessels contract into knots. Sometimes the knots can feel like small plums. You want to get past the surface tension to dissolve the "seed" knot inside. These knots pull on other areas of the body, causing contraction and pain. (Figure 5-29)

2. Techniques

If the abdomen is especially knotted and tight, do not first work directly on the knot. Instead, find an area that is loose and relaxed and work there. Extend the relaxed area to surround the area of the knot(s) with relaxed tissues. By the time you get to the knot, the area won't be as painful for the contracted area will have relaxed.

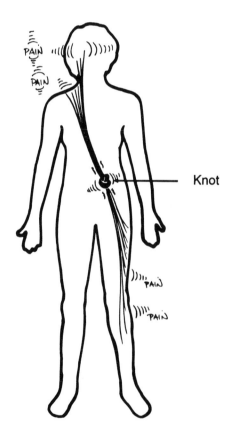

Figure 5-29. A knot in the abdomen can cause pain in distant areas of the body by pulling and creating tension

(1) Ask your student to tell you where there is any discomfort. Observe the face of the student since it will reveal the painful or uncomfortable condition.

(2) Press down gently on the knot and spiral. You may start by using the palm, then the heel of the palm, then three fingers, then two fingers, then one finger. This is not a rule, however. You can start with two fingers and go to one finger. You will discover a personal technique after having worked on several people.

(3) The process of clearing knots can continue after the session has finished. Teach the student how to do homework.

3. Tangles

Tangles occur more deeply than knots. Tangles consist of nerves, veins, and tendons that are twisted together. (Figure 5-30) They may have lymph nodes and fatty tissue inside them. Tangles, in part, are composed of small layers of connective tissue that are growing all over the organs, holding them in place. This tissue should be supple, and the organs should be able to float and move. When the connective tissues get tangled and rigid, they hold the organs too tightly.

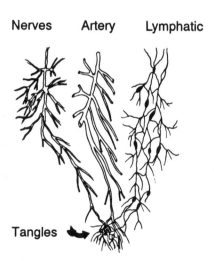

Figure 5-30. A Tangle of Nerves, Arteries, and the Lymphatic System

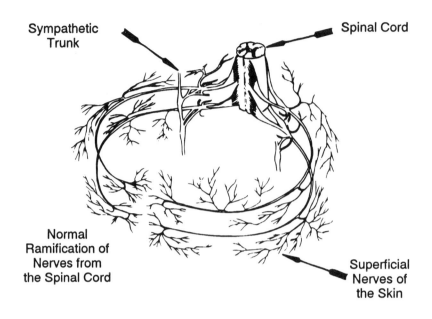

Sympathetic Trunk

Spinal Cord

Normal Ramification of Nerves from the Spinal Cord

Superficial Nerves of the Skin

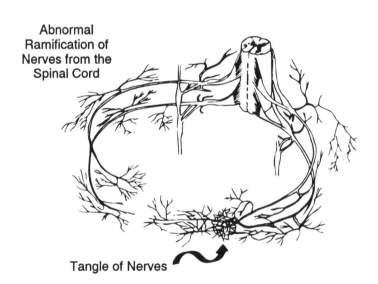

Abnormal Ramification of Nerves from the Spinal Cord

Tangle of Nerves

Figure 5-31. The nerves can get tangled

The less movement in the tissues, the tighter they will be held together. The important work here is to make the connective tissues more supple by stretching them and moving them around.

4. Techniques

a. Loosen the whole abdomen. Practice skin detoxification. Relax any knots.

b. Work at the edge of the tangle. The tangles can feel like a big ball of yarn with a head and a tail. Work on the edges of it until you feel it start to unravel.

c. When it starts to unravel, work toward the center and untangle it.

d. Be very patient. It could take weeks to attain successful results. Assign homework, and advise the student not to drink coffee. Coffee tightens the abdomen.

5. Differentiating Knots and Tangles

Knots are usually surface blockages that can appear as thickened or lumpy areas in the small intestine area. They entangle with the superficial fasciae, lymph, small nerves, and capillary beds. Tangles occur more deeply than knots and involve the larger structures of nerves, lymphs, tendons, muscles, arteries, veins, fasciae, and the organ systems and their energies. A light touch when doing CNT will keep you in contact with the knots, while a heavier touch will keep you in contact with the tangles. With a little practice you can feel the size and texture of the tissues on both levels.

6. Untangling Nerves

Freeing a tangle of nerves allows the blood and Chi to flow freely. (Figure 5-31) Numbness occurs where there is a tangle of nerves that does not permit the blood to flow. Feel for such a tangle and first work the tangled nerve upward away from the navel. If the condition does not change, work downward to the navel. (Figure 5-32)

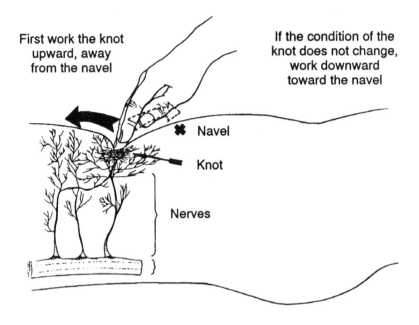

First work the knot upward, away from the navel

If the condition of the knot does not change, work downward toward the navel

Navel

Knot

Nerves

Figure 5-32. Working on Knots

CHAPTER 6

BALANCING EMOTIONS AND TONIFYING ORGANS

Emotional tension is expressed in the way you breathe. Emotional sensitivity is associated with the lungs and large intestine. The process of balancing emotions in the body is closely related to establishing good breathing patterns and insuring the body's ability to eliminate anything it does not need to carry.

The Creation and Control Laws of the Five Phases of Energy are helpful here. The lungs and large intestine comprise the Metal phase of Chi. According to the Law of Creation, Metal is controlled by Fire (heart and small intestine). This means that one way you can affect the lungs and large intestine is by working on the small intestine, the Fire organ in charge of digesting food. The small intestine is also in charge of digesting emotions; it reflects the way the mind feels. All the undigested trauma of our lives collects in the small intestine as a knot. It will hold this trauma until it is safe to release it. In most people untying the knots in the small intestine allows release through the large intestine. Clear the trauma out and the Fire energy will be stronger. Then the Fire energy can help establish powerful and abundant Metal energy in the lungs and large intestine. Establishing the ability to breathe freely and fully will allow the emotions to release.

To relieve sadness in the lungs, release the congestion all along the large intestine and then on each side between the navel and lung points. Also, release the breathing pattern of the lung points by establishing a healthy breathing pattern that fully utilizes the diaphram, thereby freeing the lateral motion of the rib cage. Finally, since Fire controls Metal, you will tonify the heart, heart controller, and Triple Warmer. (*Tonify* is a term used in acupuncture to mean tone by infusing with energy.)

You have already learned that each internal organ has a particular negative emotion associated with it. By working on the particular organ and tonifying it, you can release its negative emotion.

Before you can release any anger in the liver, you must free the breathing on the right side. Check the diaphragm to determine if it is tense and contracted. Then release any congestion in the small intestine that lies in the area between the navel and liver.

You can release anxiety in the spleen and pancreas by releasing the knots and tangles in the area of the small intestine that lies between the navel and the spleen and pancreas. You will need to re-establish healthy breathing in the middle and left side of the rib cage by releasing the diaphragm and by tonifying the liver.

To release fear and paranoia in the kidneys, work to get rid of knots, tangles, and congestion under the kidney area of the small intestine. This will help to re-establish a deep breathing pattern in the lower abdomen.

Releasing cruelty and impatience in the heart requires deep treatment all over the small intestine. First, however, you must eliminate high pressure in the middle of the chest by working very deeply on the diaphragm and tonifying the kidneys. This process could take two to three sessions.

A. Relaxing the Diaphragm

The diaphragm is a breathing muscle attached to the lower portion of the rib cage and anchored to the spine in the lumbar region. It is shaped like a dome (Figure 6-1) and projects up against the heart and lungs. Upon inhalation it pushes down against the abdomen, creates a vacuum in the chest, and allows air and Chi to fill the lungs. If the diaphragm becomes tense or stiff, which it often does when one feels inhibited, it interferes with the ability of the lungs to breathe fully and deeply.

The lungs are called the *Sea of Chi*. Chi in the lungs drawn from the air mixes with Chi derived from food (by the stomach and spleen). Together they form the blood and nutritious Chi which service all the functions of the body. The more Chi they can draw in, the healthier you are going to be. If the action of the lungs is impaired by a diaphragm that is tense or frozen, you can imagine the consequences. A deep breath also draws Chi to the lower organs, to the kidneys and bladder, and especially

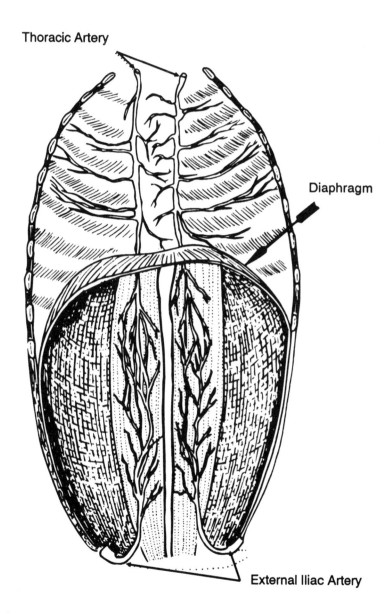

Figure 6-1. The Cavity of the Torso
The diaphragm is shaped like a dome

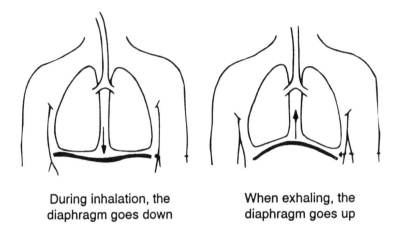

During inhalation, the
diaphragm goes down

When exhaling, the
diaphragm goes up

Figure 6-2. Front View of the Diaphragm

to the large intestine. The large intestine gets energized this way. If it does not have energy, it will not be able to do its elimination work.

Working on the diaphragm and relaxing any tension in it will help to transform shallow chest breathing into deep abdominal breathing. The diaphragm can expand fully and the lungs will be able to draw in more oxygen and Chi. The importance of abdominal breathing cannot be overemphasized.

During abdominal breathing the diaphragm lowers, forcing the vital organs to compress downward. This allows the lower lobes of the lungs to fill with air and forces the abdomen to protrude. The chest and sternum sink. Upon exhalation, the stomach returns to a flatter shape, and the other vital organs return to their original sizes and shapes. (Figure 6-2)

1. Abdominal Breathing Exercise

a. To practice abdominal breathing, keep the chest very relaxed. This may be difficult at first, but it is important.

Begin by breathing in and drawing the air into the abdomen. (Figure 6-3) It may help you to imagine that you are first breathing into the coccyx, then the sacrum, and then up each vertebrae of the spinal column.

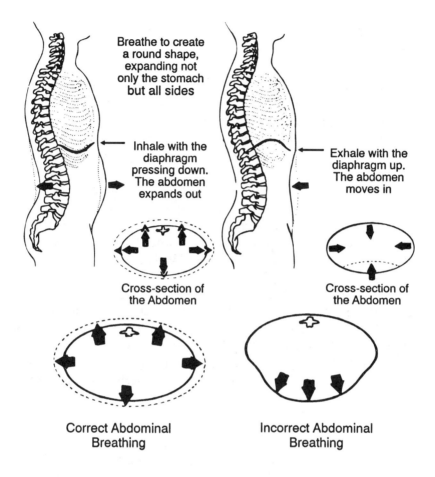

Breathe to create a round shape, expanding not only the stomach but all sides

Inhale with the diaphragm pressing down. The abdomen expands out

Exhale with the diaphragm up. The abdomen moves in

Cross-section of the Abdomen

Cross-section of the Abdomen

Correct Abdominal Breathing

Incorrect Abdominal Breathing

Figure 6-3. Abdominal Breathing

b. Make the chest hollow and drop the diaphragm down. You will feel pressure inside the abdomen which will begin to protrude on all sides in a rounded shape. Do not expand the stomach only. With the diaphragm lowered and the abdomen filled with air, the space containing the abdominal organs is minimized, and the organs massage themselves.

c. Expel the breath by drawing the abdomen up, squeezing in on all sides of the abdomen, and forcing the breath out of the nose.

2. Technique for Releasing the Diaphragm: Creating a Space

a. As in every CNT session, start massaging around the navel to loosen the tightness. This will prepare a place for the breathing when the abdomen does start to expand. Sometimes you will encounter an abdomen that is contracted and full of toxins and tension. Your student will hardly let you touch the abdomen; it hurts too much. Imagine what his or her breathing pattern is like. There is no way they can do deep abdominal breathing, even if they knew how. It's too painful. This is common. If you meet a student with an abdomen in this condition, you can be sure that you will need to do diaphragm work. This is a worst-case scenario. Even when you work on diaphragms paired with healthier abdomens, nearly every one will need some work. Observe the breathing pattern and feel the tension and toxin level in the abdomen to determine the degree of help required.

b. When the large intestine is full or constipated, it will push up into the diaphragm, lungs, and heart. Release the intestine, starting from the lower left side of the rib cage, along the descending colon, near the splenic bend. Then start working across the transverse colon, under the right side of the rib cage, loosening the area. Be conscious that you want to work back toward the beginning of the large intestine, which is at the ileocecal valve. This is done to release the congestion of the large

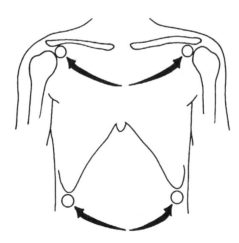

Figure 6-4. Pressing the Lung Points

intestine and allow for the expansion of the rib cage and diaphragm. Once you have opened the large intestine, work back the other way and try to stimulate its movement using techniques already learned.

c. Place one hand on the left side of the rib cage, while the other hand penetrates under the ribs to lift them while breathing in.

d. The hand on top of the rib cage will be pushing down while the student is exhaling. The range of motion of the ribs will be increased, because you will be progressively releasing the tensions in the inner costal muscles. If the tension is severe, you may have to use the technique for loosening the rib cage described for asthma treatment in Chapter 10.

e. Once the maximal range of motion is attained, find the lung points and press them as deeply as possible. (Figure 6-4) This will allow you to reach the part of the diaphragm anchored to the lumbar vertebrae.

f. Work on the right side.

g. Start at the lower left rib cage and work your way to the lower right rib cage. Use your fingers to press down all along the edge of the rib cage. (Figure 6-5)

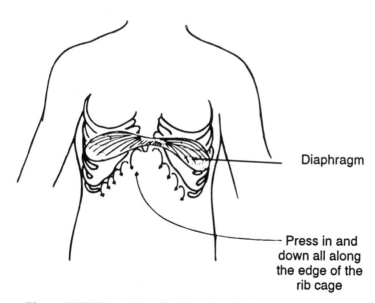

Diaphragm

Press in and down all along the edge of the rib cage

Figure 6-5. Releasing the Tension in the Diaphragm

h. Starting at the lower right rib cage, work under the rib cage using a two-thumb spiraling motion. This will loosen the diaphragm muscle. (Figure 6-6)

i. Continue spiraling along the muscle as you move up the rib cage toward the sternum. (Figure 6-7)

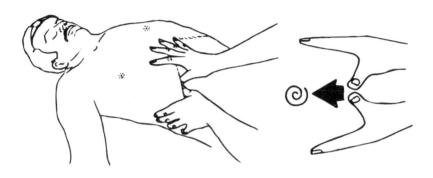

Figure 6-6. Releasing the Diaphragm by Spiraling the Thumbs

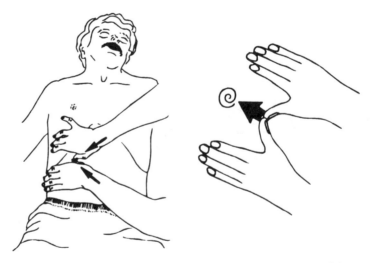

Figure 6-7. Releasing the Diaphragm on the Right Side by Spiraling the Thumbs

j. Release the diaphragm at the sternum area. Change finger technique. The ring finger supports the middle finger pressing down and forward. Spiral. (Figure 6-8)

k. Spiral and release the diaphragm at the sternum area. Use all four fingers. (Figure 6-9) You may change your finger technique until you

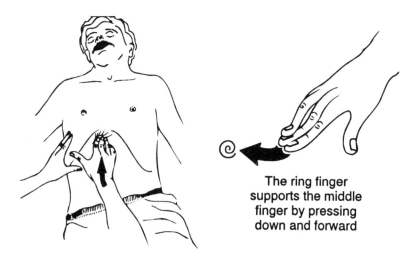

The ring finger supports the middle finger by pressing down and forward

Figure 6-8. Releasing the Diaphragm at the Sternum. The ring finger strengthens the middle finger

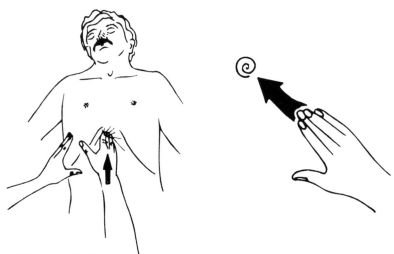

Figure 6-9. Releasing the Diaphragm Using Four Fingers

211

find one that fits your hand and allows you to do the work. Knowing different fingering techniques will allow you to select one that is appropriate for the body you are working on, i.e., thin, muscular, obese, frail, an infant's.

1. Spiral at the diaphragm to release it using the two-hand technique. (Figure 6-10)

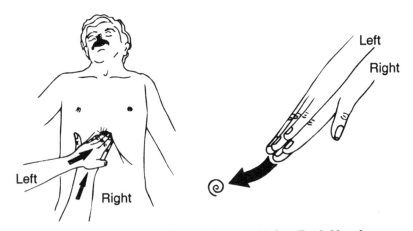

Figure 6-10. Releasing the Diaphragm Using Both Hands

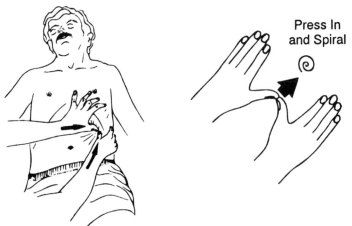

Figure 6-11. Releasing the Diaphragm on the Left Side

m. Continue releasing the diaphragm as you move down the under-side of the left rib cage, passing the spleen as you work your way down. Spiral. (Figure 6-11)

n. The result of these techniques should be spontaneous, deep, abdominal breathing with minimal motion of the upper chest.

B. Tonifying the Organs and Releasing Emotional Energy

Webster's Medical Dictionary defines tonicity as "Tonus; a state of normal tension of the tissues by virtue of which the parts are ready to function in response to a suitable stimulus." This describes the state in which you want to leave the student's body. Its systems are balanced and ready for whatever happens next. Achieving this state may involve flushing out stagnant emotional blocks, stale winds, and other decaying energies.

Tonifying the organs begins to happen automatically right after they have been detoxified. The energy spent by the organs in storing and processing the toxicity is now available for beneficial use by the organs. In CNT, points on the energy channels of those organs are also stimulated. Tonification is very soothing, and your student may easily fall asleep.

1. Techniques

These techniques should be taught to your students so that they may do them at home.

a. Lungs

(1) One hand holds the lung point, LU-1 (Lung-1) (Figure 6-12), on the chest, while the other hand is massaging the lung area marked on the CNT chart. (Figure 6-13) Massage the point on both sides, starting on the left.

(2) While you are pressing the points, your student should inhale through your hands. When exhaling the student should softly make the Lungs' Sound (SSSSSSSS) and visualize the color white. Both of you may feel sadness coming out, or a heavy sigh.

After the lungs' energy has been cleared of negative influences, try to sense whether it is strong, healthy, cool, and dry. Be aware of your particular methods of sensing. You may be very good at noticing emo-tional response, or better at determining subtle changes in organ temper-

213

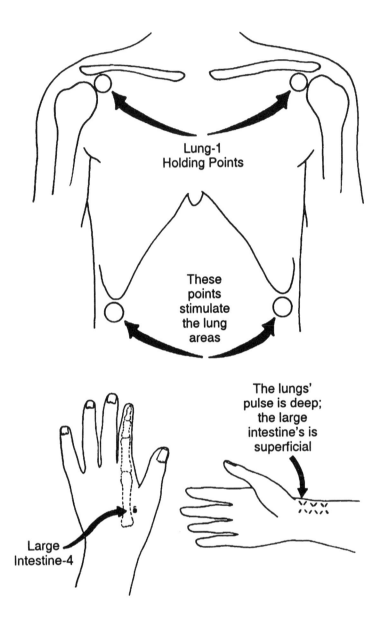

Figure 6-12. Tonifying the Lungs

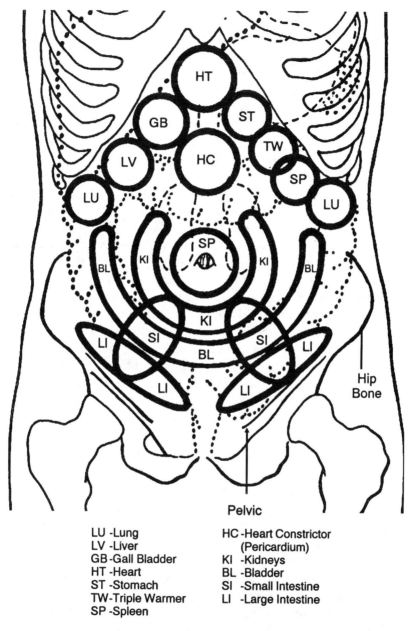

LU -Lung
LV -Liver
GB -Gall Bladder
HT -Heart
ST -Stomach
TW -Triple Warmer
SP -Spleen

HC -Heart Constrictor
    (Pericardium)
KI -Kidneys
BL -Bladder
SI -Small Intestine
LI -Large Intestine

Figure 6-13 Chi Nei Tsang chart showing areas where you can access and balance the energy of the organs
Based on drawing in *Zen Shiatsu* by Shiyuto Masunaga

atures. You might have your own method or strong intuitive feelings. Sometimes the change in energy is dramatic, but at times it can be subtle.

(3) If more energy is required, stimulate Large Intestine-4 (LI-4) in the web of the thumb and forefinger.

(4) Monitor the lungs' pulse on the wrist.

All the organs can be tonified similarly, but do not fear that a lot of unpredictable emotional energy is going to come your way. Usually one emotion will release, and this will help to relax the tension in the neighboring organs according to the Laws of the Five Phases of Energy.

You and your student can work together to forestall or lessen the impact of the emotional release. If your student loses a positive state of mind, teach him or her how to recapture it, or the negative emotion that is released could be transferred to you. If you can determine what negative emotions are predominant, both you and your student should focus on the opposite positive emotion as you begin the emotional release. Both of you should do the Inner Smile as well.

This is a good place to remember that it is important to stimulate your student's energy to avoid draining yours. Stimulating the lungs will be important in helping you figure out how much stimulation is necessary to achieve a state of balance and harmony throughout all the student's other body systems. Constantly checking the pulse and position of the navel are ways to monitor this. Since people are different, some will need more work on the lung point, others on the liver. Try to discover what energy is lacking, what is excessive, and then balance the energy. The techniques for expanding the aura of the hands (Chapter 2) will also help, for you can determine the viscera's needs when you scan the organs with your hand.

b. Spleen

(1) One hand holds the spleen channel at Spleen-10 (SP-10) on the thigh near the knee. (Figure 6-14) The other hand massages the stomach and spleen areas (along the bottom of the rib cage). (Figure 6-13) Some worries may emerge.

(2) While you are pressing the points, the student should inhale through your hands. When exhaling the student should softly make the Spleen's Sound (WHOOOOOO) and visualize the color yellow.

(3) If more energy is required, stimulate Spleen-3 (SP-3) along the spleen meridian on the foot. (Figure 6-14)

(4) Monitor the spleen pulse on the right wrist.

216

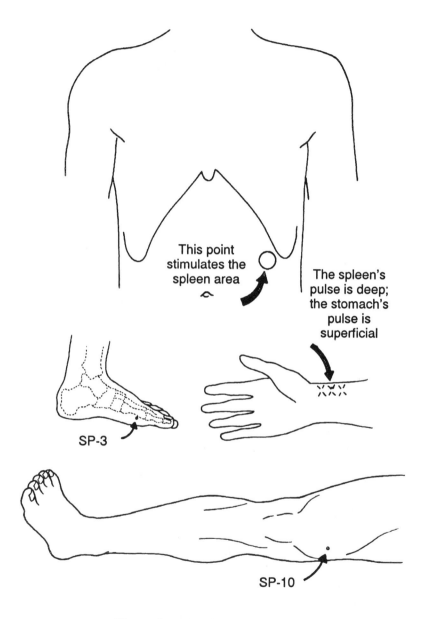

This point
stimulates the
spleen area

The spleen's
pulse is deep;
the stomach's
pulse is
superficial

SP-3

SP-10

Figure 6-14. Tonifying the Spleen

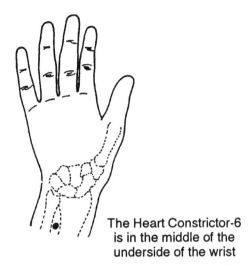

The Heart Constrictor-6 is in the middle of the underside of the wrist

Figure 6-15. Tonifying the Heart Constrictor (Pericardium)

c. Heart Constrictor

(1) Massage the Heart Constrictor point marked on the CNT chart. Be particularly gentle here, as the xiphoid process, just below the sternum, is fragile, and the whole solar plexus area is very tender.

(2) With the other hand hold Heart Constrictor-6 (HC-6) in the middle of the wrist. (Figure 6-15) This often releases spontaneous laughing in people.

d. Gall Bladder

(1) Massage the Gall Bladder mark on CNT chart and with the other hand press Large Intestine-4 (LI-4) in the web area between the thumb and index finger. (Figure 6-12)

(2) The student should inhale through your hands. While exhaling the student should softly make the Liver's Sound (SHHHHHHH) and visualize the color green.

e. Liver

(1)While massaging this area, the student may release anger. Massage the liver area of the CNT chart while holding Liver-3 (LV-3) on the liver channel near the big toe. (Figure 6-16)

(2) The student should inhale through your hands. While exhaling the student should softly make the Liver's Sound (SHHHHHHH) and visualize the color green.

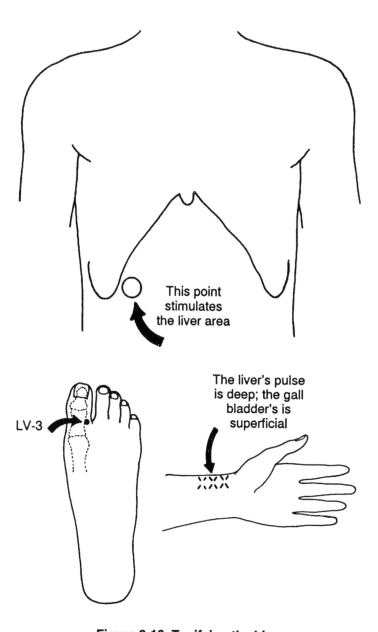

This point stimulates the liver area

The liver's pulse is deep; the gall bladder's is superficial

LV-3

Figure 6-16. Tonifying the Liver

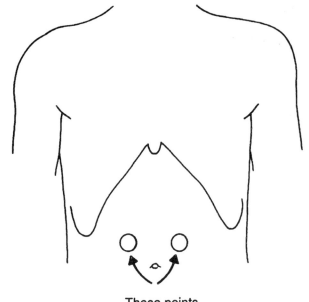

These points
stimulate
the kidney area

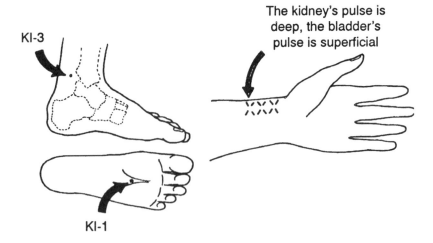

KI-3

The kidney's pulse is
deep, the bladder's
pulse is superficial

KI-1

Figure 6-17. Tonifying the Kidneys

(3) Monitor the liver's and gall bladder's pulses on the left wrist.

f. Kidneys

(1) Massage the kidneys' areas on the CNT chart while holding Kidney-3 (K-3) by the ankle. (Figure 6-17) Fears may come out. Massage both sides.

(2) Have the student inhale through your hands. While exhaling have the student softly make the Kidneys' Sound (WOOOOOOO) and visualize a dark color blue.

(3) If additional energy is needed, stimulate Kidney-1 (K-1) on the sole of the foot.

(4) Monitor the kidneys' pulse on the left wrist.

g. Heart

When a person is impatient, anxious, hasty, and/or feels hatred, the heart area will be congested, tight, painful, and blocked. Breathing can be difficult. To release the tension and tightness and increase self-esteem and confidence, massage the sternum close to the heart. (Figure 6-18)

(1) Use the one finger technique, starting from the top of the sternum working down in small spirals to the tip of the sternum. (Figure 6-18) If you find painful parts, work slowly and gently, but spend time on it. Look at the student's face. If it shows pain, just hold the point at the tip of the sternum and HT-7 for a while. Massage the tip of the sternum gently and carefully since it is soft. Work thoroughly as you massage from the top of the sternum down to its tip.

(2) Massage in between the ribs and the places at which they are joined to the sternum. Work specifically in the area below the collarbone. Here you will find painful spots on most people.

(3) If there is a lot of pain, ask the student to make the Heart's Sound (HAWWWWWW) and visualize the color red as he/she is massaged.

h. The Area Around the Rim of the Navel

If there is a lot of bitterness and hatred, the area around the rim of the navel will be tight and painful.

(1) Use the one finger technique and massage closely around the rim and the abdominal of the navel (Figure 6-19).

(2) Approach the painful part gently. Most of the time you will feel tightness on both sides of the navel. Sometimes it feels like two big tendons rising up on both sides.

221

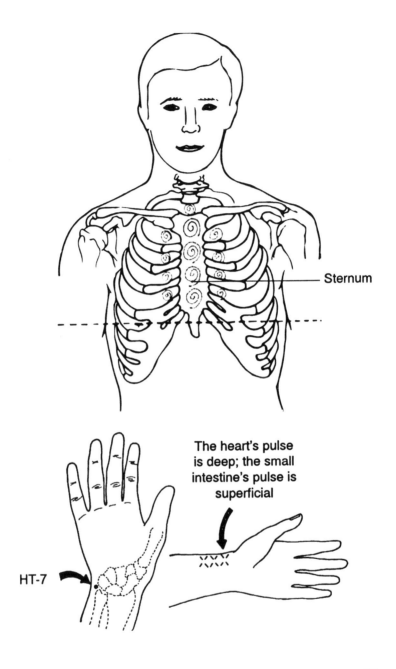

Sternum

The heart's pulse is deep; the small intestine's pulse is superficial

HT-7

Figure 6-18. Massaging in Small Spirals Down the Sternum, If it shows pain, just hold the point at the tip of the sternum and HT-7

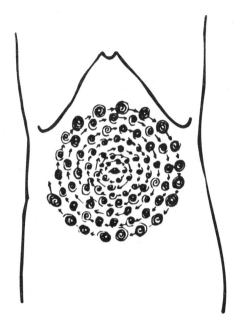

Figure 6-19. Massaging around the navel

(3) Press down on the tense points and hold for awhile, then lightly release and press down again a little more.

(4) If there is a lot of pain, have the student use the Spleen's Sound and do not work too hard or too long. It might take trying this more than once to dissolve the tension.

i. The Area in the Crease of the Legs

Tension here indicates guilty feelings.

(1) Use one or two fingers to press and spiral from one side of the groin to the other. Work slowly and gently.

(2) Press on the tight places and hold for a while, and then press deeper until you feel them release.

If there are a lot of emotions, put emphasis on the Inner Smile and the Healing Sounds. Work on the heart and increasing virtue. The feeling of love will help release emotions and avoid the problem in the future.

C. Tonifying the Navel Center Chi and Reducing Stress

This is an exercise to reduce stress and recharge Navel Center Chi.

(1) Place the right thumb on the right hipbone and spread the fingers over the kidney. The middle finger should be on the sacrum with the other fingers lying along the spine. If you have small hands and are working on someone very big, just be sure to cover the kidney with your hand. Use the hand to send energy to the kidney. A strong kidney can nourish the whole body. It is especially beneficial for the lower abdomen, since it can release lower back pain and tension.

(2) Place the left palm above the navel, just below the sternum. Press down with the left palm in a counterclockwise circular motion. Press up with the right hand. Gradually, move the left palm lower toward the navel. (Figure 6-20)

(3) Practice nine, eighteen, or 36 times. Rest and concentrate on the navel for a while. Feel the Chi energy start to move in the navel and collect at the Navel Center.

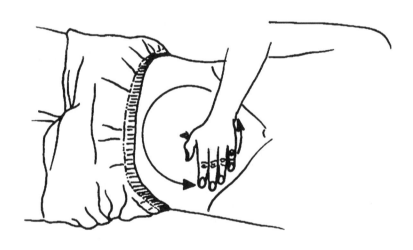

Figure 6-20. Recharging the Navel

(4) Switch hands and do the same on the left side. Place your right hand on the navel and your left hand on the hip and kidney. Use the right heel, palm, and fingers to massage the Chi of the navel in clockwise movements gradually descending from the sternum area toward the navel. You can do this nine, eighteen, or 36 times.

D. Baking the Organs

Besides tonifying the organs in the ways listed above, you can apply different techniques directly to the organs to meet their specific needs.

1. Baking Technique

Put the left palm on the back and the right on the front of the problem area. Both palms are aligned so that the healing energy can be projected from the right hand to the left through the affected area. If you need more stimulation, let the top hand vibrate and shake.

2. Baking the Liver

Hold your left hand under the lower right rib cage. Place the right hand over the liver on top of the rib cage. Bake the liver between the hands. (Figure 6-21) This soothes the nerves and stimulates cell formation to repair damaged livers.

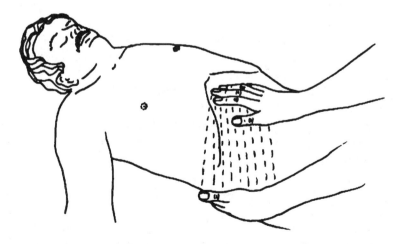

Figure 6-21. Baking the Liver

3. Baking the Pancreas, Spleen, Lungs, and Kidneys

Use the same technique used in "Baking the Liver" above.

E. Meditation

You can now understand the importance of first teaching your students the Six Healing Sounds and familiarizing them with the Inner Smile and the Microcosmic Orbit. By giving the students some self-healing techniques, you will help hand the healing responsibility over to them, and the healing process will go faster. If you teach people how to fish, then all will know how to fish, and there is no reason for anyone to come to you for fish.

Teach your students that their problems will be more easy to balance if they practice the meditations. They can concentrate on a variety of points in the Microcosmic Orbit to help with specific problems.

1. Moving the Energy through the Microcosmic Orbit for the Student

You can use your hands initially to show a student how the energy moves through the Microcosmic Orbit.

a. Start by having the student concentrate on the navel, sending all his or her attention there. When it feels warm, move the warmth from the navel up to the solar plexus. This can help with problems in the liver, spleen, stomach, pancreas, and digestive system.

b. For back and kidney pain, warm the navel as above, then move the energy and concentrate it in the back near the spine between the kidneys. This is one of the most powerful energy points in the whole system. Teach how to spiral energy there, and, when finished, how to move it back to the navel for storage.

c. If the person lacks energy or tires easily, they can move the energy from the navel, up the back to the T-11 vertebrae point, and concentrate there until the area gets warm. This will stimulate the adrenal glands. Finish by moving the energy back to the navel.

d. For high blood pressure move the energy from the navel to the soles of the feet.

e. For heart problems and depression, concentrate the energy on the spine between T-5 and T-6, which are located between the shoulder blades and opposite the heart. Remember to move the energy back to the navel when done.

f. For asthma and lung problems, send the energy from the navel to the C-7 point between the shoulders, and then back home to the navel.

g. The energy should be held in the needy area for approximately fifteen to twenty minutes.

2. The Microcosmic Orbit for the Student to Practice at Home

After showing your student how the energy moves up the spine and down the front of the body in the Microcosmic Orbit, explain how the right hand gives energy and how the left hand receives energy. Then show how the placement of the hands can encourage the energy to move in the Orbit. For example, place the right hand on the navel and the left hand on the Ovarian Palace or the Sperm Palace. Then lightly spiral out from the navel into the right hand. Send it to the left hand and then spiral it back to the area desired. Keep the energy that is coming out from the right hand cool so that the left hand can draw it in.

Chi Nei Tsang

CHAPTER 7

DETOXIFYING
THE ORGANS

Bit by bit, day by day, negative emotions, waste material, pollution, and toxins settle and accumulate in the organs. As the knots form, circulation, energy flow, and nerve impulses are blocked. The flow of the Chi through the channels to the legs and hands diminishes. When the blockage occurs at an organ, the primary generator of its particular Chi, traditional muscle massage or stimulating the organ's reflex points is like using remote control to try to correct a problem that demands hands-on attention. In CNT you work directly on the organs themselves.

The detoxification process is not immediately concerned with "tonifying" an organ that is weak, cold, and Yin. Neither is there concern for depleting an organ that is hot, overstimulated, or Yang. The primary concern is in balancing the energies to a state that is equal and harmonious by clearing the toxins and tensions from all the organs. When you are finished working on an organ, it should be able to tone and balance itself. Organs have a self-healing ability, as does the rest of the body, when blood and Chi are able to flow powerfully and abundantly. (Figure 7-1)

Always remember to use your concentration to channel your energy from your Navel Center, as well as the Earth, Cosmic Particle, and Universal energies, while you are touching another. The Chi will go where you ask; but you have to ask.

Try to follow the sequence of the practice that follows. Be creative. The techniques described are the most efficient known, but do not regard them as having been written in stone. The body is complex, and there are many techniques and variations yet to be discovered. New and effective improvements are always forthcoming from Healing Tao-trained CNT practitioners. In fact, many of them are included in this book.

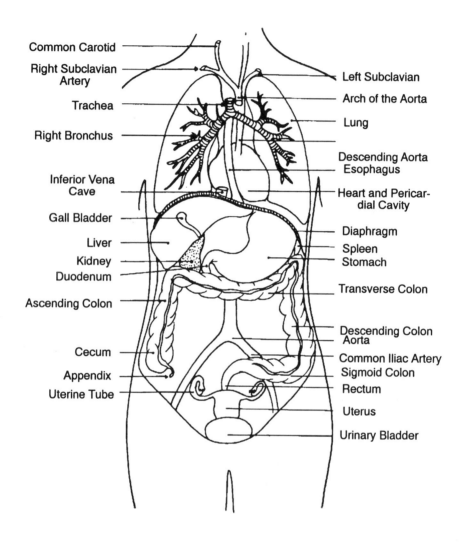

Figure 7-1. The Viscera with the Small Intestine Removed

A. The Left Lung

1. Location

The lungs are paired, cone-shaped organs located in the thoracic cavity. They are separated by the heart and by the plural membrane that encloses each lung. They are also separated from the abdominal cavity by the diaphragm.

2. Function

The lungs mix blood with oxygen, and expel used air, carbon dioxide, and other toxins. The diaphragm and intercostal muscles can control the motion of the lungs.

As previously mentioned, according to the Five Element System, the lungs are the Metal Yin organ. They have a variety of functions, the first of which is to produce Metal Chi. The lungs rule and govern this Chi and respiration down to the cellular level. It is in the cells of the lungs that Chi in the body meets up with Chi in air. The lungs also control skin and sweat.

3. Hand Techniques for the Lungs

a. Working with the Left Lung First

Always start by removing any congestion in the splenic bend under the left rib cage. Use the Figure Five Technique outlined in Chapter Five.

b. Lung Detoxification

Reach progressively under the left rib cage to stimulate the lung area. Then hold the left LU-1 or LU-2 on the Lungs' Channel below the clavicle. (Figure 7-2) Press in firmly and stimulate it with your fingertips. Have the student breathe the Lungs' Sound (SSSSSSSS) into your finger a few times, until you feel the lungs' energy activate on the meridian. When it is activated, you can feel a pulsing in LU-1.

c. Exhalation Phase

(1) Place one hand on the upper rib cage and the other hand on the lower rib cage. When working on a woman, place one hand above and the other hand below the breast.

(2) The student inhales using deep abdominal breathing. When the lungs are full, rock the rib cage. (Figure 7-3) Upon exhalation push the rib cage toward the opposite side.

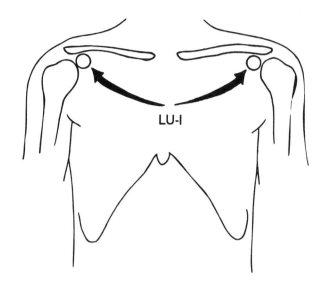

Figure 7-2. Lung Holding Points
Hold LU-1 on the Lungs' Channel near the clavicle

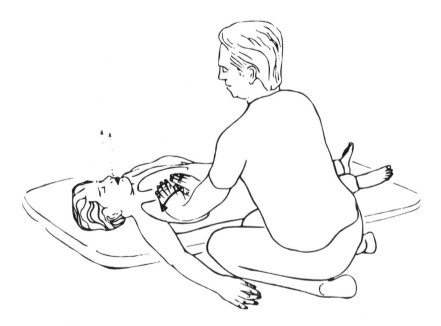

Figure 7-3. Lung Detoxification—Exhalation Phase

(3) Upon completion, hold and press momentarily. Then follow the inhalation with a gentle, but firm pressure of the hands. Return to the starting position and begin again to rock and shake.

(4) Repeat for three to five breaths. Note that you may also rock the rib cage on the complete exhalation as well.

d. Inhalation Phase

(1) Begin this phase with the same hand position. This time start in the full exhalation position. Rock the exhaled rib cage and ask the student to do deep inhalations. (Figure 7-4)

(2) While the student is inhaling, hold the pressure on the rib cage and ask him or her to breathe into your hands.

(3) When the student reaches full inhalation, keep rocking and maintaining pressure. Follow the exhalation to the starting point of inhalation, repeat for three to five breaths.

(4) On the last inhalation, ask the student to inhale deeply and quickly. When the student reaches full inhalation, remove the pressure, but not the contact of the hands from the chest. Allow the chest and lungs to overfill with air.

(5) Use this technique for the right lung as well.

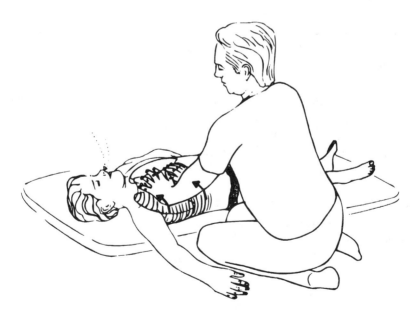

Figure 7-4. Lung Detoxification—Inhalation Phase

B. Spleen

1. Location

The spleen is located under the left rib cage, beneath the stomach.

2. Function

The spleen is the largest mass of lymphatic tissue and the largest lymph node in the body. However, it does not have any connecting vessels to the rest of the lymphatic system. It does not filter the lymph. Instead, it filters, stores, and cleans the blood. It breaks down and eliminates bacteria and worn out blood cells and recycles them into bile which is passed to the liver. Besides cleaning the blood, it stores some (about one and a half pints) for emergencies. It also plays a central role in the body's immune system. It produces B cells, which develop into antibody-producing plasma cells. When massaged, it releases extra blood into the system and bolsters the immune function.

In the Chinese system, the spleen and pancreas are associated with Yin Earth organs. Their digestive functions, associated with the digestive function of the liver and gall bladder, are in charge of "transformation and transportation." The spleen extracts Chi from food, mixes it with Chi from the lungs, distributes it according to the five tastes, and assigns it to its proper element and organ. If its function is blocked or inefficient, the blood and Chi in the whole body can be upset.

The spleen is also in charge of transporting Chi to the muscles and limbs. The muscles are the Earth tissues, and any muscular problems can be treated by working on the functions of the Earth element in the body. In acupuncture all muscular disorders are generally treated by working on the spleen, pancreas, and stomach channel, or any other Earth parts of the other channels.

3. Hand Techniques for the Spleen

a. First remove any congestion in the large intestine at the splenic bend.

b. Use your thumbs or fingers to spiral in the spleen area. The spleen is deep so add weight by pressing down on the thumb or fingers using the other hand. (Figure 7-5)

c. As you reach the level of the spleen under the left rib cage, you should not encounter any hardness because the spleen is soft tissue. It is

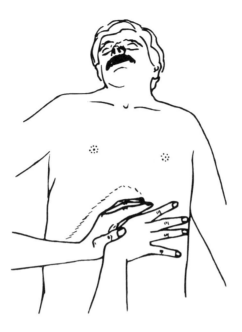

Figure 7-5. Spleen Detoxification—Spiraling with the Thumb

unlikely that you will be able to feel it. However, you should take time to work at length on it to improve its natural function and increase its pumping action. Massaging the spleen will help it to pump blood in and out and thus increase its cleansing effect on the blood. The massage will also increase the energy level in the spleen/pancreas meridian system and spread its benefits to the entire lymphatic system.

     d. Have the student push away your fingers with his or her spleen and Chi.

     e. Use the Baking Technique with one hand on top of the spleen and the other beneath it (on the back).

C. Pancreas

1. Location

     The pancreas is located behind the stomach with its head near the centerline and its tail under the left side of the rib cage near the splenic bend in the large intestine. (Figure 5-14) It is between four point eight and six inches long.

2. Function

The function of the pancreas is to manufacture pancreatic juice, which aids digestion when fed into the small intestine. Its juice is very alkaline and when combined with the bile of the gall bladder, it helps to balance acidic juices from the stomach. This is the digestive function of the pancreas.

The pancreas also has an endocrine function, which is to release insulin into the blood to allow the sugar contents of the blood to be absorbed into the body's cells. When sugar is not absorbed, the condition is called diabetes. Diabetes is caused by a lack of insulin.

Because everyone eats too much sugar, the pancreas overworks and quickly creates too much insulin. This gets dumped into the blood causing hypoglycemia. The only remedy is to remain free from sugar.

As you work just below the left side of the rib cage, you will be moving over the pancreas. You can feel the pancreas, unlike the spleen, especially if the person is addicted to sugar. Massaging the pancreas will dramatically improve its work. The massage should be done smoothly. The harder the pancreas, the softer you should do the massage.

3. Pancreas Massage Technique

a. Place the fleshy, knife edge of the palm on the head of the pancreas at the centerline, and press deeply into it. Apply as much pressure as the student can take. If possible, apply extra weight with the other hand resting on the working hand. If you are working on a sugar addict or alcoholic, the area will be very painful. (Figure 7-6) Remember the rule is to be gentle and to go slowly. The harder the pancreas is, the softer the massage should be.

b. Apply a rolling pressure with the edge of the palm and fingers. (Caution: Pump toward the body's midline so that stones or crystals do not enter the spleen.) As you get to the narrow end of the pancreas near the lower left rib cage (where the mass of the pancreas decreases), the pressure you are exerting will decrease as the tips of your fingers tail off. (Figure 7-7)

c. Together you should do the Spleen's Sound (WHOOOOOO) during the massage.

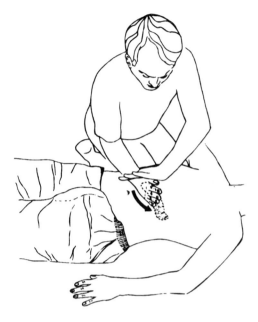

Figure 7-6. Pancreas Detoxification—Starting Position

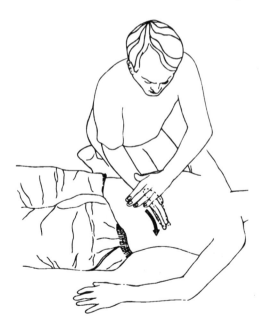

Figure 7-7. Pancreas Detoxification—Finishing Position

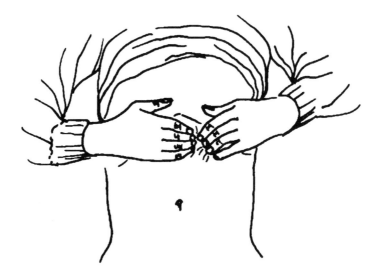

Figure 7-8. Working on Your Own Pancreas and Stomach

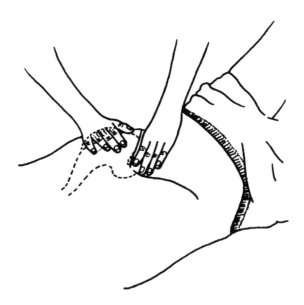

Figure 7-9. Pumping the Spleen, Stomach, and Pancreas

d. When working on yourself, use the basic two-handed spiraling technique. If you are sitting and leaning into your fingers, you can apply more pressure. (Figure 7-8)

D. Pumping Techniques for the Stomach, Spleen, Pancreas, and Left Colon

To release the toxins and tensions, first use the two-thumb spiraling technique throughout this area, then use the pumping technique for the stomach and the pancreas.

1. In this technique one hand is on top of the lower part of the left ribs, pressing down to help and encourage exhalation. The other hand progressively massages its way under the ribs. Eventually the hand working under the ribs can lift the rib cage, and increase its motion on inhalation. You can increase the pumping action on those organs to release intercostal tensions and breathing patterns. (Figure 7-9)

2. Pump several times coordinating with the exhalation of your student's breath. Pump toward the body's midline and into the body (as in the liver pump), scooping toward the navel from the direction of the spleen and stomach. This technique is very relaxing. Remember to follow the rhythm of your student's breathing, rocking your body to create the movement. Relax your body and hands.

E. Liver

1. Location

The liver is located under the right side of the rib cage, underneath the right lung and diaphragm. It passes the centerline and extends to the left side. (Figure 5-14) When empty of blood and fluids, it weighs approximately three pounds. It has four lobes. (Figure 7-10)

2. Function

The liver stores large quantities of blood, minerals, and vitamins. It prepares carbohydrates for storage in the body by breaking them down into more simple sugars. It is in charge of protein and amino acid production. It produces fats, antibodies, and most plasma proteins. It also

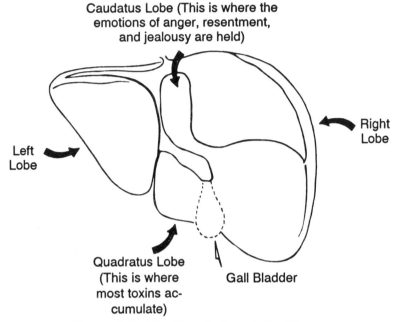

Caudatus Lobe (This is where the emotions of anger, resentment, and jealousy are held)

Right Lobe

Left Lobe

Quadratus Lobe (This is where most toxins accumulate)

Gall Bladder

Figure 7-10. The Four Lobes of the Liver Viewed from the Rear

produces bile salts which are distributed by the gall bladder into the small intestine to absorb fats from the food consumed. It produces Wood Chi.

The liver stores all the toxins, poisons, chemicals, and drugs that the body takes in. Its function is to break down poisons chemically into less toxic compounds so that they can be more easily eliminated by the rest of the body. These toxins usually stay in the liver for a long time before they have a chance to be processed. If the poisonous load becomes too high, the liver's digestive process and other functions are prevented from working properly. This also slows down the secretion of bile in the gall bladder, which crystallizes and forms gallstones.

The liver accumulates many toxins, including alcohol. Alcohol can be released during a CNT session and could intoxicate the student. Since the alcohol, drugs, medicines, or toxins have been built up over a period of time, be careful during the release. Do not release too much the first time. Liver detoxification usually accompanies detoxification of the spleen and the lymphatic system and tonification of the kidneys.

According to Chinese medicine, the liver is the Yin Wood organ. The liver is responsible for the smooth functioning of the body. Any imbalance in the liver can greatly affect all the body's systems. It is also in control of the nerves, and therefore plays a role in the thinking process and nervous activity.

The liver is also where the Hun, the spiritual souls, live. They are very skittish, timorous, and "gun-shy." They positively, absolutely do not like anger or poisonous toxins like alcohol or drugs. When these substances are present, they often flee from the body. This can be disastrous. The only way to convince them to return is to perform many good deeds, as well as more acts of compassion toward others. The Hun love this behavior and will remain with you if you behave well and are lucky.

3. Liver Hand Techniques

Liver work starts with making space by releasing the congestion of the large intestine. The large intestine, which runs over the liver at the liver bend, needs to be clear, or you will not be able to work on the liver without pain. Clear the large intestine from the ileocecal valve to the sigmoid colon. This is important for clearing the flow of the liver meridian that runs right through the ileocecal valve around the testicles or the ovaries. This is the only way to affect the part of this channel that runs deep and is not accessible to acupuncture needles.

You also need to make room by working on the spleen, pancreas, rib cage, and diaphragm. Then, finally, you can reach the liver. You can use your fingers or thumbs, whichever you find easier to work with.

a. Make small, circular motions with your fingertips on the liver, searching for the hardened spots. These hard places are areas where there are accumulations of toxins. As these toxins leave, the liver has more room and energy, allowing it to function more efficiently, and the health improves.

b. When you find a place that is unyielding, spend more time there, working until it becomes softer. Remember not to release too many toxins at once. Ask for feedback from the student. Talk, and watch the eyes for signs of pain. If the student falls asleep, listen for groans and moans.

c. To work on and drain the lower part of the liver, switch from using the fingertips to using both thumbs together or side by side. Place them underneath the lower right side of your student's rib cage. Let your fingers rest gently on top of the ribs.

d. Press in and rock up with both thumbs under the right rib cage reaching into the liver. Scoop in and down with both thumbs releasing the lower edge of the liver and creating a pumping action as you work. Move along the lower border of the rib cage. Proceed slowly and be gentle. Make small circles in a spiral motion, working upward toward the common bile duct. Move slowly, but go deep enough to meet the liver tissue. Loosen any knots or tightness. Have your student do the Liver's Healing Sound (SHHHHHHH) and breath directly into the tension. Remember to be gentle.

Use the same thumb technique to work the middle lobe of the liver. The middle lobe holds many negative emotions, particularly repressed anger and rage.

You will be working further up the liver, underneath the rib cage. Whenever you can, change the angle of your thumbs so that you can contact more of the liver tissue. Again, be cautious and go slowly. You can go over the area several times, adding more pressure and going deeper each time. Work until you reach the gall bladder.

e. To work the upper part of the liver, start with your hands positioned to the right of the xiphoid process.

f. Use one hand on top of the other for guidance and support.

g. Use the fingertips to move underneath the rib cage, sweeping toward the gall bladder. Working this area will activate the heart. The upper lobe is just beneath the heart and right on the heart reflex point. When the liver overheats, it will heat up the heart. Make sure you do not stimulate too much heat in this area.

h. Have the student do the Liver's Healing Sound through the whole process, but when you work near the heart reflex, practice the Heart's Sound (HAWWWWWW). This will counteract the tendency to overheat this area.

i. When finished ask the student to push your fingers out with his or her liver and Chi.

4. The Liver Pumping Technique

The liver is like a sponge, since all of its cells either filter or store. When you use the pumping technique (Figure 7-11), you work its sponginess and help the liver in its work. The Liver Pumping Technique is as follows:

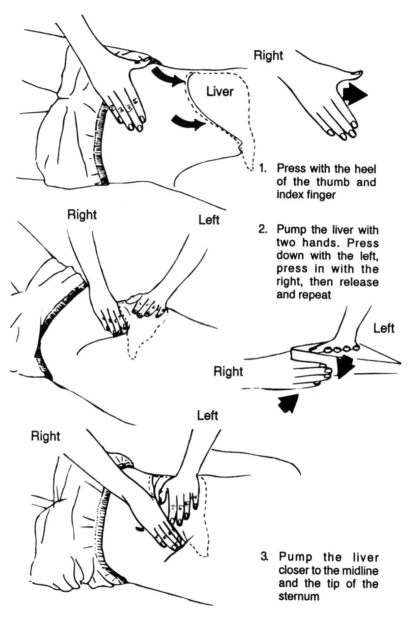

1. Press with the heel of the thumb and index finger

2. Pump the liver with two hands. Press down with the left, press in with the right, then release and repeat

3. Pump the liver closer to the midline and the tip of the sternum

Figure 7-11. Pumping the Liver

243

a. The right hand is stationary. It is positioned with the right thumb under the lower portion of the rib cage and the index finger pointing toward the sternum.

b. The left hand is placed on top of the right ribs over the liver and does the pumping action. This is a gentle downward motion toward the navel or the left hip.

c. Pump several times, coordinating with the exhaling breath. This technique is very relaxing. Remember to follow the rhythm of your student, rocking your body to create the movement.

d. Keep your body and hands relaxed throughout.

5. Working from the Rear on a Seated Person

a. Stand, sit, or kneel behind the student, reach under the arms and massage the liver. (Figure 7-12)

b. Use this technique to work on the liver and spleen at the same time. You may use this position for any of the abdominal work. (Figure 7-13)

F. Gall Bladder

1. Location

The gall bladder is a pear-shaped sack located in a depression under the liver. It is the size of the thumb and located between the two front lobes of the liver. The easiest way to locate a man's gall bladder is by drawing a line from the right nipple to the navel. (Figure 7-14) For women, you can imagine a line from the right shoulder to the navel. In either case the gall bladder is on the line near the bottom of the liver.

2. Function

The function of the gall bladder is to store and concentrate bile until it is needed in the small intestine for digestion. The bile breaks down fats in food. (Figure 7-15) The main problem with the gall bladder is that it gets too congested with bile salts; or a bacteria might arrive, and the bile will isolate it and form a pearl-like stone around it. Often many "pearls" form and obstruct the duct, and the gall bladder may then have to be removed through surgery.

In the Chinese system, the gall bladder is a Yang Wood organ and is related to decision making. When it is not working well, it can easily cause headaches, sluggishness, and indecision. It controls Wood Chi. The

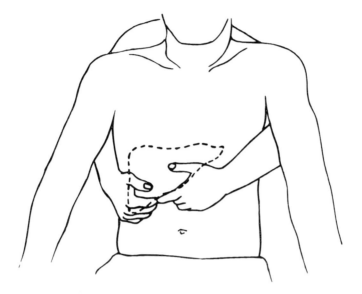

Figure 7-12 Working on the Liver from Behind

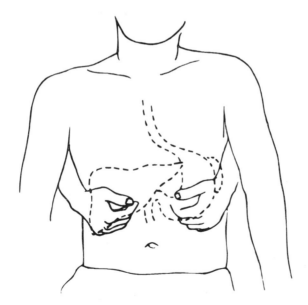

**Figure 7-13 . Working on the Liver
and Spleen from Behind**

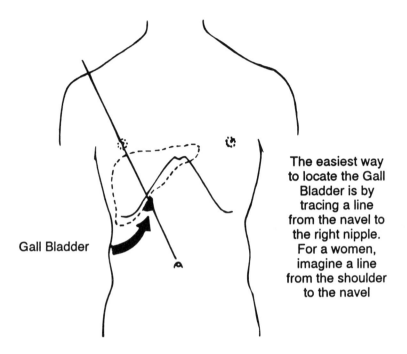

Gall Bladder

The easiest way
to locate the Gall
Bladder is by
tracing a line
from the navel to
the right nipple.
For a women,
imagine a line
from the shoulder
to the navel

Figure 7-14. Locating the Gall Bladder

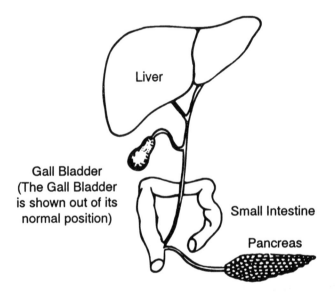

Liver

Gall Bladder
(The Gall Bladder
is shown out of its
normal position)

Small Intestine

Pancreas

Figure 7-15. The Ducts of the Gall Bladder and Pancreas

gall bladder is firmer than the liver. If there is any irritation, such as small gallstones and crystallized bile salts, it could feel tender.

3. Gall Bladder Hand Technique

a. Place your thumb directly on the gall bladder. With your thumb on the gall bladder, add weight by putting the edge of your other hand over your thumb, creating a T-shape. Press down with your hand and thumb and rotate clockwise and counterclockwise in half-turns, creating a J-shape and a reverse J-shape. Then squeeze the gall bladder and bile duct toward the midline and navel. Move any extra bile into the small intestine. This will help release the congestion from the bile duct into the duodenum. (Figure 7-16)

b. When finished, have the student push away your fingers with his or her gall bladder and Chi.

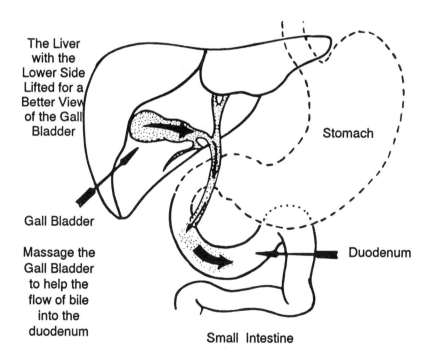

The Liver with the Lower Side Lifted for a Better View of the Gall Bladder

Gall Bladder

Massage the Gall Bladder to help the flow of bile into the duodenum

Stomach

Duodenum

Small Intestine

Figure 7-16. Flow of the Gall Bladder's Bile

G. Stomach

1. Location

The stomach is "J" shaped. It is located just on the centerline and extends to the left of it just below the sternum. (Figure 5-14)

2. Function

The stomach receives food from the esophagus, stores it, and then empties the food into the duodenum, the beginning section of the small intestine. It secretes enzymes and juices that help break down proteins and turn them into a thin liquid called *chyme*. This fluid is then passed on to the small intestine, where any nutrients are absorbed.

In Chinese theory, the stomach is called the *Sea of Nourishment* or the *Sea of Food and Fluid*, and the process of producing energy and blood begins here. It controls the Earth Chi. The spleen begins assigning some of the Chi from food while it is still in the stomach. This Chi is sent to the lungs where it combines with Chi taken from the air and turns it into blood and nutritious Chi.

3. Hand Techniques for the Stomach

a. You can work the stomach area either with your thumbs or fingertips. Start at the top and move down with the pressure underneath the right rib cage. Make this movement in small spiral circles.

b. Work on this area several times until the path seems clear of congestion, tension, and pain. This also will open this area for further work on the spleen and for draining the lymphatic system.

H. Right Lung: Hand Techniques

1. Reach progressively under the right rib cage to stimulate the lung area. Then hold LU-1 or LU-2 below the clavicle. Press firmly and stimulate it with your fingertips. Have the student breath into your finger a few times, until you feel the lung's energy activate on the channel. When it is activated, you can feel the pulse in LU-1 or LU-2.

2. Follow the directions for the "Exhalation and Inhalation" techniques described at the beginning of this chapter for working on the left lung. Use them on the right lung.

I. Kidneys

1. Location

The kidneys, like the spinal cord and the brain, are well protected. They are located above the waist in the back. They float outside the peritoneum which contains the digestive system and are surrounded by the ribs which protect them. They are the size and shape of the average ear. (Figure 7-17) The kidneys pulse and pump like the heart and are considered the deepest organs in the body which makes them the most Yin of the Yin organs.

2. Function

The kidneys filter all the fluids, removing excess water and un-needed by-products of the body's many chemical reactions. They can only move about six cups of liquid per day, including liquids that are already in the body, as well as what you drink. (This is why drinking too much fluid can be as unhealthy as drinking too little.) The kidneys regulate the mineral level in the blood and the acid balance in the body. If the moisture in the body is low, kidney stones can develop.

The kidneys eliminate toxins after they have been broken down and released from the liver. If the kidneys get overloaded with toxins, they will slow down. Loss of energy in the kidneys will cause an energy loss in the rest of the body.

The kidneys can accumulate many mineral deposits which can weaken their ability to function. If they can't function properly, then there will be too much fluid in the blood. This leads to high blood pressure. Tonifying the kidneys is part of the process of lowering blood pressure.

To the Chinese, the kidneys are the Yin Water organs. They store prenatal, reproductive energy and distribute this crucial energy, as needed, to all parts of the body. The kidneys are sometimes called the *roots of life*. They are very important in determining the level of vitality and length of life. All sexual energy comes from the kidneys. Any sexual or reproductive disfunction can be traced to the kidneys. Often, they control pain in the lower back. The kidneys also control the skeletal system, bones, and teeth. They produce Water Chi.

3. Kidneys Hand Techniques

a. To work on the right kidney have the student lay on the back and then twist the pelvic area over to the right so that the right hip is pointing straight up and the right knee is drawn toward the chest. Place a cushion behind the right knee to support it and keep it in position, or kneel behind the student and use your knee to support the raised hip. Ask the student to relax the shoulders.

b. Look at the area where the kidney should be. Look for an indentation or slight depression on the skin surface.

c. Use both hands and eight fingers to go into this area. You won't use all eight fingers to massage the kidney. Usually you will use just your two middle fingers with the others for support. (Figure 7-17)

d. Every kidney is different. If the kidney is normal and is not situated too low, you will only be able to feel the bottom of it. If it is in good shape, it might have the texture of a marshmallow or be just a little firmer. Inhale air to make your cheeks round and puffy. Feel the surface of your skin to feel what a healthy kidney feels like. It feels soft and gentle, but with a slight surface tension.

e. Use your student's assistance in finding the kidney. The student can guide you to the kidney and you may hear such comments as, "That just feels like your finger nail," or, "That feels like your just pushing

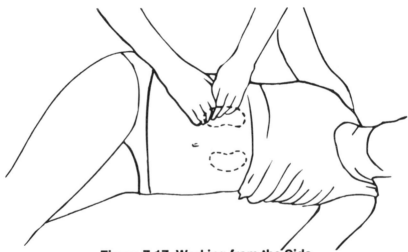

Figure 7-17. Working from the Side to Gain Better Access to the Kidneys

against my skin." When you hear, "I feel something in my back," or "You are touching it now," you can start massaging in small spirals.

f. An unhealthy kidney will feel uneven with alternating soft and hard spots. At times it is painful, and you may not be able to work on it for long. Sometimes you can't reach the kidneys because the tissue surrounding it has become very hard. In that case, gently massage this area until the congestion dissolves and you can reach the kidneys. Assign homework. Use the technique in Figure 7-17.

If working on himself or herself, the student may also sit in a chair or on the toilet, and lean into the fingers, thereby using the weight of the body to help bury them deeply.

g. When you begin to use a spiraling massage with your fingers, have the student continuously use the Kidneys' Sound every time he or she exhales. Massage very gently.

h. On the average you can spend one or two minutes on each kidney, but do not spend more than five minutes maximum.

i. The question of how long this procedure should take permits us to introduce an advanced healing technique developed by a woman who is a very talented CNT practitioner. You may attempt it when your energy is highly developed, and you are sure of your ability to recover and protect yourself. In a meditative state, she works organ to organ by uniting the energy field of her organ to that of her student. By doing this she knows when her fingers have reached the kidneys because she feels "something very respectful and valuable." If she finds a sick kidney, then her kidney also feels sick; if the kidney she is working on hurts, then her's hurts. When she begins to spiral her fingers, she can feel fingers spiraling in her kidney. She is constantly sending good kidney energy from her kidney to that of her student while constantly doing the Kidneys' Sound with her student. She determines when she will stop the massage and the healing process by evaluating the feeling in her kidney. When her kidney feels well again, then she knows she has helped her student to restore her own kidney to full functioning and a healthier state. The practitioner approaches each of the organs in this manner.

j. The release technique is very important. When you have finished the massage, have the student push your fingers out of her kidney with her energy and Chi.

k. After you have finished the massage, blow warm air into the kidney. This is an early shamanistic Taoist practice adopted by Chinese healers when they started applying burning moxa on a cold area that needed heat.

The kidneys are "cold" organs that enjoy and benefit from warmth. You may warm them by gently using your fingertips to draw back the skin over the area where you were just working.

From a distance of two to three inches, blow warm air deep into the kidney using the Kidneys' Sound as you exhale. With this technique you will be funneling healing energy directly into the kidney. This always feels very comforting to the students, and they will tell you this. Usually, they say, "Oh, that feels so good." (Figure 7-18)

When you have finished blowing warm air into the kidney, you also can use the same technique to blow warm air into the K-1 point on the sole of the foot. Use the blowing technique anywhere there is cold tissue, including a cold uterus or a lower intestine that is blocked or cold.

1. Finish the entire sequence by Baking the kidney.

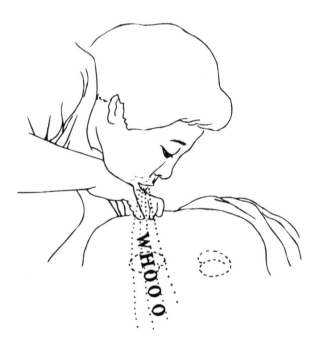

**Figure 7-18 Using the Kidneys Sound
to Blow Warm Air into the Kidney**

4. Adrenal Glands

The adrenal glands are situated in the upper sections of the kidneys. They are enclosed in common fascial layers with their respective kidneys, but separated from them by a connective tissue. Each adrenal gland weighs fourteen ounces. Often adrenal problems can cause stiff necks. After working on the adrenal glands, many of your students will notice that their neck problems have disappeared.

(1) Have the student lay on his or her side. Get behind the back.

(2) If the adrenal glands need help, they often can indicate this to you by forming a spot, pimple, or wart on the skin. Look for this spot.

(3) Put one thumb on top of the other over the spot which is usually located at T-11 (11th thoracic vertebrae). The rest of the fingers are extended and reach over the rib cage.

(4) Push the thumbs in where you think the adrenal is located. You need to ask for the student's help. Probe around until you find the right place. Unfortunately, the right place is usually painful. Have the student compare locations until you find the right one.

(5) Hold on to the rib cage with the extended fingers. Pump the back over the adrenal, using a push-pump massage. The thumbs will be pressing into the adrenal gland. Pump until the pain recedes or disappears. This normally takes about twenty to 25 pumps. (Figure 7-19)

(6) When you are finished with the massage, keep the thumb of the top hand on the adrenal. Use a sweeping motion with the thumb of the lower hand to sweep the sick adrenal energy toward and into the descend-

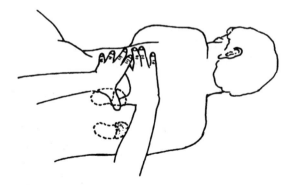

Figure 7-19. Pumping the Adrenal Glands

ing colon where it can be eliminated from the body. Use your concentration. Practice this twenty to 30 times. (Figure 7-20)

(7) Reverse the body, and work on the other adrenal gland.

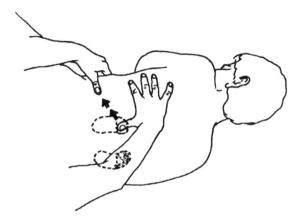

**Figure 7-20. Direct Negative Energy
to the Large Intestine for Elimination**

J. Bladder

1. Location and Function

The bladder is a hollow organ or membrane situated in the pelvic cavity. This is a Yang Water organ that receives and eliminates urine. The bladder channel is associated with almost every function of the body. It runs close to the spine and influences the sympathetic nerves. It is used quite often in acupuncture. It controls kidney Chi.

2. Hand Techniques for the Bladder

a. It is advisable to have the student urinate before working on the bladder. Locate the bladder. In a woman, it is below the uterus and just above the pelvic bone. In men it is just slightly above the groin.

b. Work with your fingers (or thumbs) in small circles over the entire bladder region until the area feels free of congestion or pain.

c. Massaging the knots and tangles out of the bladder can relieve many problems in the urinary system. (Figure 7-21)

254

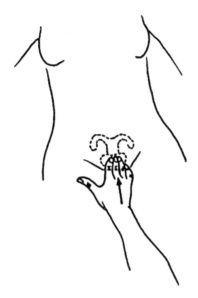

Figure 7-21. Working on the Bladder

K. Heart, Heart Controller, and Triple Warmer

As you keep moving toward the centerline, you will reach the organ points for the heart, heart controller, and Triple Warmer. (Figure 7-22).

1. Hand Techniques for the Heart

Massage the heart area with one hand while pressing Heart-7 (Figure 7-23) on the wrist with the other hand. This will sedate and slow down the heart.

2. Hand Techniques for the Heart Controller

Massage the heart controller area with one hand while pressing Heart Controller-6 (Figure 7-24) with the other hand. This will relax the diaphragm and stimulate the appetite.

3. Hand Techniques for the Triple Warmer

Massage the Triple Warmer area with one hand while pressing the Triple Warmer-5 (Figure 7-25) with the other hand to calm the nerves.

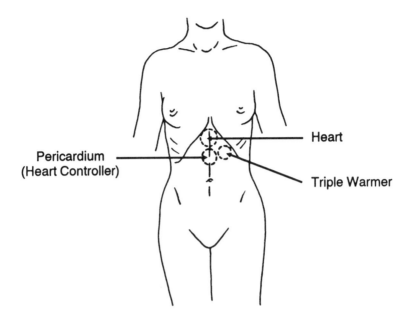

Figure 7-22. Organ Points

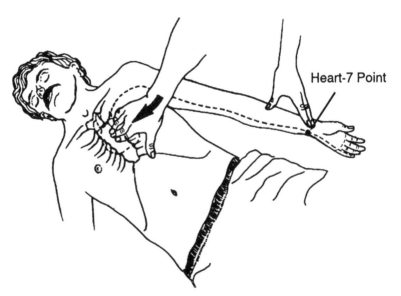

Figure 7-23. Hand Technique for the Heart

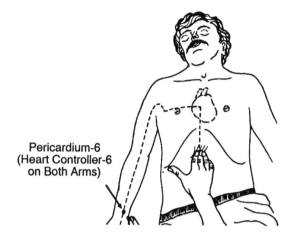

Pericardium-6
(Heart Controller-6
on Both Arms)

Figure 7-24. Hand Technique for the Heart Controller

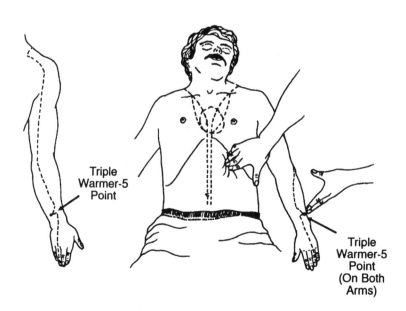

Triple
Warmer-5
Point

Triple
Warmer-5
Point
(On Both
Arms)

Figure 7-25. Hand Technique for the Triple Warmer

Chi Nei Tsang

Chapter 8

DETOXIFYING THE LYMPHATIC SYSTEM

A. The Lymphatic System

1. Lymph Nodes—the Foundations of the Immune System

Properly working lymph nodes and the proper flow of the lymphatic liquid forms the basis of our immune system. The lymphatic system is the "sewer system" of the body. Every lymph node is a purification treatment center detoxifying the lymph fluids as they move through.

Lymph is a blood plasma, except it is clear and without red blood cells. It forms in tissue spaces all over your body and gathers into the vessels of the lymphatic system. The lymphatic system consists of a network of vessels, capillaries, nodes, and ducts which function as filters and as a disposal system for toxic substances. The filtering action of the lymphatic system is very thorough, working continuously to take care of foreign matter, dead cells, bacteria, germs, and so on. When it is overwhelmed with toxicity, it becomes congested with mucus and impairs the immune system.

Lymph nodes are everywhere in the body, especially in the neck, groin, and armpits. (Figure 7-1) The largest concentration is in the abdomen, where they lay near the skin and near the spine. (Figures 7-2 and 7-3) The deep ones are large, each one about the size of a lima bean, and are close to the aorta and vena cava deep in the abdomen.

2. Lymph Circulation

The lymphatic system connects to the cardiovascular system's sub-clavicular veins near the collarbone and drains into the heart, but the

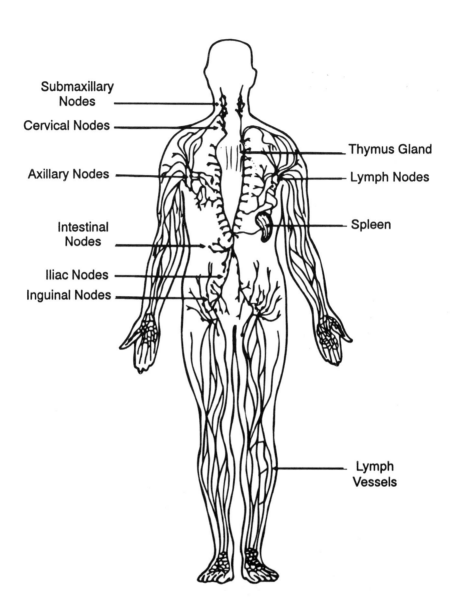

Submaxillary Nodes

Cervical Nodes

Thymus Gland

Axillary Nodes

Lymph Nodes

Intestinal Nodes

Spleen

Iliac Nodes

Inguinal Nodes

Lymph Vessels

Figure 8-1. The Lymphatic System

heart has no influence on the circulation of lymph fluid. In fact, unlike the vascular system, the circulation of lymphatic fluids is not a "closed loop system." It depends on the natural kneading or massaging action of surrounding muscles and joints as they contract and release. Contracting muscles compress lymphatic vessels in surrounding tissues. The compression of the skin from the outside, the movement of limbs or tissues, breathing, and pulsations from the arteries compress the lymph channels

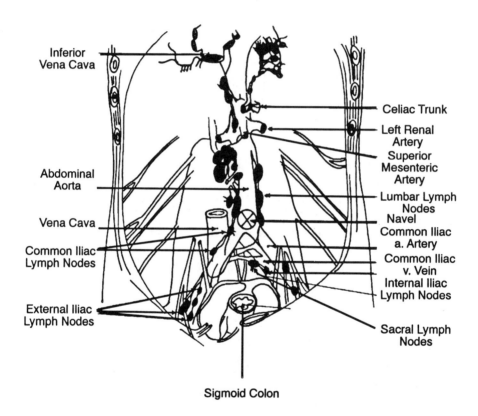

Figure 8-2. Lymph Nodes Along the Aorta

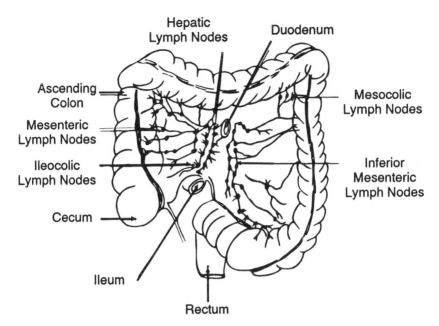

Figure 8-3. Lymph Nodes Along the Back Wall of the Abdomen

and aid in the movement of the lymph. One important reason for exercising is that it causes lymph to flow.

Since there is such a large concentration of lymph nodes in the abdomen, massaging the abdomen will stimulate the lymph nodes and cause them to drain. Massaging certain lymph nodes directly, particularly those in the abdomen, will stimulate the detoxification process.

3. Toxins and Lymph Nodes

Toxins are everywhere in the environment. Some occur naturally; human beings create others. The most common sources of toxins are food, air, and water. They can vary in size from microorganisms to large molecules of chemicals, poisons, dust, and dead cells. They are usually ingested by careless drinking and eating, normal breathing (of polluted air), and by absorption through the skin. The kidneys filter out the liquid toxins you ingest, while the liver filters out the solid toxins.

Toxins are often heavy and hard to move, especially those toxins that come from metals, such as lead and mercury. This is why they are difficult to purge from our internal organs and systems. When the body becomes overloaded with waste material, toxic matter, pollution, viruses, and bacteria, it all accumulates in the lymph nodes which swell and become painful. The lymphatic system will not function properly. The system backs up, and so the immune system is weakened.

If these small containers are unable to create enough lymph to release the accumulated toxins, they gradually harden. They become entirely inoperative, thereby diminishing the power of the lymph decontamination system. If this condition continues for several years, it can cause cancers to form.

The Chi Nei Tsang practitioner, working at the first level of the practice, can soften and clear blockages, activate lymph flow, and return these toxic substances to circulation. Then it is possible for the body to eliminate them. (Figure 8-4)

4. Feeling a Lymph Node

Since maintaining the activity of the body's immune system, much of which concerns lymphocyte production and distribution, is central to the practice of Chi Nei Tsang, acquaint yourself with the lymphatic system. Note where the many lymph nodes are and where the main ducts are commonly found.

To acquaint yourself with the feel of a lymph node, you can find one under the armpit or, since the armpit can be a very delicate area; it may be easier to find a superficial node in the groin area.

a. Locate the large nerve under the artery; it will feel like a nylon cord soaked in oil. Be gentle.

b. Next find the vein; it will feel hollow, like a water hose. You can feel the blood flowing through the vein, though there is no pulse, and the pressure is lower than in the artery.

c. Behind the vein is the artery. Here you can feel the definite pulsations of the blood.

d. Finally locate a lymph node along the artery. Practice until you can find and distinguish all four things (Figure 8-5), but take care not to massage a swollen lymph node in the armpit. (The abdomen is the only area in which swollen lymph nodes can be massaged.)

The lymph nodes feel like small glandular masses that harden when congested. If a lymph node feels like a softened bean placed in a small plastic bag filled with oil, then its condition is not too bad. If it is hard, does not move around very much, and is a sandy texture, then its condition is not good and it requires attention. (Figures 8-6 and 8-7)

263

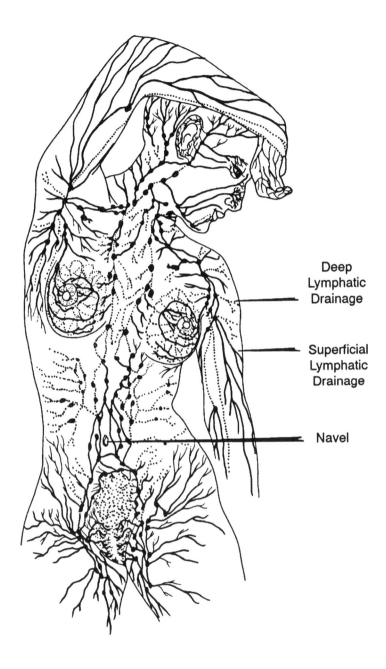

Deep
Lymphatic
Drainage

Superficial
Lymphatic
Drainage

Navel

**Figure 8-4. The Superficial and Deep Lymphatic Drainage
of the Head, Arms, and Torso**

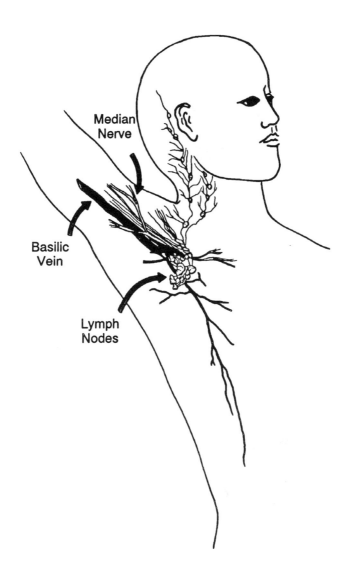

**Figure 8-5. Learn What a Lymph Node Feels
Like by Finding One in your Armpit**

265

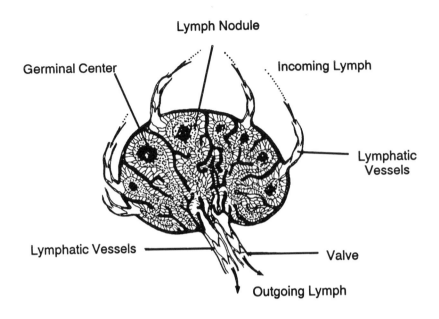

Figure 8-6. The Inner Structure of a Lymph Node

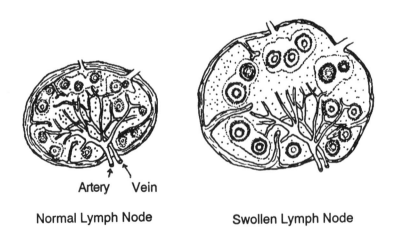

Figure 8-7. Normal and Swollen Lymph Nodes

5. The Concentration of Lymph Nodes in the Abdomen

The largest lymph nodes are near the navel. These become very clogged because the blood has picked up toxins from the body. When a lot of toxins accumulate in this area, cells can become so toxic that they begin to die. The first step in healing is to detoxify the body.

The nodes in the abdomen are positioned in two layers. The shallow group is just below the fatty layer under the skin and the other major concentration is very deep, around the kidneys and just above the backbone. (Figures 8-8 and 8-9) There is a tendency for more lymph nodes to be concentrated and congested in the lower abdomen than in the upper abdomen.

6. Lymph Drainage

The lymph drainage system covers the whole body. (Figures 8-10, 8-11, and 8-12.) The lymph from the abdomen, lower body, and legs drains into the cisterna chyli (in the lower abdomen in front of the first

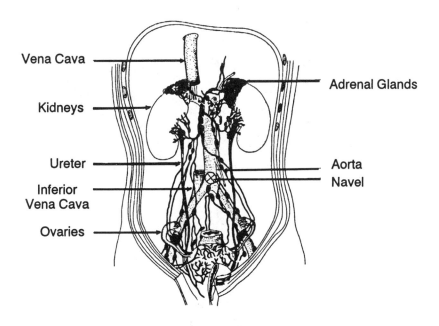

Figure 8-8. Lymphatic Pathways in the Kidneys, Aorta, and Lower Abdomen

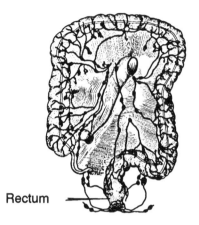

Rectum

Figure 8-9. Lymph Pathways Around the Large Intestine

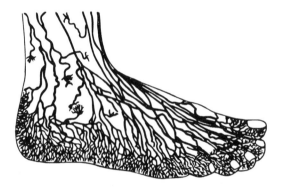

Figure 8-10. The Superficial Lymphatic Drainage of the Foot

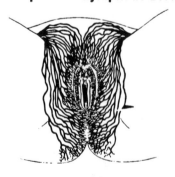

**Figure 8-11. The Superficial Lymphatic Drainage
of the Genitals and Perineum**

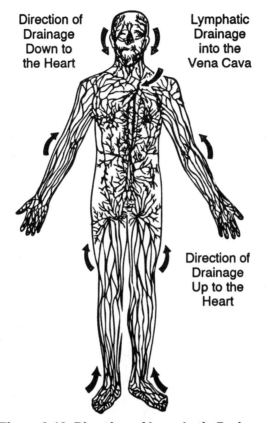

Direction of Drainage Down to the Heart

Lymphatic Drainage into the Vena Cava

Direction of Drainage Up to the Heart

Figure 8-12. Direction of Lymphatic Drainage

two lumbar vertebrae) and from there into the thoracic duct. There it is joined by the lymph from the left side of the head, neck, and chest. The right lymphatic duct drains lymph from the upper right side of the body and from the right side of the head and neck.

Eventually, the thoracic duct empties all of its lymph into the left subclavian vein and the right lymphatic duct empties all of its lymph into the right subclavian vein. (Figure 8-13 and 8-14) Together they drain the lymph into the heart and into the blood, and the cycle repeats itself. (Figure 8-15)

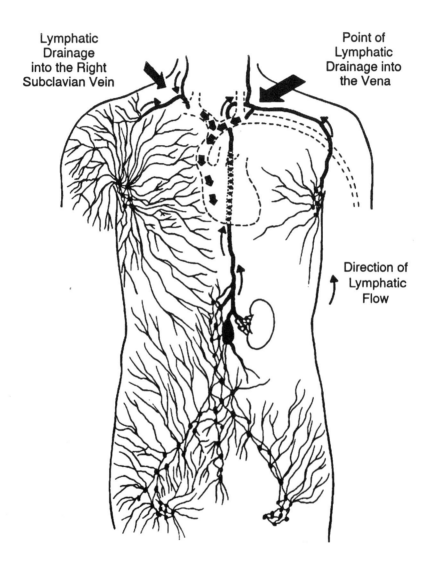

Figure 8-13. Lymphatic Drainage System

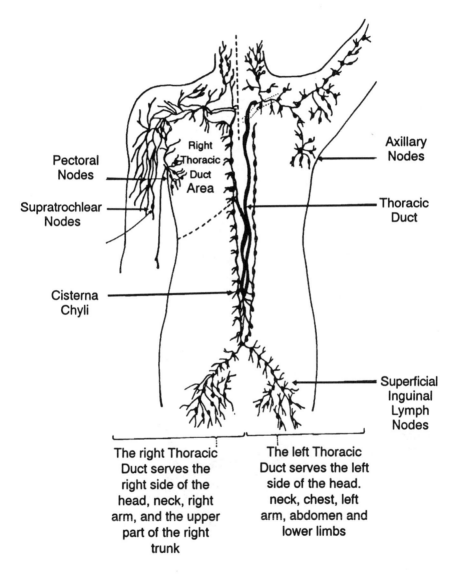

Figure 8-14. Lymphatic Drainage System

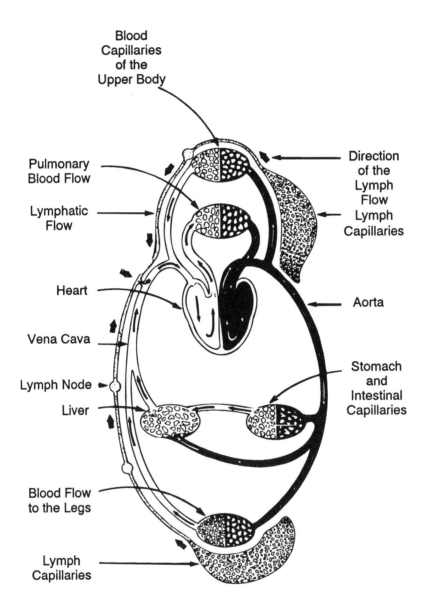

Blood
Capillaries
of the
Upper Body

Pulmonary
Blood Flow

Lymphatic
Flow

Direction
of the
Lymph
Flow
Lymph
Capillaries

Heart

Aorta

Vena Cava

Lymph Node

Liver

Stomach
and
Intestinal
Capillaries

Blood Flow
to the Legs

Lymph
Capillaries

**Figure 8-15. Schematic Representation of the Blood
and Lymph Circulation**

7. Detoxifying the Lymphatic System

As you massage the abdomen, the lymph glands will automatically be stimulated by the motion given to the tissues. This stimulation is increased by working directly and gently on the lymph nodes. Lightly stimulating the lymph in the abdomen will help to decongest the lymph nodes in this area. The abdominal lymph nodes and system are important because of their close connection with the intestines and digestive system and the detoxification system of the liver. Generally, eating loads everyone up with lymphatic waste (animal proteins, fats, milk). Bad eating habits damage the intestines and then the whole system. The remedy is a good diet and Chi Nei Tsang lymph massage.

Once you begin the process of draining the lymph, the body continues the process. It is not always necessary to continue working on a particular lymph node until it is completely clear. You may observe, in a following session, how that node has continued to soften, and how the entire lymph flow has improved. It is beneficial to point this out to your student, emphasizing the remarkable healing properties of the body and noting that the body likes a little encouragement.

a. Hand Techniques to Release Toxins from the Deep Abdominal Lymph

(1) Detoxification of the lymph toxins in the abdominal area begins by massaging the navel, first clockwise, and then counterclockwise.

(2) Do the Wave Technique until you can clear and reach deep into the abdomen. Feel for lymph nodes along the midline. They are smaller than knots or tangles. If you can feel them, then they are congested. Massage them lightly with your fingertips.

(3) Continue searching for nodes in this area especially around the aorta and vena cava close to the spine. Massage any that you find.

b. Working on the Rest of the Body's Lymph

(1) Begin by place your hands flat on the navel. Ask him/her to breathe against them while you press down. When the student exhales press down a little more, thereby activating the lymph flow into the thoracic duct.

(2) Clear the superficial lymph system in the skin by stroking the ribs. Move your hands to the lower ribs at the level of the liver. Place your thumbs underneath, pushing up from the sides in a forward motion toward the centerline. Stroke (do not rub) the skin very gently. Gradually move your way up toward the sternum.

(3) Go to the spaces between the ribs on the left side of the sternum. Place the fingertips of all eight fingers into the spaces and, with a circular and downward pressing motion, push the lymph into the body toward the thoracic duct. Work the lower ribs first and gradually move up to the upper ribs just below the collarbone. Repeat on the right side.

(4) Drain the areas above the collarbone and again direct the lymph down into the body. Place your middle and index fingers above each side of the collarbone into the hollow spaces and make a circular motion into the body, thereby draining the lymph into the vena cava.

(5) Stand at the head of your student, and turn the head to the left. When you turn the head, cradle it in your left hand and support it so that the student relaxes. Lay the head down just before you move the lymph down from the right collarbone. It is very important to use a light, feathery touch in this area since it is very delicate. Use the fingers to drain the lymph vessels from below the jaw and ear, down the side of the neck.

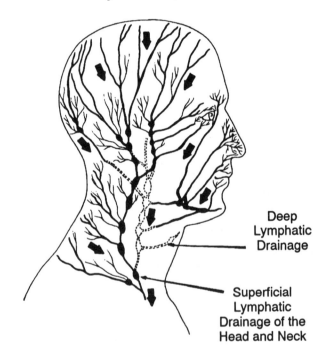

Deep Lymphatic Drainage

Superficial Lymphatic Drainage of the Head and Neck

Figure 8-16. Superficial and Deep Lymphatic Drainage of the Head and Neck and Direction of the Flow

Drain it into the space above the right collarbone. (Figure 8-16) (Do not work on anyone with a thyroid problem since this procedure can be very uncomfortable for this person.)

(6) When the lymph nodes under the armpit and around the neck are enlarged and painful, do not massage them. Wait until the pain is gone. These lymph nodes are close to the heart drainage area. Massaging them could push the infection into the bloodstream, thereby spreading it throughout the body.

The lymph nodes in the abdomen are large and numerous. Since they are far from the heart drainage area, the lymph system has a chance to deal with them. Massaging the lymph nodes in the abodmen can help inprove the overall immune system.

(7) Next, turn the head to the right, cradle the head, and repeat the massage on the left side.

You can work both sides simultaneously by placing one hand on each side of the neck (with the fingertips on the back of the neck). Make a circular motion downward, without rubbing the skin. If your hands are small, you might have to place them a little lower and do the movement a second time to work the whole neck.

(8) Using your flattened hand press the lymph nodes in the left armpit downward into the body. Repeat for the right side.

(9) Press the groin nodes towards the lower abdomen collect point near lumbar-2, also with your flattened hands or fingers.

(10) You may end by placing the students' hands over the navel and allowing rest. Thank the lymph nodes for letting you work on and disturb them.

Chi Nei Tsang

CHAPTER 9

CENTERING, BALANCING, AND FLUSHING

Ancient Chinese culture has provided us with a brilliant written record and understanding of the body's systems including natural and simple methods for correcting its imbalances. Absorbing their wisdom and techniques can help you become a better teacher. Your knowledge must include understanding the workings of the body, how to use your hands, build good energy, and practice discipline. This chapter is concerned with working on the abdomen to reposition tissues and arteries, centering energy, balancing body timing, and using the blood flow to flush out debris and toxins.

It is not necessary to practice these techniques continuously. Apply them as needed and teach your students how to use them to adjust themselves.

A. Centering the Navel

The navel, the center of the body, is the focus of this treatment. Good treatment is reflected by a change in the look of the navel. A healthy navel is round, centered, and relaxed. The thickness of the skin around the navel should be even. The shape of the navel reflects all the imbalances of the body and the direction where the imbalance is coming from. (See Chapter 3 regarding the shape of the navel.)

You are going to place pressure around the navel to see what it would take to make it round, flat, and even. Constantly referring to the shape of the navel during treatment can determine your next step. A centered navel is a result of the combined techniques listed in this book. The navel centers itself because of the whole treatment given to the abdomen. The first step is to bring the navel to the center of the abdomen by moving the skin, small intestine, vena cava, and aorta to the center.

1. Techniques for Repositioning the Navel

a. To correct the navel alignment, use a pushing, pulling, or scooping technique with the thumbs, fingers, or palms. Move the navel into the direction that makes it round and centered. Sometimes you will notice you must move the navel in many directions to make it centered and round. When you release your hands, the navel may not stay centered and round. Sometimes your adjustment is enough; usually it is not. When you see it pull out of center and reverting to its former position, observe it and try to determine what is in the abdominal area disturbing its harmony and symmetry.

b. Navels that are difficult to center will usually have a knot or tangle nearby. The navel will not center until this area releases. Sometimes these knots and tangles have a head and tail. The head is near the navel and the tail is pointed away from it. Always work the knot or tangle from the head toward the tail.

c. The navel may not center because of tension in the muscles and fasciae. If you think this is the problem, massage the abdominal muscles, starting at the lower left side near the pelvic bone. Massage all the way up to the solar plexus, spiraling clockwise and counterclockwise. Continue until you feel that the muscles and fasciae have relaxed and loosened. Do the same on the right side of the abdomen. Try to center the navel again.

d. Practice deep abdominal breathing. This will help to release the muscles and bring Chi into the fasciae.

e. To help center the navel, place your palms across the abdomen with one palm a few inches above the navel and one a few inches below. The abdominal muscles should be totally relaxed. Grasp as much of the muscle as is comfortable in each hand. This will form a small hill in the center of the abdomen. The navel will be in the middle at the top of the hill. Push, pull and hold for a while, and then release. Practice this two to three times.

B. Centering the Pulse and Aorta

To center the aortic pulse, locate it just above the navel and very slightly to the left of the centerline. (Figure 9-1) Place your fingers (one finger, two fingers, the thumb, or all the fingers, whatever way is comfortable) just above the navel and apply pressure until you feel the pulse beating into your fingertips. To feel the pulse make sure your fingers remain relaxed and sensitive. If the student is too tense or tight and you cannot find the pulse, do more skin detoxification. That will allow the abdomen to soften. Then return to the pulses later.

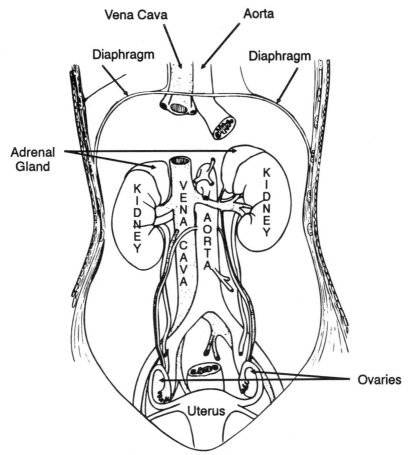

Figure 9-1. Find the aortic pulse just above the navel and slightly off the centerline

1. Techniques for Centering the Aortic Pulse

a. To center an aortic pulse that is too far off the centerline to the right, apply pressure gently with the hands from the right side and push it toward the center. Hold the navel and aorta, and the other tissues will move back to their normal position. Holding it in place for one to three minutes will release the tension in the fasciae and free the tissues so that they may return to normal.

Practice three to six times. You can trace up and down the centerline feeling for tension and congestion. Often there are tangles or knots that are pulling the aorta and pulse off-center.

The fasciae are pulled out of position any time the navel, organs, and other systems are misaligned. Once misaligned, the fasciae become dried and act as shields or splints because of the imbalance. The organs and viscera become impacted and stick together. This stops the flow of energy, forms lumps and knots, increases toxicity and heat, and pulls the aorta off-center.

Using this holding technique will help the fasciae return to a moist state and move easily. This also will free other systems of the body, lubricate the organs and tissues, and reestablish the free flow of Chi.

b. Move slowly and gently. Notice how much the aorta is moving. You may work the aorta for a few minutes before there is a change.

c. Some students may have an aorta that is on or towards the right side of the centerline. This may be anatomically correct. You may try to center it as long as you move slowly and gently. If an aorta doesn't want to move to the center line, **do not force it!** Subsequent sessions may release deeper tissues that are holding it out of place.

d. You also may find an aorta that rolls away as you work to move it. Try to notice its position when you begin and adjust it accordingly.

2. Checking the Character of the Pulse

You will find a variety of aortic pulses from person to person. The pulse can be strong and right on the skin, or it can be deep and difficult to find. It could be slow or fast. Healthy people have different pulses. There is no such thing as a standard healthy aortic pulse. You may find rhythmic imbalances by comparing the navel aortic pulse with other pulses in the body. Working with the aortic pulse is different from taking wrist pulses, which, you may remember, reflect the health of the organs.

Press and hold the aortic pulse for a minute, release, and repeat three to six times. Feel it get stronger, slow down, or even its pace. The pulse will improve its performance.

C. Balancing the Pulses

If you find a knot blocking the aortic pulse in the solar plexus, you may assume that the other pulses are out of synchronization. The idea is to compare the aortic pulse with the pulses at different places in the body. Using it as a gauge is wise because it reflects the pulse of the heart and the center of the body. Compare the speed and intensity of the pulses with each other and with the aorta. They should be nearly the same, but can be slightly different. If they are different, check the abdominal area for blockages and begin to remove them with small circular motions using both hands. You can adjust the pulses by applying pressure on the aorta with one hand while keeping contact with the unsynchronized pulse using the other hand.

Balancing the pulses and clearing abdominal blockages may take more than one session to accomplish. You may find it easy to balance and clear them in one session, only to find that the student has incurred the problem again between sessions. Give your students homework!

Remember, releasing knots and tangles in the abdominal area has a general effect on the body. Your efforts to undo these tissues induces pressure on the aorta and vena cava simultaneously. Thus, it is easy to affect many systems and organs, either directly or indirectly. For example, if you are working on the stomach at a moderate to deep level and pressure, you are also affecting the aorta, pancreas, transverse colon, and psoas muscle since these organs are aligned in layers next to each other from front to back.

1. Hand Techniques—Practicing on Yourself

a. Check the navel area. Press into it in all directions and observe the sensations. Use your thumb to move your intestines and work your way in. Sometimes you can feel your aortic pulse deep within your abdomen. (Figure 9-2) If it is off-center, try to center it using the navel massage centering technique. It is possible to align everything when you are quiet. Sometimes it may take repeated corrections before you can center your pulse. Once you feel a satisfactory aorta pulse, follow the

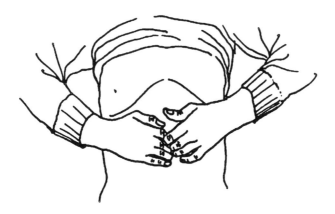

Figure 9-2. Searching for Your Own Aortic Pulse

techniques listed below and compare, contrast, and balance it with the other pulses in the body.

b. Compare it with the wrist and other pulses. Keep the left hand on the master pulse by the navel and feel the left radial wrist pulse with the fingers of the right hand. Hold the pulse until it synchronizes and beats at the same time as the aortic master pulse. Switch hands and feel the other wrist.

This will familiarize you with the technique. You may then do the other pulses as listed below.

2. Hand Techniques—Working on Another to Balance the Aorta with Other Pulses

First work on the pulses on the left side of the body, and then the right side. (Figures 8-3 and 8-4)

a. Work from the left side of the student's body. First, locate the aortic pulse and maintain your hold on the aorta with your left hand. Then place one or two fingers of the right hand on the left carotid, feel the pulse, and gently hold until the aorta pulse and carotid are synchronized.

b. Next, maintain the hold on the aorta while the finger(s) of the right hand holds the pulse in the armpit. Feel and hold until balanced.

c. Then place the finger(s) of the right hand on the pulse in the crease of the elbow. Feel, hold, and balance.

d. Then hold and balance the radial pulse in the wrist.

e. Next, place your right hand on the aorta, so that you may use your left hand to synchronize the pulses in the left leg.

f. Hold the aorta's pulse, and place the left thumb or fingers on the left femoral artery at the inguinal ligament. The left femoral artery is just below the crease of the thigh and pelvis. This pulse is very strong and not difficult to find if you move slowly and feel with your fingers. Hold

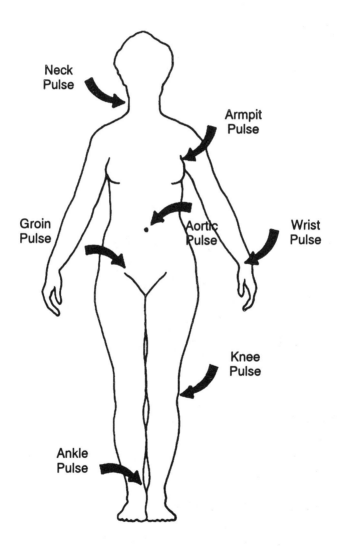

Neck Pulse

Armpit Pulse

Groin Pulse

Aortic Pulse

Wrist Pulse

Knee Pulse

Ankle Pulse

Figure 9-3. The Pulses

283

this pulse, and with the aorta pulse, feel for and synchronize the pulses of these two major arteries.

g. Next, move your left hand and place it underneath the left knee just below the crease. Feel for the popliteal pulse. Hold, and let the body adjust this pulse with the aorta.

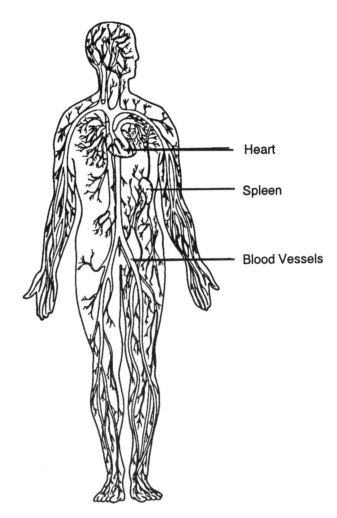

Heart

Spleen

Blood Vessels

Figure 9-4. The Cardiovascular System

h. Finally, move your left hand to the inside ankle bone and feel the pulse just below the ankle joint. Feel, hold, and wait until the pulse adjusts to the aortal pulse.

i. Move to the right side of the body and repeat the process.

3. Techniques to Balance the Pulses of the Right and Left Carotid Arteries

a. Begin by placing the thumb or fingers of one hand on the right carotid artery and the other fingers on the left carotid artery. (Figure 9-5) Hold very gently, use light pressure, and feel the pulses to see if they are synchronized.

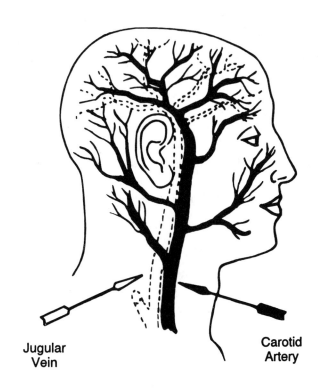

Jugular
Vein

Carotid
Artery

Figure 9-5. The Right Carotid Artery and Jugular Vein

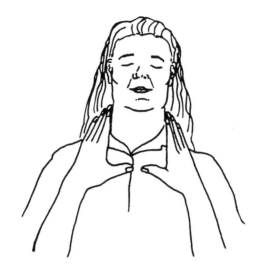

Figure 9-6. Balancing the Carotid Arteries

b. If one side is weaker, you should release the weak side slightly, and apply a bit more pressure to the strong side. Hold for a count of five pulsations. Return both hands back to the normal pressure and synchronize the pulses. (Figure 9-6)

c. If the pulses have not corrected themselves, repeat the procedure a few more times.

d. If they do not balance themselves, suspect a blockage. You might advise the student to consider talking to a doctor for an evaluation. Blockages that do not clear should be evaluated by a doctor wherever they occur in the body.

4. Aorta, Carotid Arteries, and Headaches

If your student has a headache, synchronize the aortic pulse and the left and right carotid pulse. Then gently apply pressure on the aorta in rhythmic intervals of ten to twenty seconds of holding, with ten seconds of releasing. The blood pressure will drop, the pulse will slow down. This should relieve the headache.

5. High Blood Pressure

If your student has high blood pressure, contact the aorta with one hand and place the other on the ankle pulse and use your intention to direct blood to the feet. Then make sure that the carotid arteries are balanced with the aorta using the technique above. Place one hand on one of the carotids and the other on the ankle pulse. Use your intention to direct blood to the feet.

6. Four Point Quick Check

1. Press the aorta.
2. Balance the ankles' pulses with the aorta.
3. Balance the wrists' pulses with the aorta.
4. Balance the carotids with the aorta.

D. Directing and Flushing the Blood Using the Aorta

The aorta, as a major blood vessel running deep in the abdomen in the navel area, has arteries that branch out carrying blood and Chi to the organs, bowels, and the lower limbs. (Figures 9-7, 9-8, 9-9, and 9-10)

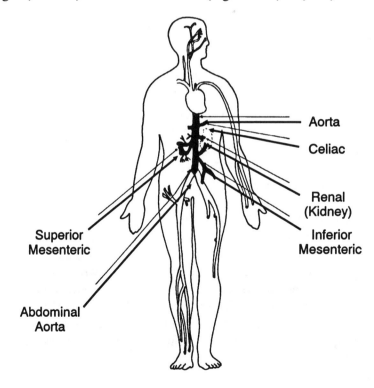

Figure 9-7. Principal Arteries of the Head, Neck, and Body

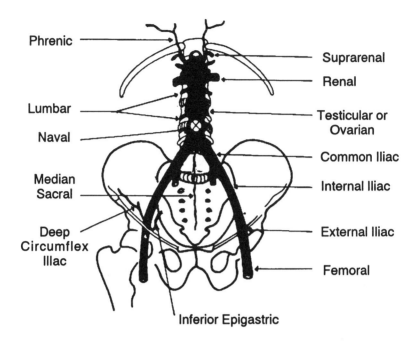

Phrenic

Suprarenal

Renal

Lumbar

Naval

Testicular or
Ovarian

Common Iliac

Median
Sacral

Internal Iliac

Deep
Circumflex
Illac

External Iliac

Femoral

Inferior Epigastric

Figure 9-8. Abdominal Aorta and its Branches

With some practice, you can direct blood to specific organs and areas of the body. This will enable you to "flush out" toxins and blockages, open restricted blood vessels, and increase blood and Chi flow through the vascular system and organs. This will help correct blood pressure and also cool down the organs.

You can check and influence the energy supply to the vital organs, depending on where and how you press on this thick, tough tube. It takes some time to learn. It is like learning to finger a musical instrument. You learn the notes and how to play, and, gradually, develop a feeling for it. Although it is not necessary, some knowledge of wrist pulse reading would be very helpful. You can direct the blood to a certain organ, then check the pulse of that organ to see what change has taken place. This will allow you make another adjustment in the organ's energy. (Keep practicing with the wrist pulses, listening for their messages, and you master the practice.)

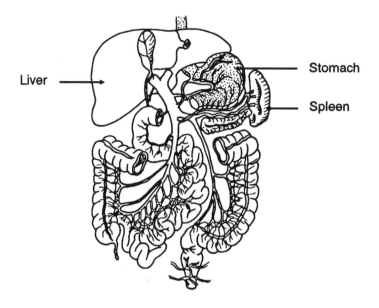

Figure 9-9. Blood Vessels of the Internal Organs

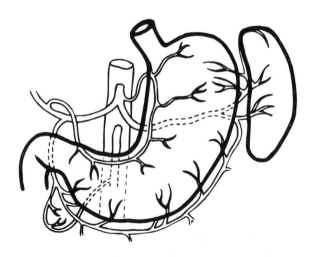

Figure 9-10. Arteries to the Stomach and Spleen

1. Blood Directing Technique

a. Begin by locating the aorta in the one o'clock position just above the navel. Use the thumb to press into the body directly over the aorta. By gently pressing *one-third* of the way into the aorta, you can slow down the blood flow. Flushing blood into the organs increases pressure as when pressing a hose. (Figure 9-11) The blood will back up slightly, creating extra pressure and volume. This increase will move into the upper aorta and its branches, and then flow into the organs and tissues. It will flush out those areas that cannot be flushed out under normal blood volume and pressure. (Figure 9-12)

WARNING AND CAUTION:
DON'T USE THIS TECHNIQUE UNTIL YOU HAVE WORKED EXTENSIVELY USING OTHER TECHNIQUES ON AT LEAST 25 STUDENTS. IT WILL TAKE AT LEAST THAT LONG TO DEVELOP ENOUGH SENSITIVITY IN YOUR FINGERTIPS TO ALLOW YOU TO WORK SAFELY WITH THE AORTA.

b. Next, move your thumb up the aorta toward the sternum, approximately one thumb's width. This will enable you to direct blood into the upper-level organs. Repeat, then press and release in this position. Continue working up the aorta, releasing each position, until you are just below the xiphoid process.

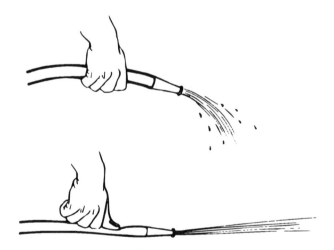

Figure 9-11. Blood directing is like pressing on a hose to increase the pressure

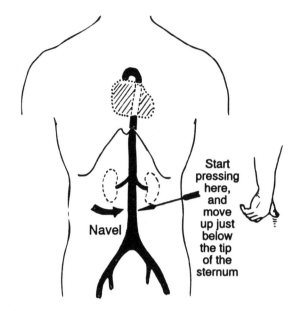

Navel

Start
pressing
here,
and
move
up just
below
the tip
of the
sternum

**Figure 9-12. Flush the blood by pressing one third
of the way into the aorta**

 c. Work gently, and slightly press it to increase the force of the flow of blood rushing into the organ. Sometimes just a little push can clear out obstructions, toxins, stones, and dead tissue. These micro particles only need a slight increase in blood flow to clear out of the systems. This is a very powerful technique.

 d. When there is sediment in an organ, you can increase blood flow to that organ and flush out the debris. Having flushed the organs, go back and check the pulses again. If you break up an obstruction, you will need to flush out the resultant particles. Usually when the obstructions are clear, the pulse gets better.

 e. After you have directed the blood in this area, your student should feel warmth in his or her back. This shows that the kidneys are being flushed. When you flush the liver, your student may feel warmth in the liver. The next position going up will flush out the pancreas and spleen. Continue to move up the aorta. You can flush all the organs and bowels, except the heart and lungs.

2. Directing Blood to the Right and Left Legs and the Pelvic Area

Using this technique to direct blood into the pelvic and sacral area can increase the blood and Chi flow into the reproductive system and lower abdominal region.

a. Start by detoxifying and getting rid of congestion in the lower abdomen and in the large and small intestine areas.

b. Feel if one femoral pulse (in the crease between the pelvis and the thigh) is weaker than the other. If so, press the stronger side first to get rid of the obstruction that is making the other pulse weaker.

c. Once the area is clear, sit or stand to one side of the student, or between his or her legs, and press the edges of both palms into the left and right external iliac or femoral arteries. Press both arteries simultaneously. (Figures 9-13 and 9-14) This will force blood back into the pelvic and inguinal area. Do this two or three times, for about ten seconds each time. If you want to direct blood into the left leg, decrease the pressure exerted by the left palm. To send blood in the right leg, let up on the right palm. (Figure 9-15)

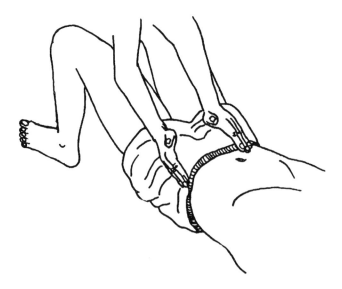

Figure 9-13. Direct the blood into the pelvic and sacral areas

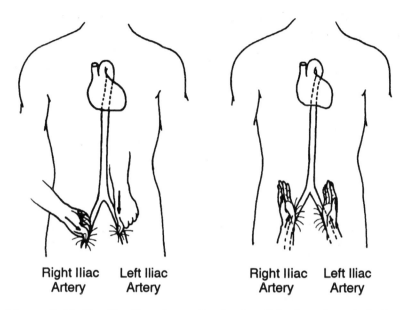

Right Iliac   Left Iliac   Right Iliac   Left Iliac
Artery   Artery   Artery   Artery

Figure 9-14. Use the thumbs or the heels of the hands to help increase the flow of Chi and blood into the lower abdominal region

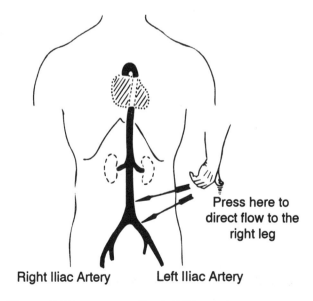

Right Iliac Artery   Left Iliac Artery

Press here to
direct flow to the
right leg

**Figure 9-15. Press on the left iliac artery
to direct blood into the right leg**

293

WARNINGS AND CAUTION:
IT IS IMPORTANT WITH ALL CHI NEI TSANG TECH-
NIQUES, PARTICULARLY IN BLOOD DIRECTING, THAT
YOU BE SENSITIVE AND GENTLE. WORK VERY SLOWLY,
AND TALK WITH YOUR STUDENT, SEARCHING FOR
FEEDBACK AS YOU ARE WORKING.

BE SURE TO REVIEW YOUR STUDENT'S MEDICAL HIS-
TORY, CAREFULLY ASKING EACH QUESTION ON THE
QUESTIONNAIRE.

DON'T DO THIS TECHNIQUE ON ANYONE WHO HAS
HIGH BLOOD PRESSURE OR WHO HAS HAD: A STROKE,
HEART CONDITION, CIRCULATION PROBLEMS, DE-
TACHED RETINAS, ANEURISM, DIABETES, NEURALGIA,
OR SLIPPED DISC(S). DO NOT WORK ON ANYONE WITH
VARICOSE VEINS, THROMBOSIS (CLOTTING WITHIN A
BLOOD VESSEL), OR PHLEBITIS (INFLAMMATION OF A
VEIN.) DO NOT PRACTICE ON PREGNANT WOMEN.

ASK THEM IF THEY CAN DO NORMAL EXERCISES, SUCH
AS SWIMMING, BIKING, RUNNING, AND WALKING UP
STAIRS OR A HILL. IF NOT, THEN THEY MAY HAVE HIGH
BLOOD PRESSURE.

CHAPTER 10

APPLYING CNT TO COMMON AILMENTS

A. Lower Back Pain

Like a suspension bridge the body works best when the torque or tension is properly set. If the tension is off, too loose or too tight, then the body will be out of balance and the structure will be affected. This will throw the center out and affect the energy in the organs and glands.

A classic "suspension-tension" imbalance is lower back and leg pain. Lower back pain is a very common complaint. Doctors treat it by administering muscle-relaxing and anti-inflammatory drugs.

Many chiropractors and orthopedic surgeons have spent their lives treating this widespread problem. Problems with the iliopsoas muscles and sciatic nerves cause most lower back problems. CNT is a powerful technique for relieving the cause of crippling back pain.

1. Releasing Sciatic Pains by Working on the Psoas Muscles and the Lumbar Sacral Plexus

Work on the iliopsoas muscles and the sciatic nerves goes together because they can influence one another. The accumulation of toxins and tensions in the abdomen presses against the nerves, muscles, and tendons that are coming out from the spine. This impairs communication between the nerves. Tension in the muscles goes on unnoticed and the muscles don't receive the message to relax. To restore the nerves to their function of controlling the muscles, the pressure has to be relieved.

First apply skin detoxification to release internal pressure. Detoxify the large and small intestines. This will allow you to go deeper and work on the lumbar sacral plexus and the psoas muscles. The abdomen has to

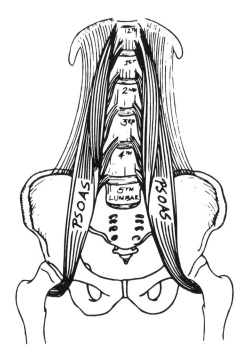

Figure 10-1. The Psoas Muscles

be softened before you can work on this area. Be careful and gentle. This is very deep work.

Major psoas muscles originate along the twelfth thoracic to the fifth lumbar vertebrae bones, descend through the pelvic region, and attach to the top part of the femur (thigh) bone. (Figure 10-1) They form part of the posterior wall of the abdomen and help support the organs in the abdomen. They are also the flexors of the thigh. On some the psoas muscles do not descend to the thighbone, but anchor to the lower brim of the pelvis.

The psoas muscles are called the *Soil of the Soul.* An imbalance between the tension on both sides of the muscles can cause curvature of the spine, malposition of the hips, one leg to be shorter than the other, and sciatic pains.

When toxic pressure builds in the abdomen, it affects the lumbar plexus and creates chronic tension in the lower back. This weakens the psoas muscles, which become spastic. In chronic cases they start to atrophy. In that state they require an overcompensation of the lower back muscles to keep the structure erect. Also, a difference in the tension between the right and left psoas muscles would automatically throw the spine out of alignment. It is very important to release, lengthen, and balance both sides of the psoas muscles. Working on them can help a variety of emotional problems, especially depression.

Be sure to do both the right and left side of the body. If you are working on the left psoas, work from the left side, and vice versa. Usually one side is normal and one side contracts and is tense. These muscles, like most paired parts of the body, have a sympathetic relationship. Work on the good side first.

2. Techniques for Releasing the Psoas Muscles

a. While the student is lying down, look at the legs and feet. One leg may be shorter than the other. This indicates tension in the psoas muscle on the short side. One foot may be naturally turned out while the other is pointing straight up. The tense leg and foot indicates tension in the psoas muscle and sciatic nerves on that side.

b. Work in the lower abdomen and pelvic area and loosen any knots or tangles.

c. Press all your fingers into the area of the psoas. The psoas is very deep, and you will need the student's help to find it. Help the student to raise the knee closest to you and pull it toward the chest. (Figure 10-2) Have him or her take over and rotate it, moving it back and forth while you search for the psoas. (Figure 10-3) The psoas muscle is engaged by this movement of the knee and leg. You can feel it moving. This is a simple way to find it, since it is so deep. When you feel it moving, lock in on it with all your fingers lined up in a row along its length. (Figure 10-4) Once you have it, the student may then lower the foot to the floor, but keep the knee bent.

d. Press down and hold your fingers still. Shake your body sideways, right and left. Be vigorous; keep the fingers on the muscle so that they can massage it. If you are working on yourself, elevate and rest your feet on a chair and use however many fingers you are comfortable with. Use a standard spiraling motion up and down its length.

The psoas muscles can easily revert to their contracted position. People develop protecting and withdrawing patterns. Teach them how to move and walk like one of their heroes, or a prince, or a queen. Unless they learn to walk with a full stride and carry themselves with great dignity and powerful expression, the psoas problem may recur. They

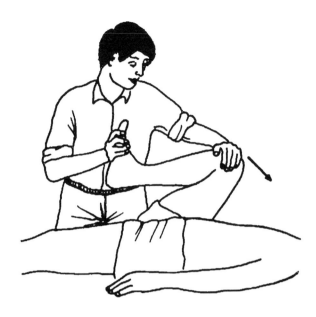

Figure 10- 2. Raise the knee to activate the psoas muscle

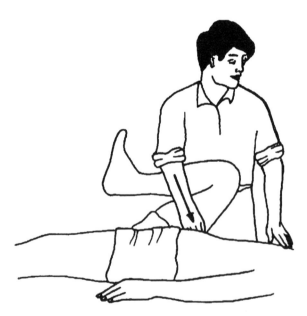

Figure 10-3. Go in deeply to locate the psoas muscle

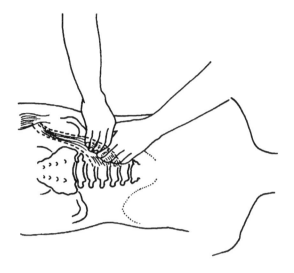

**Figure 10-4. Place all the fingers
on the psoas muscle**

have to learn how to move from the center and not just with the lower leg. Moving from the center with the pelvis and upper leg will help them to massage and stretch the psoas while they are walking. Their posture should be balanced and not leaning to one side, to the front, or to the back. Advise them to study Iron Shirt, Tai Chi, and dance.

3. Tendon Stretching to Complete the Psoas Work

This is a good technique to practice after you have finished massaging the psoas muscles on both sides. This is a technique to massage the psoas tendon that is located just below the crease of the leg. The word tendon is from the Latin word *tendere*, which means "to stretch." Tendon connect muscles to bones, muscles to ligaments, muscles to muscles, or muscles to fasciae. They allow these different tissues to stretch. In this technique you are going to help the psoas tendon stretch and relax.

4. Deep Pelvic Tendon Massage Technique

If you are both on the floor, kneel beside your student with your knees near his lower waist. If you are working on a table, sit half-on, half-off. Raise his leg and support it on your shoulder. (Figure 10-5)

299

Reach into the lower psoas area and find the tendon t the bottom of the psoas muscle. It attaches the psoas to the top of the femur bone in the area where the hip joins the pelvis. The psoas minor attaches to the lower brim of the pelvis.

Gently move your shoulder toward his head. This will cause the leg to raise further. Then lower your shoulder. As you feel the tendon lengthen, massage and gently pull on it. Feel for the psoas minor tendon as well. Be gentle, but be sure. This will help it lengthen farther and relax. Finish by massaging the area. Repeat this procedure several times on both sides.

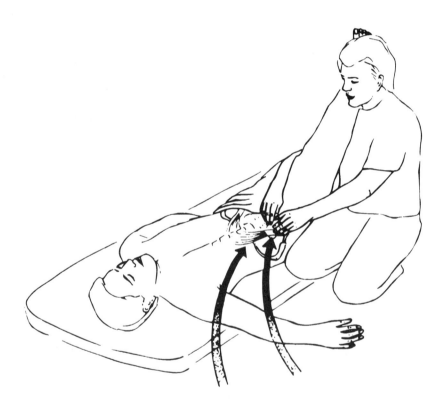

Figure 10-5. Psoas Tendon Massage

B. Sciatic Nerve Pain

You can also work directly on the nerves of the lower lumbar area. Pressure from the large intestine, or any twisting or pulling from internal tangles, knots, excess heat, dampness, or cold winds often congest these nerves. By gently going deeper from the surface down to the spine, you can become sensitive to the different levels of congestion. Once you are experienced, you can work directly on the nerves to soothe and adjust them gently.

There are many nerves that exit the spine in the lumbar plexus, or lower spine, area. (Figures 10-6, 10-7, and 10-8) These service the buttocks, perineum, and lower extremities. One of these nerves is the sciatic nerve which supplies the muscles in the legs and feet. It is the largest nerve in the body, a sheath of two nerves that exits at lumbar 4 and sacral 1, 2, and 3. It traverses the buttocks and, coming close to the surface, snakes down the hip and the thigh. At the knee it splits into two divisions and then passes on to the lower leg and ankle. At its beginning it is about as thick as the little finger. Many of your students will have

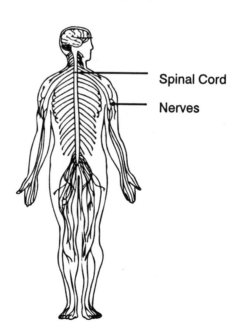

Spinal Cord

Nerves

Figure 10-6. The Central Nervous System

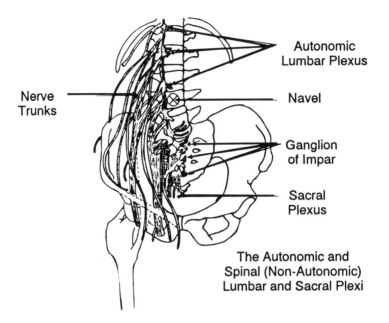

The Autonomic and
Spinal (Non-Autonomic)
Lumbar and Sacral Plexi

Figure 10-7. Nerves of the Lower Spine

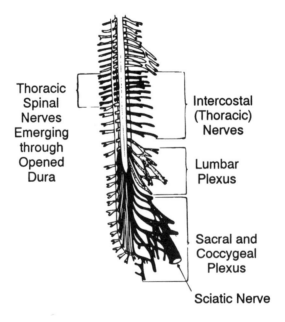

Figure 10-8. Nerves of the Spine

back and leg pains caused by problems with this nerve and the psoas. (Figures 10-9)

1. Exploring the Area and Massaging the Sacral Plexus

a. Begin at the navel and slowly work toward the backbone. When you run into the small intestine, gently push it aside. Make sure that you replace it when you are finished.

b. When you have reached the vertebral column, go to either side of it and you will be at the psoas. If this muscle is tense, it can cause back and leg pain, especially lower back discomforts. You have just learned

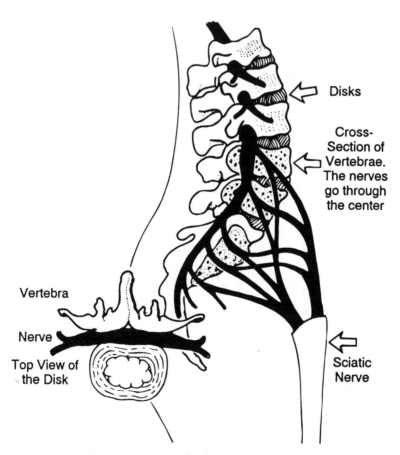

Figure 10-9. The Sciatic Nerve and the Vertebrae

303

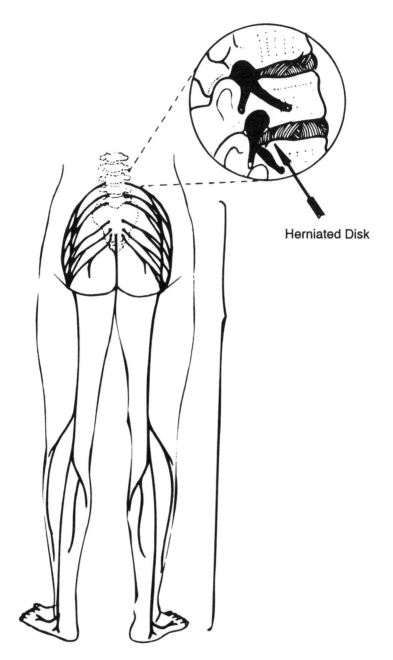

Herniated Disk

**Figure 10-10. A herniated disc can create
sciatic nerve pain in the leg**

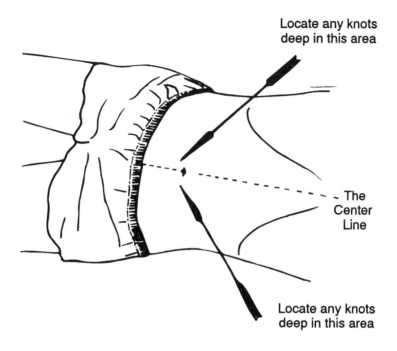

Locate any knots
deep in this area

The
Center
Line

Locate any knots
deep in this area

Figure 10-11. Search for Knots Deep in the Sacral Plexus

above how you can gently loosen this muscle. You have to go behind the psoas before you can get to the sciatic nerve.

c. The sciatic nerve branches out of the backbone in the sacral area. If the sciatic nerve becomes irritated, it can cause pain to run down the back of the leg. (Figure 10-10) This can be caused by hernias in the discs between the vertebrae, problems in the sacroiliac joint, and rigidity and congestion in the surrounding ligaments and muscles. You can relieve this pain through deep sacral massage and by pressing and massaging different parts of the body that are near the sciatic nerve.

d. Feel for knots, swelling, or tangles in this lower back area. (Figure 10-11) Massage them. (Figure 10-12)

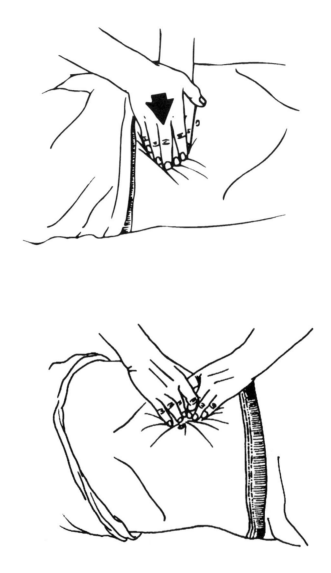

Figure 10-12. Massage away congestion in the sacral plexus

2. Releasing the Sciatic Nerve in the Buttocks and Legs

a. With the student on his back, lift the leg closest to you toward the chest and rotate it in the hip socket. This will help set the bones in the pelvic region in their right place. (Figure 10-13) You can also lift both legs at the same time. Keep the knees together and gently rotate both hips in their sockets.

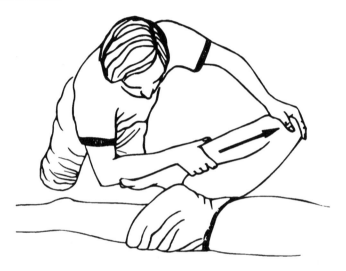

Figure 10-13. Rotate the hip joint in its socket

b. Place the student on his or her left side. Feel for an indentation or "hole" between the gluteus medius and gluteus maximus to find the piriformis muscle. (Figure 10-14) Massage and release the contracted piriformis muscle, which is close to the sciatic nerve running through the buttocks. Press straight down with the thumb or elbow. (Figure 10-15) Often this area is very painful if there is a problem. If there is no pain, there is no problem. It is important to spend some time working here. While it is painful, the massage has a "sweet ache" to it; it hurts, but the student starts to feel that he or she is going to get better. Do not forget to use your concentration to send healing energy into this area.

c. Massage down the middle line of the back of the thigh to loosen the muscle there.

d. The next position is behind the knee at the popliteal tendons. (Figures 10-16 and 10-17) Work on both sides of the knee, since the

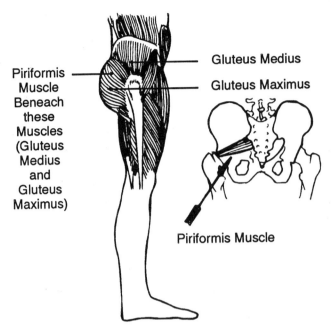

Figure 10-14. Find the piriformis muscle in the buttocks

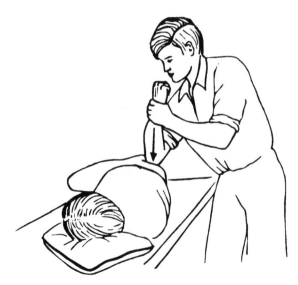

**Figure 10-15. Use your hand or your elbow
to massage the piriformis muscle**

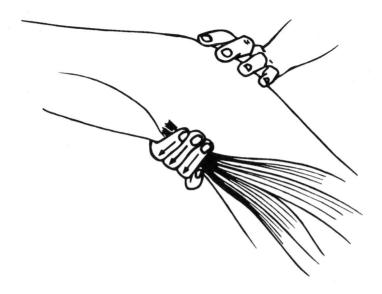

Figure 10-16. Grasp the popiletal tendons and the muscles

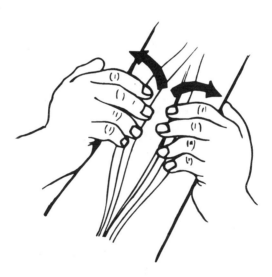

Figure 10-17. Stretch the tendons at the back of the knee apart so that you can reach the nerves

sciatic nerve branches into two divisions here. Massage with the thumbs on the left and right side and use your fingers to pull the tendons apart. This will stretch the tendons and muscles and release the pressure on the nerves.

e. The third position is under the inner ankle, under the bone. It is very close to Kidney-3. (Figure 10-18) Massage and press it with your finger(s) or thumb.

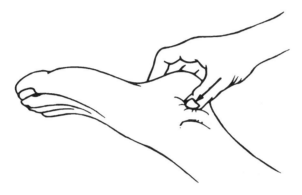

Figure 10-18. Massage the nerve area below the ankle bone

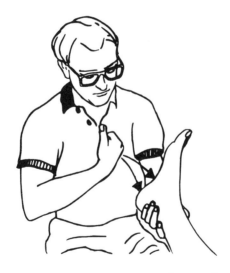

Figure 10-19. End the sciatic treatment by tapping on the heel

f. End the procedure by lifting the lower leg and tapping the heel with your fist. (Figure 10-19)

g. Repeat the procedure on the right side.

C. Neck and Related Headache Pain

For neck and related headache pain, work in the brachial plexus, looking for knots and tangles. (Figure 10-20) Tension in this area also can cause pain to extend down the arms. If the area is clear do not work it. If there is a blockage there, first work in the navel. Then, using both thumbs, massage down both sides of the cervical and brachial vertebrae. When the brachial area is tight, it can pull in on the neck and arm causing

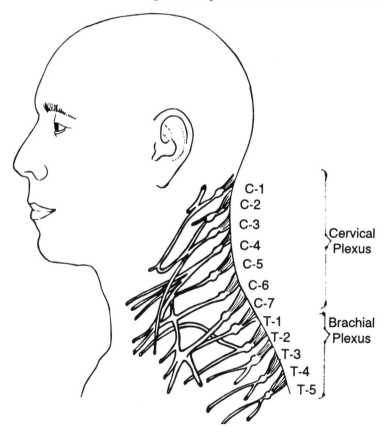

C-1
C-2
C-3
C-4
C-5
C-6
C-7
T-1
T-2
T-3
T-4
T-5

Cervical
Plexus

Brachial
Plexus

Figure 10-20. Nerves of the Neck

311

pain there and in the head. This is often a chronic problem. Clearing it up can be a slow process; therefore, it is important to spend time working in this area.

1. Working on the Brachial Plexus

(a) Have the student lay face down. Draw back the right arm and place it across the back, with the back of the hand laying on the spine. Place your right hand over his or her right hand to hold it there gently.

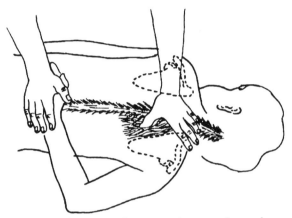

Figure 10-21. Massage the scapula muscle underneath the right shoulder blade

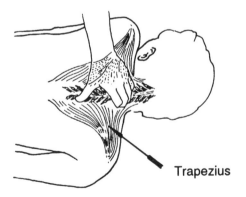

Trapezius

Figure 10-22. Grasp the trapezius muscle between the thumb and the other fingers

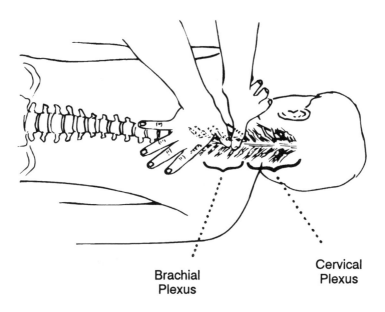

Brachial
Plexus

Cervical
Plexus

**Figure 10-23. Use both hands to massage down
the side of the vertebrae**

Use the left thumb to massage the scapula muscle underneath the right
shoulder blade. (Figure 10-21)

(b) Next, grasp the trapezius muscle between the thumb and the
other fingers. Gently massage it out toward the shoulder. (Figure 10-22)

(c) Use two thumbs to massage straight down the right side of the
spine. (Figure 10-23)

(d) Repeat the procedure on the left side of the body.

2. Serpentine Massage of the Spine

(a) Use two fingers of one hand. Place the opposite hand on the back
of the massaging hand to add weight to the fingers.

(b) Start on the right side of the spine at Cervical-7 (C-7).

(c) Cross the spine towards the left side.

313

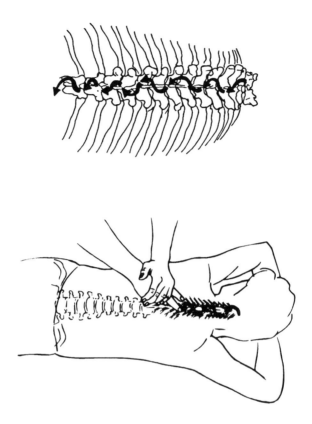

Figure 10-24. Serpentine Massage of the Spine

(d) Once you reach the left side of the spine, start back toward the right side of the spine.

(e) The movement traces a snaking "S" shape down the spine to the sacrum. (Figure 10-24)

D. Asthma

Asthma is a breathing problem of the lungs accompanied by paroxysms, spasms, and wheezing. The chest is often very expanded and tight. Those with this condition can even do abdominal breathing without ever relaxing the chest, i.e., the diaphragm can expand, but they cannot relax the rib cage.

314

The problem with asthma is that the rib cage does not move, so the lungs cannot expand. You can teach the chest to move.

Often the eyes, jaws, and hips do not move either. The eyes and hips do not move laterally (from side to side.) They are locked and tight, taking their cue from the rib cage. These body parts are inhibited. You can teach your student how to unlock, move, and breathe. All the parts can learn to move normally again. The student must practice everyday until the asthmatic condition begins to recede. You may assure the student that one day he or she will breathe and move like a graceful athlete. These techniques were discovered by a CNT practitioner who used them to cure her own severe asthma.

1. Hand Techniques

a. Start by standing or kneeling to the side of your student. Reach across with one hand and hold the chest near the lower ribs. Gently work all over the ribs with a series of quick, little pushes and jabs on the side nearest you and parallel to your far hand. (Figure 10-25)

b. Be sure to concentrate on sending Chi through your pushing hand. Feel the far rib cage (and your far hand) receive the impulse and move a bit. Move your hands up and down the rib cage. Keep pushing. You are moving and loosening both sides of the rib cage. After a while, withdraw your far hand and use both of them to do the gentle push.

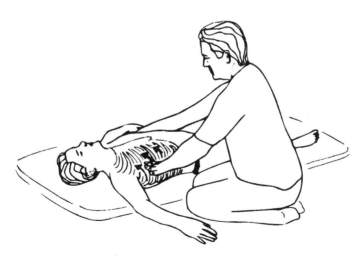

Figure 10-25. Asthmatic Massage—Working on the Ribs

315

c. Reach across the chest with *both* hands and make a series of gentle, quick, short pulls toward you with both hands pulling simultaneously. (Figure 10-26)

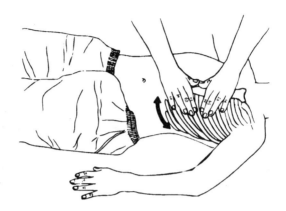

Figure 10-26. Asthmatic Massage—Working on the Ribs on the Far Side

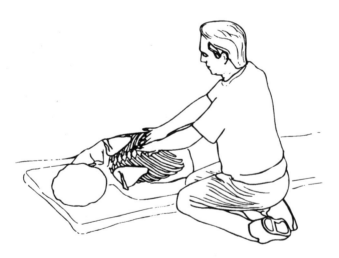

Figure 10-27. Asthmatic Massage— Working on the Back of the Ribs

d. Lay the student on his or her side and work the back of the ribs. Do the same hand motion as above. Move the student to the other side and do the other half of the rib cage. This will loosen up the back. *Relax.* (Figure 10-27)

e. Practice on yourself. Although you cannot practice on your own back, you could find something suitable to place under your back, such as a tennis ball, that would simulate fingers. Teach the student how to do homework. Stress that it must be practiced every day. Inform the student that it will hurt a bit since the chest is protesting.

2. Rib Expansion Breathing

In addition to the massage, teach the student how to do "Rib Expansion Breathing." Breathe into the side of the ribs and expand them. Breathe into the front of the ribs, the back of the ribs, and the entire rib cage, expanding in each direction as you procede. *Relax.* Impress upon the student the need for daily practice.

3. Eye Work

Teach the student how to move the eyes. Often, the person will be staring straight up. The natural movement would be for the eyes to follow the movement of the rib cage. Sometimes the body forgets these natural things. When you are doing the rib massage and are pushing to the side, tell your student to move the eyes toward the same side you are pushing. If you are pulling, the eyes should move toward you. When pushing from the back, have the eyes go forward. Have them practice at home. More practice will help unlock the energy. Fixed eyes can also suggest a back problem. They are holding in against pain.

4. Jaw Exercises

As previously mentioned, many of those with asthma have jaws and hips that are "locked." It may surprise you to know that the hips and rib cage will loosen once the mandibular joint, which hinges the jawbone to the skull, relaxes. This technique works like magic, but the magic is the energy. The free movement and motion of the activiated and exercised joint is part of the reason the Inner Smile is so powerful. Relaxing and activating this area creates a very strong energy flow because it is a crossroads for four channels or meridians: the small intestine, the Triple Heater, the gall bladder, and the stomach.

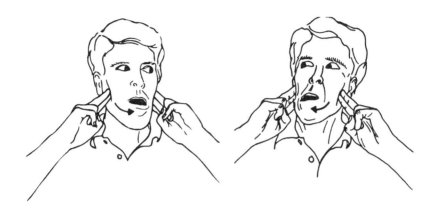

Figure 10-28. Mandibular Massage

With two fingers of each hand, massage the muscles and tendons at the mandibular joint while moving the jaw from side to side, and forward and backward. (Figure 10-28) Also, move the jaw in a circular motion. Be sure to move the eyes with the jaw.

E. Problems Women Experience

CNT has many techniques that will help with problems of the ovaries, uterus, and uterine tubes. Congestion and knots in these areas often results in cramps, PMS, ovarian pains, cysts, endometriosis, cervical and ovarian cancer, frigidity, and infertility. These techniques can be used following birth, miscarriage, abortion, or lower abdominal surgery. They will help the uterus return to its normal position and size.

It is important that this area be kept open to permit the energy to flow. Sexual or reproductive energy is one of the primary energies. Blockage, stagnation, or congestion of the sexual energy can be associated with emotional problems.

NOTE: Do not work on menstruating or pregnant women or women with venereal disease or cancer.

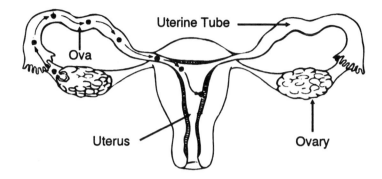

Figure 10-29. The Uterus and Ovaries

1. The Uterus

The uterus is connected within the body by tendons which frequently tighten through internal congestion and require adjusting. Problems in the small and large intestines, bladder, and kidney can account for this. If the blood and Chi are not flowing well, the uterus becomes "cold" and cysts are more likely to form.

a. Location

The uterus, located between the urinary bladder and the rectum, is shaped like an inverted pear. (Figure 10-29) It has three sections: the dome-shaped portion is the fundus, the central portion is the body, and the narrow part opening to the vagina is the cervix. The uterus has two fallopian tubes that connect to the ovaries; they pass the ova or egg to the uterus. These tubes often get twisted or tied together.

A woman may find her uterus by placing her hands together at the thumbs and index fingers in a V shape (upside down triangle). Then place the thumbs at the navel and lengthen the index fingers. The index fingers will lie at the location of the uterus. (Figure 10-30)

b. Massaging the Uterus

(1) Place eight fingers to one side of the uterus and the thumbs together on the opposite side. Keep the edges of both hands together and aligned. Apply a deep, probing, kneading motion with this combination. Massage any tangles or twists you find and hold the uterus with both hands for a while in the center.

319

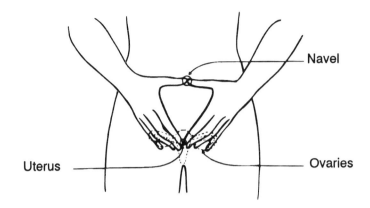

Figure 10-30. Locating the Uterus and Ovaries

(2) There are often knots and tangles in the uterus and along the branches of the uterine tubes leading to it. Trapped or excessive heat often causes this. Release the heat using the techniques for removing winds.

(3) Tightness in the muscles and fasciae holding the uterus in position can also cause this problem. This congestion may cause the uterus to be slightly tilted. Use detoxification massage techniques to clear the congestion. Then cup the hands between the ovaries, gently push in, and massage the area above the cervix, removing any congestion. If during ovulation and menstruation the energy flow through this area is disturbed, pain and cramps can occur. This practice also seems to have the very beneficial effect of helping to balance the hormones.

(4) Another technique is to do gentle circular massage on the fallopian tubes.

2. The Ovaries

The ovaries are paired glands resembling unshelled almonds in size and shape. They are positioned on either side of the uterus. Ovulation causes them to become swollen and/or scarred and wrinkled. After menopause they atrophy.

a. Location

As in locating the uterus, make an inverted triangle with the thumbs at the navel and the index fingers lengthening and falling naturally. Now spread the little fingers. The ovaries lie where they fall. (Figure 10-30) Healthy ovaries are soft, like jelly. They should be even.

b. Problems and Recommendations

(1) Make sure that the ovaries are in their correct places. When there is menstrual cramping, this area swells. Touch this area and feel the energy flow. If the egg is just beginning to move, the area will be warm. If ovulation is near, it will be hot, and, after the cycle, it will be cool.

(2) Often the ovaries are too close together and one may be higher than the other. The high one drains down to the lower one and becomes weak, dry, and tight. This can cause cramps during menstruation and make pregnancy impossible. The ova may not leave or cause great pain when they do leave. One ovary can be close to the surface of the skin and the other can be deep, sometimes so deep you cannot feel it. During pregnancy the uterus rises into the abdominal region and the ovaries go with it. After pregnancy you can help insure that they have returned to their regular position.

Moving the ovaries to their correct position may be a slow process. Be careful. You may have to do a little at a time and you may need to repeat the procedure. The ligaments of the uterus may pull the ovaries out of their correct position. If you are working on yourself, apply the thumbs to the ovaries using a circular motion. Releasing congestion in the surrounding area may help them to return to their proper place.

(3) Menstrual cramps can be caused by the ovary not releasing properly. There could be a knot in the area. Shaking will loosen surface congestion. Perhaps the fallopian tube is not in the right position or is crimped. Sometimes the ovary and tube become twisted. You cannot feel the twist, but the surface of the skin looks uncomfortable, and the area is very painful to touch. If the fallopian tube is very tight, pregnancy is impossible.

The blood supply to the area might not be adequate. Surgery near the ovaries may cause menstrual problems. If the lower sections of the large intestine or bladder press against the ovary, it may cause pain. Loosen up the area first and get rid of any congestion in the sigmoid and cecum colon, otherwise you cannot reach the ovaries. (Always work with the sigmoid colon first.) You must clear space to reach them. Very often that is all that must be done to relieve pain in the ovaries.

Practice liver detoxification. Pump the liver. Do the Liver's, Kidneys', and Spleen's Sounds two or three times.

(4) The arteries and veins of the ovaries may have become tangled together. There are frequently many little knots, tangles, and blockages near the ovaries. These must be removed. The ovaries can get twisted

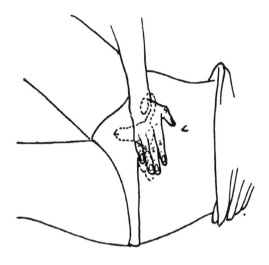

**Figure 10-31. Ovarian Massage: Start
with the heel of the hand**

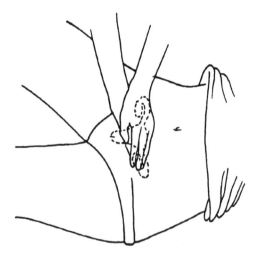

**Figure 10-32. Rock your hand to the ovary farthest from you,
and apply your other hand to add extra weight**

with their connective tissues; this can cause infertility, cramps, and early menopause.

(5) CNT is also very effective on ovarian cysts, as long as they do not develop into cancerous growths. Massage adds to the circulation by breaking down the congested matter. If the hardness does not release, you should advise the student to have a medical check-up. If there is a medical problem, work only with the authorization of the doctor. You should teach her how to stimulate and raise the energy level of the organs and tonify the tissues of the abdomen. This should eventually get rid of the problem.

(6) One technique for balancing the energy in the ovaries is to place the tips of the fingers toward the ovaries, gently press down, and massage. Check for tightness on the left and right sides and for sensitivity to heat and winds.

3. Ovarian Massage Technique

a. Have the student pull her knees up. Search for the ovaries. (See Figure 10-30)

b. Use the fingers and heel of the hand in a rocking motion. If working from the right side, the heel of your hand massages the right ovary. (Figure 10-31) As your hand slowly sinks in, the fingers massage the left ovary. You can add your other hand for extra weight, although one hand is heavy by itself. (Figure 10-32) Do this for five minutes (or longer) and many of the conditions listed above will correct themselves. Push and pump. Do a soft rock and roll. Send them energy, talk them back to health. This is very comfortable to the student, and she will feel serene and trusting.

c. This technique works better if is it is done by another person. It is much faster than working on just one side at a time. Nevertheless, you should teach your students to work on themselves at home to maintain the work you have done. (Figure 10-33) If the student doesn't do homework, the ovaries will revert to their old position after a few days. They are used to being in the same place and would like to go back. Its like an old habit. Make them feel comfortable in their new situation.

4. Frigidity

Frigidity, or sexual unresponsiveness, is a difficult problem. While it may be caused by problems with the organs, emotional tensions

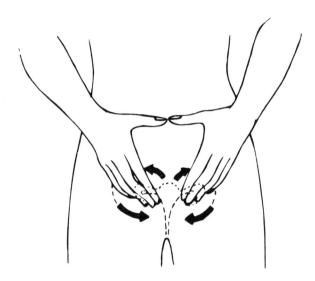

Figure 10-33. Ovarian Self-Massage

frequently cause it. The problem is often a "two person" one and is beyond the scope of this book.

Nonetheless, CNT techniques may help. Start by releasing the diaphragm. Then detoxify and do emotional release and balancing. Tonify the sexual organs. Work on the kidneys first, and then the Triple Warmer and the pericardium (circulation sex) points on the CNT chart. Tonify the liver.

5. Menstruation

The above techniques may be applied to menstruation problems with success. They will help the student remove the toxicity that accumulates in the lower abdomen. It can also help relieve nervous tensions. Regularly applying CNT to women with menstrual problems, with particular attention on the lower part of the abdomen, can help to reduce and prevent menstrual cramps, water retention, and bloating.

6. Endometriosis

CNT may also help in controlling endometriosis, which is caused by an abnormal growth of the lining of the uterus. It grows through the wall of the uterus and creates tangles in the small intestine, lymphatic system, and sacral plexus. It also can contribute to circulation problems in this area. This is a very common problem and is only temporarily halted during pregnancy. The moving embryo massages the walls which causes the endometriosis to recede. CNT massage mimics this motion.

If you have a student with this problem, teach her how to work on herself. If the student is facing surgery, you may consult with her doctor and recommend an alternate procedure. If surgery corrects an advanced case, CNT massage may help as a follow-up and prevent recurrence.

7. Healing Tao Practices for Women that Complement CNT

Other practices that are recommended for women to practice at home are: Ovarian Breathing, the egg exercise, breast massage, the Orgasmic Upward Draw, and the Pulling-Up technique used in Iron Shirt Chi Kung. (Refer to the following books: *Healing Love through the Tao, Cultivating Female Sexual Energy,* and *Iron Shirt Chi Kung I.*) These are long term and continuous aids for good sexual and reproductive health.

F. Male Problems

Taoists believe that letting the vital sexual energy drain out during ejaculation causes many male sexual problems, such as impotence and prostate problems. Whether or not you believe this, you may successfully apply CNT principles and techniques to these aliments.

1. Impotence

(a) If the student is impotent, first work on the liver. The liver channel goes through the testicles. Any weakness of the channel in this area can cause problems in the sexual organs.

Check for knots and tangles in the lower abdomen and along the creases in the legs. Study an anatomy chart of that area and note how the nerves and blood vessels pass into the penis. If there is any kind of blockage here, it could affect the ability of the penis to become erect. Clear the area with massage. This area can be very sensitive and working here can cause some pain. Be gentle and careful.

(b) Teach the student how to do the testicle and duct massage, as explained in the Healing Tao book, *Bone Marrow Nei Kung*.

(c) Pull the urethra out from the perineum and squeeze it to loosen or dissipate any plaque formations.

(d) Work just above the pubic bone, massaging in circular motions with two fingers until you locate a depression that is directly above the bladder and prostrate. Massage this area a little longer.

(e) For knots and tangles in the pelvic area, find the hole where the testicles ascend and descend. Insert a finger into this hole to locate and loosen such obstructions.

(f) Bake and massage the kidneys and adrenal glands.

2. Prostate

Blockages near the prostate gland can cause impotence. When these blockages are removed, virility may return. Toxins in that gland are usually another cause of this problem.

The prostrate is right above the perineum, between the anus and the testicles, just under the skin. Massage this area as well as the testicles.

G. Some Common Abdominal Problems

Kiiko Matsumoto and Stephen Birch in their book, *Hara Diagnosis: Reflections on the Sea*, have identified some common abdominal complaints. Descriptions of some of these symptoms are outlined in this section as well as Healing Tao techniques for resolving such problems.

1. Tension in the Muscles that Cover the Gall Bladder and Pancreas

a. Symptom Description

(1) Hypertension of the muscles that cover the gall bladder on the right side and the pancreas on the left is often a reflex used to protect the weakness of the underlying organs. These areas are tight and inaccessible to the fingers. Such hypertension can be accompanied by chronic anxiety.

Pressing hard on these tight muscles can cause difficulty in breathing, discomfort in the chest, reactions that run from the neck to the shoulder, and pain dispersing in the arm and running down the face into the arm.

b. CNT Application

(1) Start on the left side if both muscles are involved.

(a) Brush and press the left side of the rib cage with both hands, working alternately.

(b) Continue exerting pressure and bring it to the sinking points on the rib cage.

(c) Practice the Figure Five and Reverse Figure Five Techniques (see Chapter 5) to chase the pressure from under the rib cage.

(2) Repeat for the right side.

(3) Practice deep and soft massages of the muscles.

(4) Detoxify and tonify the corresponding organs.

2. The Umbilical Region

a. Symptom Description

The area is swollen and soft superficially, but hard on a deeper level. Very often the area under the rib cage on the left side feels tight and hard.

b. CNT Application

(1) Detoxify the skin.

(2) Apply the Wave Technique (see Chapter 5) until the abdomen softens.

(3) Brush and chase the fluids under the left side of the rib cage with the Figure Five Technique.

(4) Tonify the stomach, spleen, and pancreas area.

3. Small Tangle in the Left Umbilical Region

a. Symptom Description

The area feels hard and tight, and bulges from the surface of the abdomen. It is painful if touched and feels like a hard stone. Pressing it deeply can bring shooting pains to the chest, face, head, arms, legs, or anywhere in the back and neck.

b. CNT Application

(1) Do skin detoxification around the navel. Make sure you spend a long time on this to release internal pressure.

(2) Use the Wave Technique on the large intestine.

(3) Work deeply with both hands to untangle the knot.

(4) Reach deeply toward the spine and induce a rocking motion from that area to the rest of the body.

(5) If you find a tangle on the right side, apply the same technique. Detoxify and tonify the liver.

4. Severe Tension in the Lower Abdomen

a. Symptom Description

The lower abdomen is tight and hard. This is often associated with constipation, fluid stagnation in the stomach, kidney problems, lower back pain, lung weakness, and gynecological problems.

b. CNT Application

(1) Detoxify the skin.

(2) Open the Wind Gates. (See Chapter 4.)

(3) Do the Wave Technique.

(4) Chase the fluids from under the rib cage with the Figure Five Technique.

(5) Work deeply under the rib cage until the tissues are soft.

(6) Do the Wave Technique.

(7) Tonify the lungs.

(8) Tonify the liver.

(9) Tonify the kidneys.

(10) Apply more Wave Technique until the lower abdomen softens completely. It can take up to an hour and a half from the beginning of the procedure.

(11) Work on the psoas muscles.

(12) Work on the lumbar plexus.

5. Pain in the Lower Right or Left Abdominal Regions

a. Symptom Description

There is pain in the lower right or left abdominal regions, close to the hip and extending into the groin. The area is tight, and you can find string-like muscles. You can feel hard matter and gas bubbles trapped in the small intestine.

The area is painful if touched. There is pain in the legs, and there are lower back problems.

b. CNT Application

(1) Detoxify the skin.

(2) Do the Wave Technique. Detoxify and tonify.

(3) Detoxify the liver.

(4) Detoxify the lungs.

(5) Detoxify the kidneys.

(6) Loosen the psoas muscles.

(7) Work on the lumbar and sacral plexus.

(8) Release the pressure on the sciatic nerve.

6. Pain in the Lower Back Part of the Abdomen Near the Spine.

a. Symptom Description

The area is hard and painful to touch. If soft, there is a feeling of bundles moving inside. The lower abdomen is cold. The student has constipation or diarrhea, gynecological problems, or lumbar pain.

b. CNT Application

(1) Detoxify the skin

(2) Do the Wave Technique. Start close to the navel, where it is easiest to work without causing excessive pain.

(3) Rock the body while holding the lumbar region.

(4) Do more of the Wave motion until the pain and tightness clear.

(5) Work on the psoas muscles.

(6) Work on the lumbar and sacral plexus.

7. Pain on the Right Side under the Rib Cage

a. Symptom Description

The area is very tight. The rib cage is sunken and feels softer than the left side. The area withdraws when touched. The stomach is painful and burns.

b. CNT Application

(1) Detoxify the skin.

(2) Do the Wave Technique.

(3) Do the Reverse Figure Five Technique.

(4) Work deeply on the left side under the rib cage.

(5) Do gentle and soft work on the right side, under the rib cage. Work your way in progressively until you can reach under the rib cage and lift it. Ask your student to push your hand, which is holding the rib cage. This will help to expand this area.

(6) Release the diaphragm. Teach abdominal breathing.

(7) Tonify and detoxify the liver.

(8) Tonify and detoxify the spleen.

(9) Tonify and detoxify the kidneys.

(10) Tonify and detoxify the lungs.

8. Pain on the Left Side under the Rib Cage

a. Symptom Description

The area is tight. If touched, the student becomes anxious and withdraws.

b. CNT Application

(1) Detoxify the skin.

(2) Release the fluid from under the left side of the rib cage by brushing the chest using the Figure Five Technique.

(3) Detoxify the lymph.

(4) Detoxify and tonify the liver.

(5) Detoxify and tonify the lungs.

H. CNT After Surgery

CNT may help those who have recovered from surgery. A surgeon, upon entering the body, has to cut through many layers of skin. As the surgeon is leaving the body, he or she stitches the internal as well as surface layers. This may cause problems.

If you remember the descriptions of fasciae, they were described as watery linings that covered most organs and muscles groups and allowed everything to slide around easily. Any irritation of the fasciae can cause serious problems by stopping the energy from flowing. This can start an internal jam. An internal abdominal scar acts like a grain of sand in an oyster; lots of tissue forms around it to isolate it. This can throw off the center. Massaging the internal scars will eventually cause them to disappear (unlike the external scar). CNT, therefore, may be employed to overcome very real post-surgery trauma, including the psychological tension from surgical intrusion.

I. More About Headaches

Headaches are a pain. Any pain has to be taken as a warning signal that something is wrong. If you take a pain killer, you are only suppressing the signal (symptoms) and are ignoring the cause of the pain. Your body is alerting you; do not ignore it. In CNT pain is a guide to the source of the problem. Respect this pain and rest. You can save the body's energy which it can then use to strengthen the organs. Of course, people do not want to hear this; they want to keep working or playing, so they take pain killers in the belief they have no time for preventive measures.

Often, the pain is expressing itself along a specific channel when it involves a specific organ. Most channels run through the head. If the head pain is localized, study a chart of the head channels. Then you can figure out the organ that is involved with the problem. The most common causes are heat in the liver, blockage in the gall bladder, and constipation.

Tension and stress are also causes. Fear gets trapped in the kidneys and weakens them and the adrenal glands. This can create tension which causes heat in the heart. The heat rises up and creates tension and pressure in the head.

You can alleviate this pressure as follows:
1. Detoxify the skin.
2. Release the large intestine.
3. Detoxify the liver, gall bladder, and kidneys.
4. Work on the adrenal glands.

J. The Dropped Bladder Technique

Many women suffer from a bladder that has dropped, but men can also have this problem.

1. Stand at the student's head and have him raise both legs up with the knees bent. Keep the feet on the floor.

2. Have the student drop the legs down on the count of three. Practice this for a few times so that the legs will drop quickly and remain totally relaxed. Return the legs to the starting position. (Figure 10-34)

3. Reach down to hold the bladder with a two-handed, eight finger scoop. On the count of three, have the student drop the legs (as rehearsed) while you hold the bladder in position. Be sure to scoop deeply from below the bladder and under the pubic bone. (Figure 10-35) Usually, this procedure is only necessary once.

4. This technique is not advisable for people who have bladder infections. When the infection diminishes, this movement will bring the bladder back to its natural position.

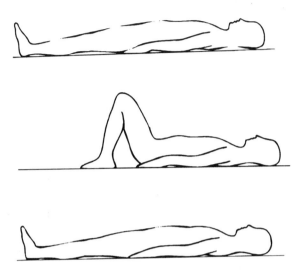

Figure 10-34. Practice for the Dropped Bladder Technique

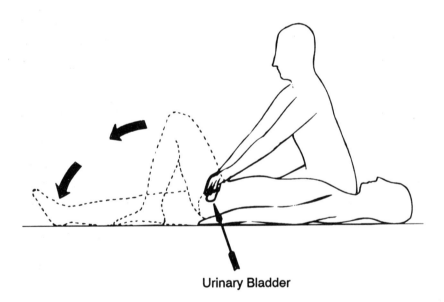

Urinary Bladder

Figure 10-35. Dropped Bladder Technique

K. Arrhythmic or Congested Heart, Angina Pectoris, Heart Attack, Asthma

Two major problems can occur with the heart: the heart loses its rhythmic beat, or it becomes very congested and tight. Severe congestion and tightness of the arteries and heart causes heart attacks. The heart is choking (to death sometimes). CNT can help loosen the congestion around the heart. It also can reset the beating of an arrhythmic heart.

The abdomen of a heart attack victim or one close to a heart attack is extremely congested and tight. The small intestine is the paired organ of the heart and they each effect the other. This situation clearly reflects that connection, and you have to spend a lot of time releasing the small intestine and rest of the abdomen.

1. Place the right hand (or you may use the left hand) on the aorta at the navel. The right hand moves up with the aorta pulse. It jumps when the pulse jumps and rises when it rises. (Figure 10-36)

2. Place the left hand on the heart. When you feel the right hand "pushed up" by the impulse of the beat in the aorta, gently push down on

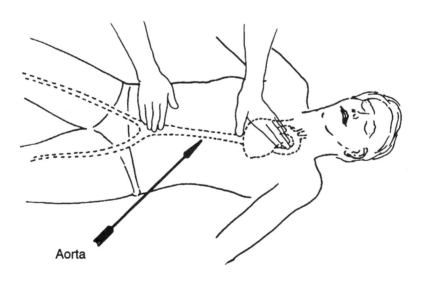

Aorta

Figure 10-36. Working on the Heart

333

the heart with the left hand. The left hand pumps the heart between its pulsations.

3. When done correctly, the hands will move in an alternating motion. When the right hand is rising, the left hand is descending, and then when the left hand starts to rise the right hand should have already started descending.

4. You probably will lose the pumping rhythm. When you do, just stop and start again until you get it back.

5. After a few tries the heart will start beating with an even rhythm.

L. Preparation for Death

In the case of impending death, the Taoists observed the abdomen and found that at this time it is usually tight and blocked. At the moment of death, many knots form. Since at the moment of death the soul and spirit either leave through the navel or travel up to the crown, they will have to struggle through the knots to exit the body. Such a struggle wastes time and energy, and the soul and spirit can miss the light or not have enough energy to follow the light that appears at death to take them.

In addition to this problem, some people who contracted diseases or who experienced extensive medical procedures face death with a great deal of their energy already depleted. Sick and dying people need to clear blockages and reserve some energy in preparation for their deaths.

Abdominal release will clear blockages in the navel to help the dying person's soul leave the body. After the knots and tightness are loosened, the CNT practitioner can place his\her hand over the navel to give the dying person some reserve energy. The person should be aware of or concentrate on the navel area in front of the kidneys.

Also, the dying person should be aware of the back of the crown and the mid-eyebrow. (The soul and spirit dwell behind the crown at the back of the head and not in the crown. Here they connect to the pineal gland.) (Figure 10-37) Also the person should consciously feel the sexual organs and anus lightly closed so that the soul and spirit will not go down and out these openings. (Figure 10-38)

Use the following procedure.

(1) Use the opening of the Wind Gate to activate more energy.

(2) Start with the one finger technique from the navel and slowly move in a spiral out, spending more time on the knot.

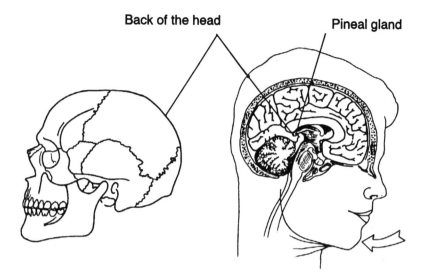

Figure 10-37. The soul and spirit exit from the back of the head

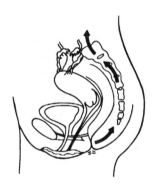

**Figure 10-38. The sexual organs and anus should be
lightly closed**

(3) Massage the whole stomach until the knots clear. You will find the knots will continuously return to form each day after you massage, but each day you will find it easier to untie the knots.

(4) Teach the person to be conscious about closing the sexual organs and anus to conserve sexual energy.

335

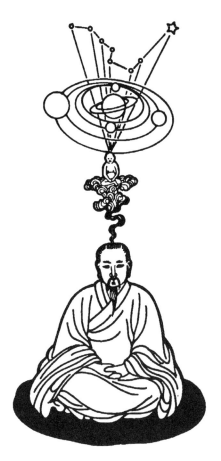

Figure 10-39. Be aware of the North Star and the Big Dipper

(5) Teach the person to turn his/her awareness of all the senses into the navel area so that the soul and spirit cannot go out through the openings of the senses.

(6) Find the point at the back of the crown that connects to the pineal gland and place your finger there. Tell the person to concentrate on that point.

(7) Be aware of the North Star and the Big Dipper. Tell him/her to envision flying toward the North. (Figure 10-39)

(8) It is very important to help gather the force in the navel and Door of Life area.

CHAPTER 11

WORKING PROCEDURES

A. Precautions

1. Chi Nei Tsang is a healing art; like any art you will need time to cultivate and develop an expertise. Always work carefully and gently. The first rule is to apply the techniques correctly so you will get the best possible results.

Remember, you cannot diagnose. Leave medicine to the doctors. Only doctors practicing CNT are permitted to give diagnosis. For obvious health problems, it is sometimes necessary to work in coordination with the medical establishment. Recommend a medical consultation with a doctor when you are in doubt about the use of CNT for a particular problem, or when you cannot find a source for the problem. Chi Nei Tsang works well with all the body's systems in prevention and maintenance. It clears the toxins and obstructions in the organs. If it becomes evident that the problem is with the skeletal system, the person should be referred to a chiropractor or an osteopath. If sickness or acute infection develops, a doctor should be consulted. A psychiatrist or psychologist should be consulted if the problem is in the mind.

2. Ask students for a history of their health before working with them. Find out if there is any contraindication for any of the techniques of CNT. If any such problems appear, let the student talk to a doctor to say that he or she is learning CNT. Sometimes physicians may regulate medications to allow for various massage therapies.

WARNING
- **DO NOT WORK ON THE FOLLOWING CONDITIONS: CANCER, INFECTIOUS DISEASES, THROMBOSIS, ACUTE INFLAMMATIONS, SKIN INFECTIONS, ANEURISM, MELANOMA, LYMPHOMA. YOU MAY WORK ON**

THOSE WITH PSYCHOLOGICAL PROBLEMS UNDER A DOCTOR'S REQUEST, OR UNDER THE SUPERVISION OF A LICENSED PSYCHOTHERAPIST.

- DO NOT WORK ON WOMEN WHO ARE USING I.U.D. BIRTH CONTROL DEVICES. THESE DEVICES ARE IMPLANTED IN THE UTERUS. YOU COULD TEAR OR RIP THE UTERUS. THE UTERUS IS CONNECTED WITH THE KIDNEYS AND LIVER, AND YOU MIGHT ALSO EFFECT THEM IN A NEGATIVE WAY.
- DO NOT WORK ON MEN OR WOMEN WHO HAVE IMPLANTED PACEMAKERS. THESE ARE ELECTRONIC DEVICES USED TO ACTIVATE THE HEART. IN CNT YOU WILL BE MOVING ELECTRONIC FIELDS AND IT IS POSSIBLE TO AFFECT THE PACEMAKERS.
- DO NOT WORK ON THE PSOAS MUSCLE OR SCIATIC NERVE OF ANYONE WHO HAS AN ARTIFICIAL HIP OR KNEE. IF NECESSARY, WORK ON THE OPPOSITE HIP OR KNEE, PROVIDED IT DOES NOT ALSO HAVE AN ARTIFICIAL JOINT. (MANY TIMES BY WORKING ON THE OPPOSITE SIDE YOU CAN CAUSE A SYMPATHETIC REACTION THAT IS BENEFICIAL TO THE PRESCRIBED AREA.)
- DO NOT WORK ON PREGNANT WOMEN. YOU CAN HELP BY TEACH ING THEM HOW TO IMPROVE THEIR BREATHING BY RELEASING THE DIAPHRAGM.

B. Caring for Yourself

In Chapter 2 the exercises described are designed to raise your own energy level and protect you from the sick energy of anyone you work on. What follows are ways to care for yourself while you are working on someone, and what to do immediately afterward.

While you are working on someone you should activate all your energy processing "turbines." Do the Microcosmic Orbit, the Six Healing Sounds, Fusion I, and Kan & Li. This will offer you and your students maximum protection.

If you are unfamiliar with these practices, you may, nonetheless, drain off any negative energy you might have picked up. You should wait until you are out of the presence of your students. This is a courtesy and kindness. Most of the time people will come to you because they are ill.

You don't have to embarrass them by revealing just how "sick" you think their energy is.

1. After you have worked on someone, do not wash your hands right away. First, shake your hands and concentrate on your navel. Feel the navel, hands, and palms become warm. If you have been practicing with a tree and have a connection with it, you can picture the tree and thereby transfer the energy to it. When you have a chance to touch and meditate on a tree, you can pass the energy to it directly. (Figure 11-1) Trees and Mother Earth have the power to transform sick energy into good energy.

2. If you do not have a good connection with a tree (or if no tree is available), you can use a wall and pass the sick energy to the ground. First, shake your hands loose and feel them become warm. Then touch a cement or brick wall until you feel the sick energy drain away into the wall. (Figure 11-2) If you cannot find a wall, use a drain pipe that runs into the ground. You can pass the energy to a large rock. Don't touch a

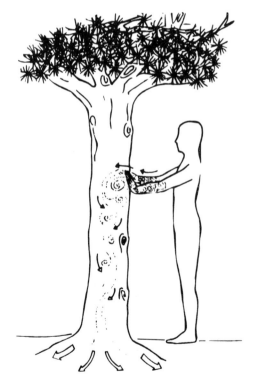

Figure 11-1. Passing Sick Energy to a Large Tree

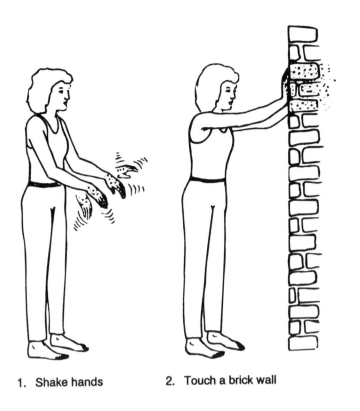

1. Shake hands   2. Touch a brick wall

Figure 11-2. Removing Sick Energy

metal door or a window handle. Anyone touching the door afterward can pick up the sick energy.

3. Remember, these are real energies you are dealing with; they are not products of the imagination. When your energy is higher, you will not be so vulnerable. Then you can block the sick energy with mind power. Train your mind to burn the sick energy by growing your aura using the sun at the navel. Also, bring the sun into the palms to help burn out the sick energy.

4. After you ground the sick energy, you can further balance yourself with meditation. Put your hands together in the sitting meditation position and meditate until you feel your navel become warm. Feel the warmth spread to your hands. The warmth shows that the sick energy is coming out of your skin.

5. If you want to wash your hands, use tepid running water. If you wash your hands in still water, you will not eliminate the sick energy and it will quickly absorb into your bones. Sick energy entering your system in this way is difficult to get out.

6. Meditating after a session is crucial and cannot be taken lightly. Ignore this advice and you may discover (the hard way) why there is a warning. You could develop a fever, a rash, or awaken in the middle of the night and need to vomit. It will only take a few minutes. When sick energy gets into you, you are of no use to anyone, not even yourself. When your energy is higher, you can meditate after seeing a few people, or at the end of the day.

7. Cosmic Chi Kung and Healing Hand Chi Kung are very important to practice because energy leaves and enters mostly through your fingers. Energy routes become strengthened through these practices. Your ability to sense what is happening in your hands is also greatly magnified. Cosmic Chi Kung and Healing Hand Chi Kung meditations will place you in a better position to deal with sick energy. You learn a means of forcibly moving energy out through your fingertips and strengthening all your energy systems.

8. During the session it is very important to remain in touch with the outer energy sources. Feel the Universal force on the crown, the Human Plane (Cosmic Particle) Force coming through the mid-eyebrow, and the Earth Force through the soles of the feet and the perineum. Feel the power of your personal star, or the North Star and the Big Dipper. (Figure 11-3) If you do not feel the energy, stop and reconnect with the force. Then continue.

9. Whether you work on the floor or at a table, it is important to keep the back straight, the head pulled up, the chin tucked, the shoulders relaxed, and the chest sunk. (Figures 11-4 and 11-5) The posture is important and is based on the same posture principles seen in Tai Chi and Iron Shirt Chi Kung. The correct posture allows the energy to flow into you and through you. If your back or neck is bent or you are tense, you can block the free flow of the energy.

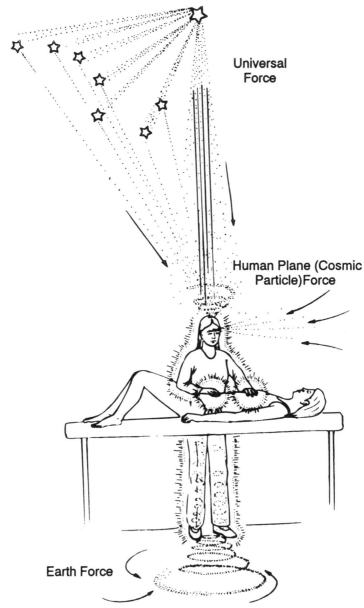

Universal
Force

Human Plane (Cosmic
Particle)Force

Earth Force

**Figure 11-3. When touching another, remain in touch with the Forces.
Draw down the Universal Force through the crown.
Draw in the Human Plane Force through the Third Eye.
Feel the Earth Force coming through the soles
of the feet and the perineum**

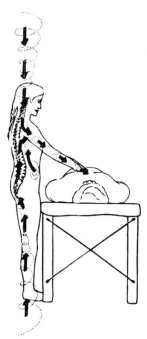

**Figure 11-4. Good posture allows the energy to flow.
Keep the back straight, the chin tucked in,
the shoulders relaxed, and the chest sunk**

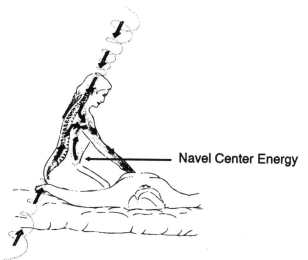

Navel Center Energy

**Figure 11-5. When working on the floor, try to maintain
an erect posture so the energy can flow**

C. Session One—Hands-On Procedures

Five one-hour sessions are usually required to teach the basics to a student. It is necessary to teach the fundamentals so the student can do homework. The more toxic a person, the more time this might take. You should teach the person until he/she can take full charge and responsibility for his/her own health. This is the basic purpose of CNT and this book. The Healing Tao Organization wants to help create a culture in which people can care for themselves both physically and spiritually.

1. In the first session interview your student using the Questionnaire in Chapter 3 as your guideline. Remember, in particular, to note the shape of the navel and the areas of tension near the navel and in the abdomen.

2. If the student is a male, sit or stand to his right. If a woman, sit or stand to her left. This is not a rule, but it is the traditional way. Elevate the knees by placing a pillow(s) under them. (Figure 11-6) This will take some of the tension from the abdominal muscles.

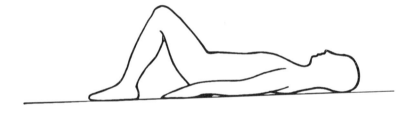

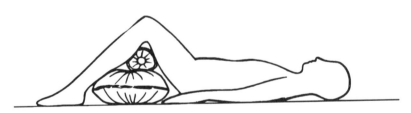

Figure 11-6. The abdominal muscles are most relaxed when the legs are bent. A pillow can be used for support. Keep the arms by the sides to prevent pulling the abdominal muscles up

3. Remember that you are giving the person life-force. It must be of a better quality than his or hers. Do the Microcosmic Orbit and Fusion of the Five Elements meditations.

4. It is important to center yourself and balance your energy. Sincerely and respectfully wish your students well. Extend your aura to cover each of their auras. Feel that you are in touch with the Universal, Human Plane (Cosmic Particle), and Earth Energies.

5. Always start by opening the Wind Gates, beginning with the points in the groin. Sometimes the navel may be very hard and painful, and the student cannot take the finger pressure needed to open the Wind Gates. In that case you will need to release tension and congestion first.

6. Tonify and balance the lungs, teach abdominal breathing, and teach the Lungs' Sound. Begin emotional release in the lungs. Emotion can be released through gentle, shallow massage of the organ holding points. Hold the point until you feel the release. When working on the lungs, for instance, do the Lungs' Sound together with the student.

7. Detoxify the skin and superficial lymph nodes. Use gentle and shallow massage. Begin in the navel and work outward in a clockwise direction in tight spirals. Explain what is known about the navel, including how to detoxify the skin around the navel. Do not frighten students with what you see or feel. Use sensitivity, but teach them what you are doing so that they may know how to detoxify themselves. This is very important. If they do not begin to soften up the abdomen, you cannot go deeper in subsequent sessions.

8. Detoxify the large intestine. Check the state of the sigmoid colon, the cecum, and the ileocecal valve. Use the Figure Five, Scooping, and Wave Techniques.
    a. Use both thumbs or two-four fingers.
    b. Use the double finger cupping technique.
    c. Spiral clockwise.
    d. Shake and knead to loosen toxin formations.
    e. Pat the abdomen.

9. Center the navel. Center the aortic pulse. Balance the pulses.

10. Assign homework. When you find a knot or tangle, use a non-toxic marker to mark the problem area(s) for them, or mark it on the CNT sheet and teach your students how to work on the knot or tangle. Ask them to work on themselves in front of you. Offer advice, if needed.

11. Spiral to collect energy in the navel.

345

12. Cover the navel with your hands as each student you work on meditates to keep it warm. The warmth will help to burn out some of the sick energy.

13. Teach all of your students to shake the hands and legs before getting up. This will help to activate their blood circulation and lymphatic flow. Also teach them to do this every morning before getting out of bed.

14. Allow your students to rest, then have them rise from their right sides.

15. Teach the Lungs' and Kidneys' Healing Sounds. Introduce your students to the Microcosmic Orbit. Teach them to meditate on the navel area so that they learn how to turn their awareness into their navel areas to make them warm. Also teach them to do the basic Inner Smile.

D. Session Two

1. Repeat steps one through eight from Session One.

2. Detoxify, tonify, and balance the emotional energy in the spleen and pancreas. Teach the Spleen's Sound. Pump the spleen and pancreas.

3. Clear the congestion in the small intestine. Search for and massage any knots and tangles.

4. Teach about the lymphatic system, massage, and detoxify the lymph nodes in the abdomen. Congested lymph nodes tend to be rounded and somewhat ellipsoidal. Gently massage the nodes until they become soft. Use the one-finger technique on the nodes. Shake the nodes and let the student breathe against your hand to help release their fluid into the thoracic duct. Remember that each lymph node is composed of delicate tissue, so be gentle.

5. Work on specific problems.

Teach women to work on the ovaries if cramps are felt. Teach men to work on the testicle massage. (The techniques for testicle massage are listed in the book, *Bone Marrow Nei Kung*, pp. 104-112.)

6. Assign homework. Let them feel any knots, tangles, or other problems that you have located. Show them how to do the massage.

7. Spiral to collect the energy in the navel.

8. Cover the navel with your hands as each student you work on meditates to keep it warm.

9. Allow your students to rest, then have them rise from their right sides.

10. Teach the Liver's and Heart's Healing Sounds.

Teach them how to meditate on the navel area. Teach them to turn their awareness into the navel area and make it warm. Expand the warmth to the Door of Life (the Ming-Men) opposite the navel.

11. Teach more of the Inner Smile. Extend the smile to the eyes, the face, and down to the heart. Feel love and joy and happiness. Spread the love and joy to the lungs. Enhance the smiling energy in the lungs as it transforms any sadness and depression into righteousness and courage. Finish by having them collect the energy in the navel.

E. Session Three

1. Repeat one through five from Session Two.

2. Do deeper work on the intestines, searching for knots and tangles.

3. Activate the heart and heart controller areas.

4. Detoxify, tonify, and balance the energy in the liver and gall bladder. Teach the Liver's Sound and do it together. Pump the liver. When the liver is cleansed, more toxins automatically replace those removed until the body is completely detoxified.

5. Loosen the structure of the rib cage and the diaphragm.

6. Balance the pulses.

7. Work on specific problems.

8. Assign homework.

9. Spiral to collect the energy in the navel.

10. Allow for rest, and have students rise from the right side.

11. Teach the Spleen's and Triple Warmer's Healing Sounds. Continue teaching how to turn the awareness into the navel area and make it warm. Expand the warmth and awareness to the Door of Life, opposite the navel. Expand the concentration to the sexual center. Connect this to the navel and the Door of Life. Feel the whole lower area warm-up and expand.

Continue teaching the Inner Smile. Let love from the heart and courage from the lungs spread to the liver and transform any anger in the liver into kindness. Spread the love, courage, and kindness to the spleen/pancreas. These energies and a healthy smile are strong enough to dissolve any worry in the spleen and turn it into fairness. Next, send all the positive energies generated thus far to the kidneys. In the kidneys they will help dissolve any fear and transform it into gentleness. The Inner Smile works instantly. You and your student can feel its effect immediately.

F. Session Four

1. Repeat one through seven from Session Three.
2. Detoxify the stomach and bladder.
3. Teach the Heart's Sound.
4. Search for deep knots and tangles.
5. Tonify and detoxify the kidneys. Teach the Kidneys' Sound. Work on the adrenal glands.
6. Flush the blood and clean out the organs.
7. Chase the Winds to the abdomen. Bake them.
8. Work on the psoas muscles only if there is a problem related to them.
9. Work on specific problems.
10. Assign homework.
11. Spiral and collect the energy in the navel.
12. Allow for rest, and have the student rise from the right side.
13. Review the Six Healing Sounds and demonstrate how to warm the entire lower abdominal area. Continue to teach the Inner Smile. Smile to the organs. Bring the smile back to the eyes and do the Inner Smile on the Middle line, the digestive tract. Start by swallowing the saliva. Follow the saliva with a smile. Send the smiling energy to the stomach and the small and large intestines. Smile through the anal canal to the anus. This will help strengthen the digestive tract.

G. Session Five

1. Repeat one through nine from Session Four.
2. Practice the Triple Warmer's Sound.
3. Search for and release the deepest knots and tangles.
4. Work on the lumbar and sacral plexus if there is a related problem.
5. Release any sciatic nerve pain.
6. Work on specific problems.
7. Spiral and collect the energy in the navel.
8. Allow for rest, and have students rise from the right side.
9. Review the Six Healing Sounds.

Teach your students again how to meditate on the navel area and demonstrate how to turn the awareness into the navel area and make it warm. Expand it to the Door of Life. Expand the concentration on the sexual center and connect it to the navel and the Door of Life center. Tell them to feel the whole lower area becoming warm and expanding. Show your students how the energy moves up the spine and down the front of the body in the Microcosmic Orbit. Teach them how to spiral and collect the energy in the Tan Tien at the middle of the body.

Continue to teach the Inner Smile. Smile to contact the energy. Smile down the organ line, come back to the eyes, and then swallow the saliva. Smile down through the digestive system. The last part involves smiling to the brain and down the spine and ribs, and then smiling to the whole skeleton, including the pelvis, hip, and leg bones. The final teaching of the Inner Smile involves smiling down through the whole body at once. Smile to yourself, you are going to help a lot of people learn how to help themselves. Good luck.

H. Commonly Asked Questions

Q: What do you do when someone's abdomen is too hard?

A: Relax the abdominal muscles by massaging the skin while giving a soothing, rolling and rocking motion to the whole body. While massaging the skin let the fingers slowly sink through the muscles as they start to relax. The fingers have to be very soft. The harder the abdomen, the softer the fingers. It may take twenty minutes of rocking before you can start the Wave Technique. Then apply the Wave Technique as long as necessary to smooth out any remnants of muscular tension.

Q: What do you do when someone's abdomen is too painful?

A: Never work a spot that is too painful. Work around it instead to dissipate the congestion that creates pain. Work on knots and tangles as if you were untangling a piece of yarn. First work to loosen the area around the knot. When the knot area is loose, it is easier to untangle. If the yarn's knot is too tight and you pull at the center, it will break. Loosen up any secondary knots before you get to the main knot or tangle. This will make it easier to work on.

Q: What do you do if the abdomen is painful everywhere?

A: If the pain is acute and includes a fever, you should advise the student to seek medical care. Otherwise, with one hand over the navel, use the rocking and rolling motion of the whole body, and ask the student to do deep abdominal breathing. If it is still too sensitive, turn the student onto his or her stomach and work on the sympathetic ganglia along the spinal column and on the intercostal muscles to relieve pain from nervous tension.

Q: What do you do if the person is too ticklish?

A. Ticklishness is a sign of tension. Try the rocking and rolling procedure described above. Work from the top to the bottom. This could take some time.

Sometimes you can just have the student do deep abdominal breathing while laying on the back in the standard position. Massage only during the exhalation phase. Use the rolling and rocking motions to soothe the nerves.

Q: How about colitis and other forms of inflammations?

A: Take care of the inflammation and/or infection medically first, then apply CNT to prevent further attacks.

Q: What can I do for a hernia?

A: A hernia is a protrusion of tissue or a part of an organ through an abnormal opening. It is caused by internal pressure and weakness of the tissue. A medical dictionary might list over 90 different hernias in all parts of the body. You can correct abdominal hernias over time. First release the pressure in the area by releasing pressure in other parts of the abdomen. This will allow the pressure that is creating the hernia a place to flow to and dissolve. Do not work on the hernia itself for that would be very painful. Instead work all around the abdomen, especially in the healthiest areas. Gradually extend the healthy area and allow it to "intrude" upon the unhealthy tissues involved with the hernia. The idea is to relieve pressure in the abdomen and to strengthen the tissues slowly. When the hernia's pain dissolves, then it will be possible to work very close to the protrusion and to strengthen those tissues.

Q: What about ulcers?

A: An ulcer is a defect on the surface of an organ or tissue caused by an inflammatory liquid produced by that organ or tissue. They can occur in many parts of the body, but are often seen in the stomach. First advise the student to seek medical help. Chi Nei Tsang's purpose is not to cure diseases or acute or chronic problems directly. The purpose of Chi Nei Tsang is to reverse the degeneration of the organs and tissues and improve and strengthen their condition. Your work and your student's work can reverse the process of bad health by repairing the organs and modifying the life style that caused the problem. The energy in the organs will then be strong enough to guide the student toward the healing of an ulcer or any other problem.

Most ulcers are caused by stress. Never work directly on an ulcer, or any other painful area, or you will cause more pain and problems. Instead, work where the body feels good and extend the diameter of the healthy area. Make the good area feel even better. Work on the whole body and relax it. Practice emotional balancing and tonifying, particularly concentrating on anger in the liver, fear in the kidneys, and worry in the stomach and spleen. Learning Fusion I is crucial. Encourage students to intensify their work with the Inner Smile and the Six Healing Sounds. Strengthen the organs and put them in control of the ulcer. The energy coming from healthy organs and a vitalized Navel Center can balance out any problem in the body.

Q: What about a herniated or fused disk between the vertebrae?

A: Problems with the disks between the vertebrae can be caused by a weakening of the disks' tissue, which allows the supporting fluid to leak out. Such problems are further complicated by weak muscles and bad posture. It is necessary to improve the quality of the tissues in the whole body. Detoxify everywhere, and remove internal pressure. Search for tangles deep in the sacral plexus.

Q: What can CNT do about cancer?

A: Generally, cancer is not worked on. Sometimes when people are subjected to chemotherapy, however, the treatment is such a shock that special healing techniques may be needed to replenish their bodies. Talk to their doctors and get medical advice about contraindications. If a student is going to receive chemotherapy, you can help strengthen the body to withstand the treatment. Do not work directly on tumors. Teach the Six Healing Sounds, the Microcosmic Orbit, and the Inner Smile. Inform the student about daily exercises, meditations, books, and tapes. It is highly recommended that anyone with cancer read Deepak Chopra's extraordinary book, *Quantum Healing*, and apply the full range of Healing Tao meditations.

351

Chi Nei Tsang

CHAPTER 12

CHI NEI TSANG AND STRESS MANAGEMENT

A. Definition of Stress

Among the different stress situations that modern men and women encounter in their lives, the ones that affect them most quickly are emotional and work-related stress. In both cases the first organ system to be affected is the small intestine, which is in charge of not only digesting food but also emotional traumas. This creates a tight, painful, bloated stomach, poor digestion, constipation, PMS problems, and other symptoms. This in turn causes problems in the liver and gall bladder.

Emotional stress can come from a bad relationship or the idea or anticipation of the end of a relationship caused by separation, divorce, or death. This stress affects the heart, the heart controller, and the lungs. Besides the obvious action on the heart, the lungs are involved because of the grief and sadness resulting from the loss or the lack of affection and companionship.

Work-related stress is the most frequently encountered health problem. In modern commercial life the pace demanded by the always increasing need for growth, expansion, and financial survival requires executives, entrepreneurs, and the work force to be alert longer than their biological rhythms would allow. The result, besides fatigue from the constant draining of the life-force energy from the kidneys and the adrenal glands, is an anger and frustration that severely hurts the liver. Fear of losing a job, money, or business damages the kidneys. Shady or unethical business practices rebounds on the lungs and heart. Working in unpleasant locations weakens the functions of the stomach, pancreas, and spleen.

1. How Emotional and Work-Related Stress Affect Each Other

Emotional breakdown negatively drains the lung's energy causing sadness and grief. This causes confusion in the nervous system, prevents clear mindedness, and negatively shocks the liver, causing frustration and anger. (According to the Control Cycle Law of the Five Elements, Metal (lungs) controls Wood (liver).) This emotional state causes a lack of concentration, making any work situation untenable. People become accident prone and are quick to fight with co-workers and managers.

People who are stressed at work return home tired, angry, and full of negative emotions. They are easily provoked and often dump their emotions on their loving partners. Couples fight all the time because they have so much anger to release. Wood nourishes Fire (Creation Cycle), and this means that negative energy coming from the liver will feed the heart. Since anger is feeding the heart, the heart expresses impatience and cruelty instead of love, joy, and respect. It is common for couples to fling angry words at one another, creating a self-perpetuating situation that sometimes turns violent. Such an exchange often carries through the night, possibly causing alcoholic drinking and a liver that is so intoxicated that it becomes brick hard, perpetuating the foul mood. Intoxication of the liver eventually causes the anger level to drop, until the person collapses and finally goes to bed. Soon the relationship is finished and one or both of the lovers is an alcoholic, addicted to drugs, overeats, or is prone to some other dysfunction.

2. The Main Causes of Stress

a. Apprehension

Most negative energy generated by stress is often created long before any stressful situation occurs. People get stressed by "living in the future" and projecting their concerns to problems that are not even appropriate. People dwell in fear of "the worst possible case." Taoism teaches you to live in the moment, especially since you have little control over future events anyway.

b. Lack of Method

People want to do everything at the same time and go faster. They disperse their energy and are unable to do anything. This results in frustration from the loss of time and inefficiency.

c. Self-Consciousness

Very often people are obsessed with the idea that everybody is watching their every move, so they want to please everybody. Actually, since everybody is so similarly self-conscious and thinking the same thing simultaneously, nobody is watching anybody. This common state of mind not only increases isolation between people, but creates an atmosphere of suspicion, and unrealizable and unnecessary goals.

d. Artificial Self-Confidence

We often lack the necessary self-confidence to carry off assigned projects. As people reach for more prestigious positions and higher paying jobs, they often assign themselves roles that are beyond their capabilities. Often the work is poorly done and the result bad. This creates fear of negative remarks by supervisors and poor performance reports. Sometimes it just takes knowing your limits.

e. Social Isolation—Lack of Support Systems

Because today's societies are based on individual performance, we are often surrounded by people whose lives and survival are energized by competition and not cooperation. We are born into societies we did not make and it is very easy to find oneself all alone. Often, all we have is our family. It seems today, however, that even members of the family are easily disturbed and unable to offer the love, care, and concern needed. During the last ten to fifteen years there has been an explosion of neighborhood self-help groups, such as Alcoholic Anonymous, Overeaters Anonymous, Adult Children of Alcoholics, Love and Sex Addicts, and many other similar groups. Here the isolated, overstressed, and addicts of all sorts can drop in for an hour at any time throughout the day and evening to share their problems and find support. Thus, people in communities throughout the land have established stress "pit-stops" where the displaced and disoriented can go to get balanced and recharged. There is something very appealing about this. Perhaps this is proof of how easily and effectively we can help one another and ourselves. This is what Chi Nei Tsang is concerned with.

f. Dumping Stress

Overloaded garbage dumps are a big problem everywhere. People, through custom, force of habit, and carelessness, turn their natural resources and treasures into garbage. Similarly, as a result of living in societies that have "trashed everything" for centuries, many citizens, through spiritual and social atrophy, have lost their natural ability and facility to process love, joy, and respect. Instead of having the skills to process and recycle any pain or stress that enters their lives, they dump it into the closest vulnerable places, the family and work environment. In return, stress accumulated during work or from emotional situations is often the reason people act so disrespectfully toward nature. If you cannot dump it at home or at work, dump it on the Earth.

B. Symptoms

To aid in observation and instruction, the symptoms are divided into five categories according to the element to which they belong.

Under Metal are all the symptoms related to breathing and elimination. Water encompasses the symptoms related to energy level and fluid control. Under Wood are symptoms related to nerve problems. Under Fire are symptoms that involve high pressure and heat. Under Earth are symptoms that belong to food, the habitat, and the environment. The symptoms are interrelated, but for the purposes of teaching, we are breaking them down individually. For example, high blood pressure is under Fire and Water. Though high blood pressure affects the heart, it is a fluid problem resulting from kidney weakness. Degenerative diseases are under the Water (kidney) category because they result from a breakdown of Ching, but the symptoms can appear anywhere in the body. This includes cancer, multiple sclerosis, AIDS, arthritis, Parkinson's disease, and others.

1. Metal—Lungs and Large Intestine

- Breathlessness
- Asthma
- Constipation
- Diarrhea
- Colitis
- Depression

2. Water—Kidneys and Bladder

- Fears
- Phobias
- Constant tiredness
- Impotence
- High blood pressure
- Degenerative disease

3. Wood—Liver and Gall Bladder

- Dizziness
- Insomnia
- Nightmares
- Nail biting and tics
- Headaches
- Neck and backaches
- Skin rashes
- Anger and violence
- Allergies
- Intoxication and addictions
- Accidents

4. Fire—Heart and Small Intestine

- Palpitations
- Heart diseases
- High blood pressure
- Impotence
- Strokes
- Foot and finger tapping
- Intestinal Cramps
- Diverticulitis
- Acute indigestion

5. Earth—Spleen, Pancreas, and Stomach

- Nausea
- Vomiting
- Loss of appetite
- Craving for food
- Bulimia

- Anorexia
- Chronic indigestion
- Ulcers
- Chronic anxiety
- Claustrophobia
- Agoraphobia

C. Anatomy of an Over-Stressed Body

1. The "Fight or Flight" Response

When confronted with an emergency stressful situation, the body reacts as follows:

- The brain becomes super alert.
- Adrenalin starts to flow.
- All the glands release extra hormones.
- The pupils dilate.
- The heart rate increases.
- The muscles tense.
- The blood vessels of the skin and limbs constrict as all the blood flows to the center of the body.
- All other blood vessels dilate, i.e., the muscles, the heart, the brain, and the organs involved in fighting off danger.
- Breathing becomes rapid.
- Blood sugar level rises.
- All the normal processes of the body, such as digestion, are slowed or even stopped, and the body collects and conserves all available energy for the perceived threat.

In an emergency, when your life is on the line, you should be grateful that the body reacts as described above. Nevertheless, when the situation lasts too long, or is repeated too often in a short period of time, it results in a chronic condition that prevents the body from resting. This is stress.

The first result of this is that the "fight or flight" response is going to be triggered by situations that are less and less threatening. A self-perpetuating situation, it pushes the person to imagine danger when there is none at hand. This can develop into paranoia and "adrenalin addiction."

Caffeine, nicotine, and sugar all help to activate and maintain the "fight or flight" response.

2. The Body's and Mind's Responses to Stress

a. Body

After a certain period of stress accumulation, the body gives some warning signals (ulcers, nerve problems, depression, colds, etc.). Those warning signals will vary from person to person according to their energy balance, tendencies, and physical condition.

b. Mind

The first reaction of the mind is the same in everyone—DENIAL. Everyone says, "I feel fine." The result is an accumulation and increase in symptoms until they reach a point at which the mind reluctantly starts to admit that there is a problem. That is when the person affected starts to worry about a particular symptom.

3. Anatomical Description of the Symptoms of Stress

a. Rib Cage

Breathing becomes restricted because of chronic contraction of the intercostal muscles and the diaphragm, preventing the rib cage from expanding and contracting freely during normal breathing. It requires great effort, and sometimes is impossible, to open or close the rib cage. The upper torso is "frozen."

b. Abdomen

The abdominal muscles become hard and tight, and the whole abdominal cavity is under a tremendous amount of pressure. The whole surface of the abdomen is like a closed door, or even like the massive, impervious front of a walk-in vault. The body knows enough to protect its weakened organs from external life-threatening influences. Under the impressive muscular surface, the viscera will reflect the different abuses they have been through.

(1) The Small Intestine

We have learned that tension in the various quadrants or sections of the small intestine suggests the organ involved is causing the congestion. Often in cases of chronic stress, the entire small intestine is very hard. This shows that all the organs are getting weakened by the situation and are unable to process toxins or negative emotions.

In addition, hastiness during meals and lack of appreciation for food will prevent normal digestion and increase the accumulation of toxins.

(2) The Large Intestine

The lack of movement in the abdomen, when added to the accumulated pressure, will prevent normal peristalsis and cause constipation in the large intestine. The splenic and liver bends, which are near the lung points, will feel extremely sensitive when touched.

(3) Pancreas

Sugar and alcohol consumption will make it feel hard and sensitive if touched. Intestinal bloating with air and fluid around the pancreas indicates the accumulation of anxiety.

(4) Stomach

A tight and oversensitive stomach, especially near the duodenum, is a sign of repressed nervousness and anxiety, and will often accompany gall bladder and pancreas problems.

(5) Liver and Gall Bladder

A hard liver and gall bladder that are painful when touched indicate accumulated toxins or intoxicants. Any stagnant or repressed anger will affect the range of motion of the right side of the rib cage when compared to the left side.

Prolonged cases of anger and/or violence and any overworking of the liver will start to drain the kidneys (Water feeds Wood). The emotional result is a build-up of fear accompanied by violent reactions. In extreme cases this will lead to phobias.

(6) Kidneys

An oversensitive kidney area of the abdomen around the navel (see CNT chart, Chapter 6), especially when accompanied by extreme fatigue or exhaustion, indicates that the adrenal glands are running "wide open" and are continuously pumping and draining. When fear and paranoia are present, and the lower abdomen above the public bone (the sexual center) is cold and congested, this indicates that the kidneys themselves are drained. The life force, the prenatal Chi, is uselessly leaking out of the body. This is why "stress kills."

D. CNT Applications

1. Hand Techniques

a. Untie any knots close to the navel.

b. For emotionally caused stress, detoxify the liver and gall bladder.

c. If there is a loss of appetite, detoxify the spleen, pancreas, stomach, and liver.

d. Use the Six Healing Sounds.

2. Recommendations

The best recommendation you could give to a victim of stress is to tell them to take as much time off as possible, and to use the free time to learn about stress management. This would include how to change behavior while working, driving, and eating. They should learn how to manage interpersonal relationships and improve communication and expression at home and at work. Of course they should learn how to integrate relaxation techniques into their daily routine.

E. Healing Tao Techniques for Overcoming Stress

1. The Inner Smile
2. The Six Healing Sounds
3. The Microcosmic Orbit
4. Fusion of the Five Elements

These ancient methods continue to be the most efficient ways to recycle stress. Stressful situations are going to come at you day-after-day, year-after-year. But you do not have to let modern life damage your health. If your defenses are weakened, Chi Nei Tsang and the meditation techniques and formulations of the Healing Tao will help you to recycle bad energy into positive energy and transform stress into vitality.

Chi Nei Tsang

CHAPTER 13

CHI NEI TSANG AND CLINICAL PSYCHOLOGY

Chi Nei Tsang can greatly benefit the clinical practice of psychiatry, psychology, and general counseling. It is fortunate that the Healing Tao can offer you the experiences of Dr. Nicole Tremblay, a psychologist and Healing Tao instructor. She is a dedicated healer who has successfully integrated this system into her innovative work. CNT has a wide range of possible applications. If this is your field, hopefully you and your patients will benefit from her procedures. If you adopt her methods, you are encouraged to share your experiences with the Healing Tao and with your colleagues.

The following description of her procedures was composed from interviews with Dr. Tremblay that were conducted during the 1990 Chi Nei Tsang workshop held in Phoenecia, New York. She spoke from memory and without her clinical notes:

"I, Nicole Tremblay, am a psychologist, acupuncturist and massotherapist with specialized training in Shiatsu, Jin-Shin Do, and Chi Nei Tsang. I have practiced in Quebec, Canada since 1983. As a psychologist, it is my profession to heal the emotionally distressed. They come to me because fear, anger, worry, hatred, and sadness have confused their lives. My training in Western style psychology taught me to listen to their complaints, pinpoint their negative emotions, and form an interpretation that will allow them to explore those emotions that limit their personal growth. This procedure leads to lengthy treatments and an emotionally exhausted therapist. I have developed an approach that integrates both the Eastern and Western medical traditions to help the emotionally disturbed accelerate their healing and, at the same time, to build up my own strength to meet the challenges they bring. I believe it is important to give both physical and spiritual support to the patients to help stabilize their emotional lives.

I typically begin the therapy with a combination of Western style psychology and massage interwoven with the approach of traditional Chinese medicine to reduce the patient's immediate stress and help him/her control his/her emotions. This initial phase of the treatment is followed by confidence and responsibility building, during which I expose the patient to a variety of Healing Tao techniques. It is important at this stage of the therapy to develop confidence and a sense of responsibility. This is necessary for the patient to integrate these techniques of self-healing and spiritual growth into his/her daily life. Patients are screened to insure that the technique used is appropriate (e.g., psychotics are not given any practice that will raise the sexual energy.)

I build their confidence in me as a healer by interacting with them on a physical level with massage and acupuncture while I listen to their complaints. Chi Nei Tsang is a valuable tool at this stage of therapy because it lets the patient feel immediate stress relief. Conventional Western psychotherapy that relies primarily on verbal communication is not as effective when the problem also manifests itself in the physical body. The patient makes a quick association between the application of massage and acupuncture and an improved sense of well-being. Teaching elementary techniques for self massage and appreciation of one's own body is possible once this connection is made. With the beginning use of these techniques and the positive results they produce, the patient develops a sense of power over any emotional disorder.

Developing good habits of nutrition is critical in establishing good health. I review the patients' eating habits with them and make recommendations for improvement according to theories of traditional Five Element Nutrition. During treatment I emphasize the idea that for healthy minds, they need healthy bodies.

I usually expose my patients to two traditional Chinese medical concepts. The first is that emotional disorders typically occur coincident with physical disturbances in the major organ systems of the body. Second, all human beings can be categorized by type as having certain strengths and weaknesses of the major organ systems. I discuss body types and show the relationship between the body's weaknesses and emotional disorders. I encourage them to improve their mental and physical health by pursuing a program directed at strengthening the weakened organ systems. The program for self improvement is recorded in a series of taped sessions. The patients have cassette tapes that they bring to each session when a new installment of the self improvement program is given to them.

The program presented to them includes dietary changes directed at strengthening the weakened organs (Five Element Nutrition), positive visualization of organ health (the Inner Smile Meditation), physical manipulation of their body (Chi Nei Tsang), and mental exercises for stress relief of the organs (the Six Healing Sounds). In the pursuit of this program the patient is required to regularly attend to his/her own physical and emotional needs. A positive and aggressive health-conscious attitude is encouraged, and the patient begins to feel responsible for himself or herself.

Eventually the patients begin to see themselves as energetic beings with a responsibility to continuously monitor their emotional condition. Stress has to be constantly released. The patient comes to understand that emotional disturbances tend to amplify themselves and should be balanced as soon as practical. Positive emotions can be cultivated by establishing habits of physical and mental behavior that correspond to a positive world view and gratitude for life itself. I teach my patients that the physical being is the foundation of the energetic one. A holistic approach to mental and physical health is established during treatment so that they can continue through life by acting as their own healers. A few examples will serve to illustrate the development of this procedure."

A. Case One—Severe Depression

Description: Woman; 52 years old; single; no children; a telephone receptionist. She was one of a family of twelve children and close to her father who died during her adolescence. She was referred by a physician for severe depression and psychosomatic problems. At the start of her treatment she had not worked for six months.

Medical History: Tuberculosis in adolescence, operation and amputation of one lung and kidney. Complains of lack of energy and persistent cough and colds. Takes antibiotics and sleeping pills constantly. She is constipated and has cold hands and feet. She is tired of the telephone and of her job.

Habits: She has no friends, does not socialize or get out, does not eat well, cannot cook, and lives and works in a dusty environment.

Traditional Chinese Medical Observation:
- Type: Tai Yang, tall, slim, brown hair.
- Pulses: Kidney, hyperactive; lung, strong; heart, strong. All pulses are false yang type to compensate for weak yin.
- Emotions: Sadness, fear, worry.

Treatment: This woman was treated with one year of psychotherapy and acupuncture treatment at one week intervals. Initially, I listened to her fears about tuberculosis and her need to have a man and some friends in her life. I identified her tastes and desires, which included concerts and classical music, literature, theater, and writing.

I helped her modify her behavior. This included eating at regular intervals, drinking more juices, reducing the quantity of antibiotics and sleeping pills, and learning to cook. For her lungs she installed a humidifier at home, and placed eucalyptus oil in the water to be humidified and on the clothes she wore to work. I taught her dietary changes based on her typology and sickness and based on Five Element cooking.

She went back to work after the first seven months of treatment and she was more secure and ate and slept well. The persistent cough was reduced and intervals between respiratory problems increased to three or four months. The frequency of her therapy was reduced to once a month.

In the second year of her treatment, I introduced her to additional ways of caring for herself. She was offered various methods of self-relaxation and she selected the Healing Tao practices of the Inner Smile and the Six Healing Sounds. She practiced for six months without any of her symptoms reoccurring. She began to study literature at the university. As a part of her therapy, I taught her how to build an energetic lung and energetic kidney. She learned how to channel the energy from those organs. She only had two colds that winter. Six months later I offered her CNT, a self-healing massage therapy that she can use on herself. I started by balancing the navel and Wind Gates and proceeded to skin detoxification. I then detoxified the lungs and kidneys using the Six Healing Sounds. Then I worked on the large and small intestines, heart, liver and spleen, and finished by working on the lymph system.

The patient developed an increased feeling of control over her life and health. She continued working and studying, and joined a group in a museum. She developed a circle of friends and became confident that she could handle the emotional and physical problems in her life.

B. Case Two—Schizophrenic Paranoia with Catatonic Periods

Description: Male; 35 years old; single; no children. He is working on a Masters Degree thesis that is incomplete. He is unable to live a conventionally complex life and is not able to complete his university work while living with someone. He was not referred by a physician but came by himself. He felt unable to continue his therapy with another woman psychologist who had rejected his offer of love.

Medical History: He had previous treatment for depression with a psychiatrist after the death of his father when he was 20 years old. He complains of pain and cramps in the abdomen and the navel area, insomnia, constipation, bad digestion, and constant fatigue.

Habits: He has lived alone for five years and has no friends. He stays in contact with his family. He does not cook or eat regularly. He does not do exercise or sleep well. He takes drugs, anti-depressive and others.

Traditional Chinese Medical Observation:
• Type: Yang Ming, average size.
• Pulses: all low (weak by blockage); the body is not weak.
• Emotions: Anger, fear, and hatred.

Treatment: This man was treated with psychotherapy, acupuncture, and massage each week for two years to help him express his emotions.

At the beginning of the treatment, he expressed all of his emotions by grimaces and other physical behavior. His dreams also portrayed his disturbed emotions vividly. As the treatment progressed, the patient expressed a lot of anger and hatred against his father who didn't care for his desire to be a hockey player, and instead wanted him to work on the family farm. He was angry with his mother whom he accuses of neglect and lack of expressed love. He discussed the fear and belief that every woman has had an incestuous relationship: his grandmother, mother, sisters, niece, girlfriends, and his previous psychologist. He often expressed a desire for suicide. The therapy and acupuncture treatments have had some success. He had good periods but, in general, he still refused to do anything for himself or for others. He slept all the time, was not active, and had no outside interests. He did not want to succeed in anything that would have pleased his father. He repeatedly asked his therapists to send him to a hospital so he could be completely dependent. As an alternative his mother agreed to live with him. Afterwards he could not support the idea of his sister visiting with her children. If his mother prepared for a trip, he would stop eating and taking care of himself.

During the second year of his treatment I discussed the possibility of doing some relaxation exercises at home. I started to teach him the Inner Smile and the Six Healing Sounds. I introduced him to the practices very slowly, one organ at each session. I took special care that he thoroughly understood each practice before advancing to the next. I did not allow him to come to the group session and practice the Microcosmic Orbit because of the intensity of his sexual disorder.

As he practiced the Healing Sounds and the Inner Smile, he gradually stopped grimacing and began to be able to speak about his real emotion. He wanted to kill himself because he had always wanted to kill his father. When his father died, his subconscious dream was realized, and his feeling of culpability blocked his ability to strive for success or self-realization. It stopped his work, his research on his thesis, his personal relationships and resulted in him living more and more in isolation. With all his problems he still wanted to work his way out of his sickness. This was manifested by his asking for information on the medical drugs he was taking and by his intention to follow a program of physical activities that would be difficult to maintain because of the pain and cramps in his abdomen, lack of appetite, and constipation.

I recommended Chi Nei Tsang as a kind of massage that he could practice on himself each day to accelerate his healing. I started slowly to teach him how to balance the groin and navel area, and I told him to practice it for two weeks. After this we worked on skin detoxification. We realized that all the organs were hard and blocked, particularly the liver, heart, and spleen. To get rid of the tension in these three vital organs, the patient and I decided together to work on the lower organs, the small and large intestines. I taught him to massage the Chi in the abdominal area. He practiced the massage on himself in conjunction with the Six Healing Sounds that he previously learned. I then gave him a diet to aid his digestion and to help with his constipation. After this we started to work on the gall bladder, liver, heart, spleen, and stomach. The tension and blockages were so deep that we worked for two months on those organs. Finally, the kidneys were the most difficult to reach and massage because of the muscular tension in the abdomen. There was a lot of burping and yawning during these treatments. He often cried and expressed his fear of staying sick all of his life, and his fear about not wanting to work.

After four months of sessions, the pain and tension in the abdomen started to release. He began to accept the idea of eating the food that he needs at each meal. He began to take a walk each day for fifteen minutes, and increased it until he was walking an hour a day. The patient developed a greater interest in the drug treatment he was receiving from his psychiatrist and, after some discussions and reading about his particular condition, he requested his psychiatrist to reduce the drug dosage he was taking. During the last two months he has taken better care of himself, his clothes, and his health. He is now more aware of what is around him. He is beginning to help his mother with the dishes. He washes his own clothes and goes by himself to his therapy sessions. Finally, he has resumed work on his thesis.

C. Case Three—Anguish, Neurosis, and Paranoia

Description: Woman; 43 years old; one of eleven children; single; one child. She worked as an artist and educator in a national museum. She was the oldest daughter in the family and was abused by her mother from childhood until she was nineteen. Her mother was an artist who ended her career when she was married. Her father was a teacher who never interfered with the behavior of his wife. He provided no emotional support to his abused daughter, but at the age of eleven he told her he was praying for the death of his wife.

Medical History: Blockage in the intestines, insomnia, pain in the neck, shoulders and upper part of the back. The patient had an extremely negative image of herself, she saw herself as a bad mother and found it difficult to keep friends or a lover. She still worked but complained of a lack of energy and difficulty in finding the emotional support in her environment for her creative work.

Habits: She lives alone, visits her daughter every two weeks or so, and has a boyfriend that visits her occasionally. She has some friends in other cities. She does not eat regularly and has no physical activities or hobbies.

Traditional Chinese Medical Observation:
- Type: Shao Yin, large bones, white skin, cold feet.
- Pulses: Weak kidneys, spleen, stomach and lungs.
- Emotions: Worry, sadness, anger, hatred and fear.

Treatment: This woman was treated with acupuncture and analysis combined, followed by Chi Nei Tsang. At the beginning of the treatment, during the acupuncture sessions, the patient expressed a series of negative emotions. Primarily she feared to be touched, to suffer, and to have pain. She related these fears to the ill treatment from her mother. She remembered many specific experiences. We could not proceed quickly but waited two weeks between each treatment to allow her time to express the negative emotions liberated by the treatment. After she expressed the fear of pain, she was able to talk about her sadness at not being respected by her family or helped by them. The sadness was related to the stomach cramps and other difficulties in the intestinal tract. The third emotion to appear was anger at having been in situations of abuse, and at having to do things by herself again without any help. She refused any kind of responsibility in this emotional pattern. "I've been beaten, and I am responsible for that—NO!," she would yell. The fourth emotion that surfaced was hatred of her mother.

She dreamed about killing her and could not support this idea. She started to ask for another kind of help such as relaxation techniques because she knew she could not go to the point of acting out these dreams. I tried to teach her the Inner Smile, but she was not able to smile at herself. She still had a very poor opinion of herself and too many negative emotions. I started teaching her the Six Healing Sounds, so she could learn how to transform the destructive emotions in the organs into positive ones. She felt that the negative emotions were not being released because they were too intense and deep. To help her with this, I suggested to her that when the negative emotion appeared, she could surround it with a ball of light and try to look at the emotion as it is captured and surrounded, not overflowing and out of control.

During this stage of the treatment she began to associate specific emotional memories with her present emotions. We continued these exercises each week for three months before she felt comfortable enough to do them by herself at home. During those three months she gradually overcame the fear of what other deep emotions she would discover within herself. She elected to take a seminar on the Microcosmic Orbit Meditation, but was unsuccessful. She was not yet able to tolerate group participation because of her poor self image of being unloved and socially undesirable. She was also still rejecting the concept of self responsibility and still carrying some of her negative emotions.

Then she received individual instruction in the Microcosmic Orbit Meditation. The purpose was to activate the energy trapped in the lower abdomen and help the transformation of negative emotions such as anger and hatred, and particularly sadness. Her self image was still very poor. Her language was expressive. Some analogies she uses about herself were: garbage bag, dirty pig, or a poor dog that nobody can love. I suggested that she identify a positive animal image within herself that she likes and then seek out these qualities within her behavior. She selected a dolphin, and I asked her to find one thing a day to do so she can enjoy life like a dolphin. At this point in the treatment I discussed the concept of integrating a self-administered massage therapy, Chi Nei Tsang, into her program of self-help. I explained that Chi Nei Tsang helps to release tension in the center of the abdomen and in the organs; this would help her to release her grip on the negative emotions.

Initially the navel was very cold and the pulse of the navel was empty. The major tension was located in the heart and liver. The other organs were weak, but did not have as much tension in them. We started the massage at the navel, opened the Wind Gates, and then moved on to skin detoxification. It was still very difficult for her, she would twist and voice her fear. We talked about it and decided that she would practice the massage by herself for one month. We would then continue at the clinic with a more gentle massage to help her get in touch with her body so that she could integrate a good experience of being touched softly with a better awareness of her body.

When she began the work at the clinic, she started to feel a deep pain in the neck and shoulder. I taught her a way to channel that pain out by using the bladder and gall bladder meridian. She questioned, "What will I do without the pain? I only have that." She finally accepted the responsibility of taking the pain out. We started again with Chi Nei Tsang and deeply massaged the liver, heart, spleen, stomach, and kidneys. She was more receptive and readily accepted responsibility for performing the practice herself. I emphasized the importance of taking time after massaging each organ to leave her hands over the organ and let the energy of the associated color enhance the area. Subsequently, we added the balancing of the pulses.

She eventually acquired a full range of self healing practices, including Tai Chi, the Six Healing Sounds, the Inner Smile, the Microcosmic Orbit, and Chi Nei Tsang. She now has a new "toolbox" of meditations to work with. She has to use these "tools" to have results and has to accept the responsibility for her own healing.

D. Summary

Each human being that comes to me is unique. There are no formulas for introducing each one to the responsibilities and practices of self-healing. Most of them come with habitual behavior that requires them to distance themselves from their emotions, to look at these emotions mentally, and then forget them. They came to me for help because this behavior has been unsuccessful.

Some people do not just forget disturbing emotions. They can begin transforming negative emotions to positive emotions after fully remembering and then confronting the life experience that started the problem. Western psychoanalytic techniques help these individuals to retrieve their disturbing life experiences. The therapist can help the patient to understand the associated emotions and then capture them in a positive image. In agreement with the energy techniques of Tao Master Mantak Chia, I use a large ball of good energy, a Chi ball, to surround the bad emotion. The technique of capturing the negative emotional energy for transformation to positive energy is typical Taoist methodology. It is based on the principle of conserving life-force energy, which advocates the preservation of emotional energy. According to this concept, an individual who goes through life releasing large quantities of negative emotions often becomes progressively weaker and less able to preserve the emotional stability necessary to function effectively in society. Alternatively, if the negative emotions can be transformed and used to strengthen the individual, then that individual is less likely to fall victim to physical and emotional disorder.

The transformation of the emotions is a Taoist extension of the traditional Chinese medical concept of the theory of five emotions. This theory, in one of its more simple expressions, states that: fear produces anger, anger results in hatred, hatred leads to worry, worry increases sadness, and sadness causes more fear (the Law of Creation). This model for the sequence of the emotions is then superimposed on the five major organ groups: kidneys, liver, heart, spleen, and lungs. The meditative techniques of the Tao taught by Master Chia begin at this point and show how to transform the emotions from negative to positive.

The problem with using these techniques directly in my work is that the Tao transformation formulas are intended for use by the emotionally stable who seek to further purify their lives. I use Western style psycho-analytic techniques to bridge the gap between the deeply disturbed and safe use of the Taoist transformation techniques.

I am the first patient in my clinic each morning. I work on myself and make the Healing Tao System an essential support in cleaning the negative emotional energy I receive from the people who come to my clinic. At the same time the Healing Tao System is an excellent tool for transformation for them. The Taoist spiritual disciplines I practice insure that each day I start my work with a strong and healthy body, a clear mind, an open heart, and a clean Spirit.

Chi Nei Tsang

CHAPTER 14

INTERVIEWS AND CASE HISTORIES

A. INTERVIEWS

1. Interview One with an Acupuncture Therapist and Chinese Herbologist:

Q: Tell us your experiences.

A: I have been using CNT in my practice. I incorporate it with acupuncture sessions, and I do have many cases that have very good results. There are so many that I don't know where to start. I'll offer the most recent one.

A woman in her 60's had several severe surgeries on her neck, on her lower back, and for lung cancer. She just came to me two or three weeks ago. When she first came in, she had to be carried upstairs to my office. She used a cane to walk with. She has been under the care of a hospital. They've given her all kinds of drugs, medications, and training in pain management. She said often the pain would be so bad that she could just jump out the window and commit suicide. Basically the pain was in the head, neck, and back.

In her first session I was very cautious, so all I did was CNT without any needling. After I worked on her abdominal area for about ten minutes, I suggested that she try to stand up to see how she felt. At first she was very afraid of moving her body, especially her back. So I encouraged her to trust in herself and to try to move just a little on the table. She did this and then tried bigger movements. She found she was much looser. So I worked on her a few more minutes and asked again that she try to get up off the table. She finally did. She

375

got up and walked around not needing her cane. She was so excited and had a big smile. When I asked her about her level of improvement, she said she felt about 40% better.

In a second case I worked with a woman in her 30's. She was a very capable and successful business woman. Once she came to me complaining of a lump in her breast. She was afraid she would need surgery. I started using CNT and, as expected, I found a very sensitive spot on the abdominal area. While I was working on it, she could tell that the lump was getting softer and, gradually, flatter. I worked on this sensitive spot of the abdomen for about ten minutes and then needled the spot. After the sessions I gave her some herb tea. In all, it took about three sessions. After that, the lump was gone.

2. Interview Two with a Massage Therapist:

Q: Please tell us your history.

A: Last year I came for the first time to the CNT workshop. I had been to several workshops with Master Chia, and I thought that this would be very interesting to add to the Reiki work I had been doing. When I came back from the workshop, my father suddenly became very ill. He had been on some heart/circulatory medication and suddenly they decided that he needed open heart surgery, a quadruple by-pass. They found that all his peripheral arteries where blocked as well as his coronary arteries. He decided that he had been on medication for too long and he wanted to do something about this. He asked, "Is there anything that you can do?" I asked him to come and see me right away. When he arrived he was very grey. I had never seen anybody that grey who was still alive. He was very weak, very frail, and had lost a great deal of weight.

I found that what the doctors had said apparently was true. There was very little blood flow. When I checked the pulses around the body, there seemed to be very little blood flowing anywhere except in one arm. Everything else seemed completely clogged.

I worked on that for some time using Reiki, CNT and the Buddha Palm. Eventually I saw his face become pink, and I thought that something is now happening. His first reaction was to tell me he was very tired when he came in, but now he didn't feel as tired anymore. He also did not feel cold anymore. When that session was over, he was feeling warm and his skin was pink all over. Before he went home I taught him some skin detoxification, because I didn't want to work too deeply on him with the massage. He was so frail at that point. I told him to do skin detoxification, the Heart's Sound, and deep breathing to relax. He had experienced terrible problems with angina, so I used my training in hypnotherapy to work with the fear he had about it happening again. Half the problem with the angina was that he was afraid it would happen again and this would cause everything to become tense. Therefore, it happened more often than it would have.

Q: Did you feel there was any particular aspect of CNT that worked well for him?

A: I could feel that the arteries were clearing, and that the blood flow was there again. It hadn't been there when I started, but it was there when I finished. Something had happened.

Q: So were you doing general CNT massage?

A: I didn't do everything the first time. I did a little skin detoxification. What I worked on primarily were the arteries and veins. I was trying to get the blood circulation to improve.

Q: You worked with the aorta then?

A: Yes, basically a lot of that was because it was not functioning properly at all. I wanted to get the blood to go into the peripheral arteries and veins to try to flush the areas because everything was clogged up. It was caused partly by diet, by lifestyle, and by all those other things that happen to people. He said he felt a lot better, and he seemed to have more energy. He went home and my mother said he was working on things. The next week when he came in, he looked better. He said he had more energy, and he wasn't tired as often. He had been to the doctor who checked his peripheral veins. He told the doctor that he didn't feel the same as he had felt before. But the doctor didn't believe him. My father said "I want a different doctor." He's been working with the techniques for about ten months now, and he's much better. He doesn't have the pain or angina anymore.

Q: How many hours of CNT would you say you gave him?

A: I gave him about four hours over a period of three weeks. He says he's still working on the detoxification and sometimes he does the Healing Sound. He was also told that he had trouble with his liver and that he had cancer there. I didn't want to work too much on that. They said it was just a matter of time. That was last winter. After this trouble with the heart, they told him about the liver because he kept losing weight. Now he's stopped losing weight and seems to be okay. That's my experience with my father. I've had some experiences with other people as well.

A lady came to me about three months ago who was told that she had cancer of the jaw. It was a lump that was visible on the x-ray. She hadn't been able to heal it because it had been growing, and she was frightened it was growing too fast. They were going to do a biopsy. I didn't want to do the actual manipulation, because I didn't want to take the chance of spreading the cancer. So I did some Reiki and a double beam of Buddha Palm on her jaw. She said suddenly that she didn't feel it as much anymore, and when I finished, she said she didn't feel it at all. She felt as if it had been cauterized with this intense heat, but she didn't feel the heat on the surface of the skin. Instead she felt it in the jaw, in the bone itself where the growth was

Q: Did she get any clinical examinations after that?

A: I don't know; I've lost contact with her. But I saw her twice, and the second time she said she hadn't felt that bump in the week between her first and second visits. She said she had been feeling it constantly before that. She felt it had been burned out of her by the energy. I don't know if that's been clinically confirmed or not. I do know that my father's case is documented and that they are taking him off the heart medication now.

3. Interview Three with a CNT Student:

Q: What was your experience with Chi Nei Tsang?

A: My experience with CNT was quite incredible. I didn't know what to expect, but I went in with an open mind. It was really a very simple session; it wasn't complex. It began with spiraling around my navel area. I was worked on first by Larry Tupper. He explained to me that the navel area connects the organs and different functions of the body and coordinates them. So any blockages would, therefore, be reflected in that area. As he began to work on me, he explained that there were small knots, twists, and pea-shaped knots that could be released through gently spiraling and lightly shaking them.

The pressure was light. At first I didn't feel anything other that a very mild amount of pressure on my abdomen. Then, one by one, I felt the little peas that he was working on melt and disappear. He continued to spiral circularly, working on different areas around the navel. I could feel deeper tension there in the connective tissue, the fasciae, surrounding the muscles. He explained to me that there was an imbalance. My navel was pulling slightly to one side. To correct it, it would be necessary to relieve the tension in that area.

After a while the pressure felt a little more intense as he went deeper working on releasing deeper blockages. I began to feel the effect of the spiraling and the release of those points on my navel. I could feel the sense of energy moving around my navel area more than I ever had in any of my meditations. I was concentrating and working with the Microcosmic Orbit to keep the flow of energy moving.

As the session progressed I could feel the strength of my experience with the Microcosmic Orbit Meditation and an increased perception of the energy flowing in a spiral around my navel. It was not until the end of the session that I started to feel a tremendous state of relaxation that gradually increased as the session ended. He had circled often in a gradually wider area around the navel. I felt light. I felt my shoulders were relaxed; I felt the tension dissolve in my neck. I felt any lower back tension I had release. When I closed my eyes, I could see a spiral coming from my navel that suddenly had grown immense and very strong, almost like a large wave circling my entire aura.

Larry told me after the session to get up slowly and sit up carefully. After a few moments I stood up and started to move around. I felt such an incredible experience, as though I was in a different plane and incredibly light.

Q: Besides having these wonderful sensations right after the session, do you feel the experience has had some lasting physical effects in terms of any problems, ailments, or the like?

A: Yes, I can say that I've had increased strength in my meditations and that I've continued to maintain a relaxed state. The tremendous effect of the session that I felt within the first few hours of its completion—an intensity of relaxation and state of almost floating—gradually wore off. That was partially due to the Tai Chi and Chi Kung class that I took very shortly after the session which caused me to enter another mode.

Q: When you mentioned relaxation, you said you were more relaxed than ever before. Before the session, did you have problems relaxing?

A: Yes. I had chronic tension in my shoulders, and I had pain in my lower back that would come and go in spite of being athletic and involved in many sports and in good health. I couldn't alleviate tension in those parts of my body. The session really had a profound effect on that.

Q: You mentioned your lower back. Did the discomfort continue in any way after the session?

A: The discomfort didn't return, but as I exercised intensely over the next few days, particularly working with the Tai Chi and Chi Kung exercises, I found myself creating a large amount of energy flowing through my body. I could feel the deeper blockages in the sacral and abdominal area. I could sense my lack of complete harmony. The imbalances I had became more evident, and even though the effect of the session stayed with me, I became more aware of those areas that needed further attention.

Q: I take it that it really heightened your sensitivity and awareness of your body. Would that be a correct statement?

A: Absolutely! Incredibly so. It very much heightened my sensitivity to my organism and the energy flow within my body.

Q: Now you mentioned the first time you were treated by Larry. Where have you been treated subsequently?

A: I've been treated, but not by a practicing CNT teacher or an experienced practitioner. That was a unique experience, and I can't compare anything else I tried to it.

Q: Do you have anything else to add to this statement?

A: Well I'd definitely like to say that through this experience of working with Larry Tupper, I realized the profound potential of CNT. That is a very important aspect of the session that will stay with me for the rest of my life.

4. Interview Four with a CNT Student:

Q: How did you get involved with the Healing Tao and Chi Nei Tsang?

A: Four years ago I took a course in Cambridge and a couple of other courses with Mantak Chia. I thought they were very interesting. Last year (1989) I attended the Chi Nei Tsang retreat and enjoyed it quite a bit.

Q: Have you practiced other forms of massage in the past?

A: About five years ago I attended a healing massage course, and I participated in many different types of massages. This gave me an overview of several different methods.

Q: How do you find Chi Nei Tsang relates to the experiences you had with the other techniques?

A: The others treat the full body, and they are a little more pleasure oriented. Mantak Chia's system goes right into the stomach area, and it might be more powerful.

Q: Did you have the opportunity to practice with people, or did you practice it on yourself? How have you used the techniques you have learned?

A: Mostly just on myself. Larry Tupper, a practitioner in Boston, has done several sessions over the last year. They have been fantastic.

Q: So you practiced Chi Nei Tsang sessions on yourself with a certified therapist?

A: Correct.

Q: What sort of experiences and results did you have with that?

A: When I had a hectic week, it was very balancing. I run a business, and we have up to twelve crews running around. So I go in many different directions. When I get a session, it fully centers, balances, and grounds me. It has always worked out very effectively.

Q: Have you had any health problems where you really needed therapy?

A: I have had severe mood swings for the last eight years. In the last six years, I have checked out different things that have helped to balance out things. The Healing Tao practices have been the most effective.

Q: Have you incorporated Chi Nei Tsang into the general spectrum of the Healing Tao practice, and is that an easy thing for you to do?

A: Certainly. The easiest thing in the world to do is to wake up in the morning and go right into your belly area and start massaging it. When you feel tightened areas, loosen them and get any excess heat out. This balances you right away and feels good.

Q: Do you have anything else to add?

A: Yes, it is a very nice system and a good way to balance oneself. It's very effective. I'd like to see it spread.

5. Interview Five with a CNT Student

Q: I understand that you had the opportunity to be involved with some sessions given by some instructors. How did it feel, and what sort of experience did you have?

A: The first experience with Master Chia was very new to me, and he worked very deeply in the area round the navel. It was very painful. I had an operation ten years ago, and everything in that area was knotted up, but I was not aware that there was still tension remaining there. I have had therapies such as massage, acupuncture, and other sessions to help release it, but there was still work that needed to be done. I could feel the effects of Master Chia's demonstration for about three days.

Later I had a session with Ron Diana. I was suffering from sciatic pain for the last three years because of the operation, and my left hip was bothering me. During the session with Ron, I relived the experience of the operation in detail, and I was crying as I went back through this memory in my body. A tremendous amount of cold energy came out of my hip; it was a cold wind that surprised both of us very much. After the session I felt completely empty and tired, and I just wanted to go to sleep. Since this session my belly has been smooth and free of tensions. This has helped me a lot, and I have improved in my Tai Chi and Iron Shirt practices. Previously, I was not able to hold the postures since I was too tense and could not practice the form smoothly.

6. Interview Six with a CNT Student

Q: Have you taken the Chi Nei Tsang workshop?

A: Yes, I attended a workshop in Europe for four days with Master Chia. That was two years ago.

Q: Did you learn a lot from that workshop?

A: Yes, I feel I learned a lot, but I have practiced mainly on myself. I have had some great experiences with it, but I saw that you need to practice it every day, as it seemed new knots and tensions accumulated that needed to be worked out. I like to practice in the evenings before I go to bed. It helps soothe and relax me and helps me fall asleep. The work I have done on myself has helped me to get in touch with my organs and inner structure. I have medical student friends who find it amazing that I can palpitate my abdomen and find my kidneys, liver, and other organs. For me Chi Nei Tsang is a very nice experience.

Q: Do you find that the Chi massage benefits you in your other Tao practices?

A: Oh, yes, because it is difficult to release all the tensions and blockages using only the Microcosmic Orbit. Chi Nei Tsang helps me to get more of a feeling for what's going on.

Q: Do you find that it helps you as a Healing Tao instructor?

A: Yes, of course. It is helpful in guiding other people to learn how to get in touch with their bodies, and it gives me an awareness of where people may have knots or tensions.

Q: Have you worked with anyone other than yourself?

A: Yes, I have done some work with members of my family, especially with my little five year old brother. It was very nice and relaxing for him. It seems that this massage is very beneficial and enjoyable for younger children.

7. Interview Seven with a CNT Practitioner and Senior Instructor

Q: Master Chia says that when people have high blood pressure we should be careful of using the blood flushing technique because too much energy blood can go to the head. What do you do to avoid that? Where do you press down?

A: That's a good question. The first thing is your intention. Just as you can direct the energy up or down in the Microcosmic Orbit, you can also influence the direction of energy in this practice by your intention. But that's something that comes with practice. You can also have the person use his or her intention to work with you in directing the energy down. You can also open the areas it could flow down to, especially the legs, and femoral arteries. So, if it's not flowing down or if there are blockages, open them in the navel area so that there is less congestion. That's why we stress the importance of the pulse at the femoral artery and the pulses at the back of the knee and ankle. The whole body has to be freed of congestion gradually so that the pressure can be normalized. Then you use your intention and gentle pressure in the beginning to bring the energy down.

Q: So it's usually safe to work first on the lower pulses. Many people have tendencies toward high blood pressure.

A: Yes, sometimes the blood pressure rises. But determining this comes with experience, so it's hard to generalize. Often there is a lot of tension at the center, basically because all the blood is flowing through the center. If there is a lot of tension here and those large vessels and arteries (the aorta and vena cava) are congested, they will begin to squeeze and the pressure will rise. So just by releasing the center, you can affect the pressure and normalize it to some extent.

Q: So it might take more than one session.

A: Definitely, there is no rush; you can take your time. By affecting the surface you will also affect beneath the surface. Because wherever you touch the body, the effect is felt deeply. In another, more advanced level of the Healing Tao practice called *Cosmic Chi Kung*, you can deeply affect the body without ever touching it.

Q: When you start working with new students, how do you determine how often they should come to you?

A: It depends on your assessment of how much the students can detoxify, and how much they can handle emotionally, physically, and spiritually. Another important consideration is their willingness to participate in their own healing to gain deeper knowledge of their own bodies. If they do their homework by practicing the Inner Smile, Six Healing Sounds, and Microcosmic Orbit techniques to quiet themselves down and circulate the energy, you may be able to work at a faster pace. Ultimately you have to assess several factors to determine the frequencies of their visits with you.

The most important thing is not to make people dependent on you. Each one must participate in self-healing. They shouldn't feel that they always have to come to you. This system is set up for people to help themselves grow and become independent. I don't know of any other healing system that so conscientiously tries to teach people how to care for themselves. If they don't use it, what can we do?

Q: But you can't tell people not to come if they don't do anything for themselves; you have an established practice, but they don't.

A: You get better and better at making this assessment. For example, you might notice that some come back more often. Don't try to get everybody to come back to you. Continue to teach those people how to become more independent, more empowered. In my experience this allows your practice to grow more.

When you're good, people will attend. So you don't have to worry about it. Your purpose will become more and more clear to them. Your purpose is not to take care of everybody, not in this system as opposed to many other systems whose common purpose *is* to take care of people. The idea, like all parts of Taoism, is to teach people how to take care of themselves.

There are so many people in the world who are never going to receive any decent health care. Do you know how expensive Western medicine is? Even doctors do not necessarily receive good health care.

This system can serve the basic health needs of the whole world. It's all in there. I've been doing Chi Nei Tsang for a long time, and I'm still amazed by how effective it is. But first people are going to have to develop confidence in the whole system, and understand their own body energy. They must build the confidence that they can apply the system to themselves. That is our role. How often do you have the opportunity to help people in such a way? It's the best feeling you can have. Chi Nei Tsang offers a great deal.

Q: What do you do for emotional problems?

A: The Inner Smile and the Six Healing Sounds are very helpful. That surprises a lot of people because these exercises are so simple. People wonder, "How could something so simple as some vowels and a smile be so powerful?" Those two meditations are very, very simple and very, very powerful.

Before treating a person, talk to that person about what you're actually going to do so that they have some kind of a framework to go by. Have them come to classes; give them a list of books that are available so that they can go home and practice. Start by explaining simple kinds of feedback; give them something to take with them. People like to have something when they go home. Don't open more than the person can handle. Finding that level comes through sensitivity and experience.

Q: How can people work on themselves?

A: I think an easy way for people to work on themselves is to sit in a chair, bend over, and lean their weight into their fingers. You can work directly on the abdomen this way. You also can work on yourself lying down, but be sure to elevate your knees. Find out how to release knots, blockages, tangles, and emotional stress. It's so important and so simple.

Q: Can you work on the nerves of the spine?

A: It all can be done, but I wouldn't start with telling a person that you can adjust the nerves or the disc since this work is extremely deep.

Q: Practitioners agree that it is healthy to work around the navel. You work the energy up, free the blood and Chi, and then just let it take off and do what it has to do. Has this been your experience?

A: Yes, it's that simple. Every single day you should rub your belly. This is a good practice to give to the general public.

B. CASE HISTORIES

1. Charles

Charles is a middle-aged man. He is a chef in a fancy Italian restaurant and lives with Zoe, whose case history follows. He came on the suggestion of Zoe. His mental and physical health were weakening from non-stop work, from early morning to late night, seven days per week. He felt compelled to go to work even on his single day off. Because his relationship with Zoe was suffering a great deal, he believed that he was on the verge of a nervous breakdown. One day at work he started crying for no apparent reason and had to take the rest of the day off. I saw Charles the day after this event; he came with Zoe.

a. First Session

Charles is not the talkative type. Zoe started to talk about how he didn't eat in a healthy and regular manner, and how he drank too much champagne. He said that he could not eat because he was around food all the time and he denied drinking too much. When I touched him, the liver area was pretty hard and swollen. The whole stomach was distended, and the entire ventral cavity looked congested to the point of being ready to burst.

I began with skin detoxification while simultaneously softly massaging the gut to give some internal motion. After about ten minutes we heard the first gurgling sounds. I then moved to the rib cage, working first under the left side and subsequently under the right. The hardness gave way allowing me to work on tonifying the organs and cleansing the emotions.

Soundless tears started to come profusely and, as I worked on the lung points there was a great sob of release. As the pressure released it became easier to work in the abdominal cavity. I then worked on the peristalsis of the intestine, releasing tension and pressure from the gut.

At the end of the first session, Charles looked very rested and remarked that he was "floating in his pants." He could tighten up his pants a good three more notches. I told him that I could not do anything for him if he did not take some time off from work for rest, start to eat properly, and cut down on drinking and eating sweets.

b. Second Session

This time Charles came by himself. He told me that he could not work on himself very efficiently. He did, however, take a day off from work and did not think about the restaurant at all. He went fishing with some friends and had a great time. I easily got deeper this time, working on tangles and knots. I worked on winds and spent a long time on the liver and gall bladder area.

2. Zoe

Zoe is a middle-aged Belgian who has an eighteen year old daughter and a six year old son. She is visiting the United States with her son and is currently living with Charles, the chef described above. She was referred by Christine, another Belgian woman, who is a regular student. Her main complaints included a tight stomach, and always feeling nervous to the point of being very easily irritated.

a. First Session

Her muscles were very tight, so I did Shiatsu for her shoulders, neck, and back, having her breathe into the abdomen. She had a hard time here, as her chest automatically pumped the air up, making her shoulders rise with every breath.

She started to breathe calmly after I worked on her stomach region for fifteen minutes. I then worked smoothly but deeply under the rib cage in her left side, freeing loud gurgling sounds.

I found a lot of tension throughout the gut and worked on moving the intestines rhythmically in a calming motion. I baked the liver for a long time.

b. Second Session

She reported feeling very good after the first session. She felt less anxiety and more rested after sleep. She still feels discomfort in her abdomen. This was a general session. We worked on winds and emotional clearing.

c. Third Session

Zoe feels better and better. She is less irritable and more relaxed, has decided to look for a job, and wants to be more active and worry less.

This session involved the same work as session two.

d. Fourth Session

Zoe's gut feels looser. She had a little bit of diarrhea during the week which made her feel lighter in the abdomen.

e. Fifth Session

Her doctor told her she had a dropped bladder. This was a general session, focusing on deep kidney work and the bladder technique (i.e., dropping the legs while holding the bladder up from behind). The bladder went back into place with a big gurgling sound.

f. Sixth Session

Zoe feels better and better. She is talking about the "bladder miracle." Her mood is definitely better, and her breathing is fuller.

We had a general session.

3. Ted

The student is a doctor in his early 50's who has generally been in good health.

a. First Session

His pulses reveal an energy deficiency in the bladder, liver, and lungs. His tongue is loaded with "white moss," indicating a Chi deficiency. I taught him how to smile down to the organs and thank them for all their work over the years. I taught him the Lungs Sound. Then I did general detoxification of the skin and activated the lung holding points. I noted some hard knots and marked them on the chart. He said he enjoyed the session. I was very relieved since he was a doctor, and I dearly wanted to impress him and make him feel better.

b. Second Session

I focused on clearing the digestive track, the large intestine, and the ileocecal vale. I taught the Lungs and Kidneys Sounds and did the Inner Smile. The doctor said, "This is a great technique, and I seem to be feeling better."

c. Third Session

His pulses were normalizing. The pain and soreness were alleviating. I taught him the rest of the Healing Sounds, and how to Smile Down the midline and spinal column. He continues to feel better.

d. Fourth Session

All the pulses show Chi deficiency. He may be having a healing crisis. I intend to allow more space between this and the next session. We did all three parts of the Inner Smile, detoxified the spleen, and did some lymph drainage. At the end he said he felt much better and more energized.

e. Fifth Session

I detoxified the kidneys and the gall bladder. All his pulses are strong. He feels that this massage has improved his overall health. I told him to keep practicing.

4. Olga

a. First Session

She has a very large belly with the navel off center to the right. All the pulses were weak. She had extreme pains in her back, left knee, stomach, and was experiencing headaches. After session one her left knee felt better. I taught her the Lungs Sound.

b. Second Session

She experienced more energy for a whole week after our first session. Her knee felt better, but her headaches were worse. We worked on session two and energized the lung points. Her pulses were much stronger and there was more energy in the belly. I couldn't find any lymph, perhaps I didn't get deep enough. She said her headache was much better. I gave her homework and Healing Sounds to do.

c. Third Session

She had pains all over her belly on both sides. She is very fidgety, and her central large intestine is full and sensitive. Her headache was better after the session. I worked on the Healing Sounds.

d. Fourth Session

Her knee, head, and back were all better. There has been a general improvement. Her head is clearer, and the pulses are even. I did deep work. Her large intestine was full and hard. I worked on that a bit. It was painful, but she eventually fell asleep.

e. Fifth Session

She said that she felt great the day after the last session, and was feeling pretty good all week until she found out her good friend died. I massaged her colon and worked deeply all over her body. Eventually she fell asleep.

f. Sixth Session

There is only one tender part left in her belly. Her pulses are even. Her skin is itchy "on and off." She says her knee and her leg are much better, and her headaches have gone. She is more cheerful and active and her memory has improved.

5. Larry

Larry is in his thirties. He is lean, but of muscular constitution. He broke up with his girlfriend two months ago, with whom he was living for three years. He had been drinking heavily and taking too many drugs. He was distressed and depressed to the point of feeling suicidal. He quit his job and became apathetic. He was seeing a psychologist, who urged him to start a program of detoxification at once. He came for sessions because of poor sleep, anxiety attacks, and poor digestion and appetite.

a. First Session

I first worked on his shoulder and neck, chest and diaphragm to release the breathing process. Then I worked at length on the lung points. He fell deeply asleep, with deep and heavy snoring that vibrated all the way down the chest. While he was asleep, I worked on the digestive tract for an hour. The liver and ascending colon were particularly crowded. The small intestine felt hard and tight. Since he didn't wake up, I worked deeply, though he could have felt pain. Big gurgling sounds came out all over the digestive tract. He woke up as I was finishing and patting his stomach. He called me about two hours later, telling me that he hadn't felt so well in months and that he could eat with an appetite again.

b. Second Session

The superficial layer of the abdomen was no longer tight. This allowed me to reach a deeper level of tension in the small intestine that I couldn't feel during the previous session. I did a general CNT session, concentrating on the liver.

c. Third Session

Larry told me that he had recovered from his apathy and that in a week he had found a new job and a new place to live. He's also taking long walks every day. I gave a general session.

6. Denise

Denise is a young woman in her early thirties. She is working as a head nurse in a hospital. She's also teaching in a nursery school. She's

391

working lots of hours on different shifts and is under constant stress, caught between patients, the administration, and doctors. She came in because of tensions resulting from stress accumulation and pain in the back.

a. First Session

I worked on the diaphragm and released the breathing process, working on the lung points.

b. Second Session

I gave a general CNT session, working on the digestive tract that felt hard and bloated. I worked on the stomach, Triple Warmer, spleen, and two big knots or tensions located approximately at five and seven o'clock around the navel.

c. Third Session

Her tension released more that sixty percent. She reported feeling much better, having better digestion, appetite, and cleaner energy. During sessions she had an emotional release and reported experiencing unusual feelings. There were big gurgling sounds in the liver, gall bladder, heart constrictor, spleen, and Triple Warmer areas. I released hard matter in the small intestine.

d. Fourth Session

I gave a general session, and there was more release everywhere in the stomach. I worked on the wind that attacks the liver and the heart.

e. Fifth Session

She reports feeling much better. The previous session released tensions that allowed uncovering what feels like older tensions in the lower abdomen. I gave a general session, working deeper on the large intestine, small intestine, bladder, and kidneys.

7. Eva

a. First Session

Eva, who is 40, has a lot of tension in her belly. Her energy is very loud, and emotionally she is very quarrelsome. I did a general first session. She wants to get pregnant but can't because her abdomen is totally blocked. I taught her the Inner Smile and encouraged her to massage around her navel.

b. Second Session

She did her homework well. It's incredible how I was then able to touch her belly. She couldn't handle anyone touching the scar on her right side. As I neared her rib cage, she would get nervous. She was not able to breathe or relax as I gently tried to massage and pull down her diaphragm.

c. Third Session

She came back from the holidays with a stiff neck. I did a normal session with her. I did a lot of belly massage, and we did the Inner Smile and some of the Sounds. I gave her homework.

d. Fourth Session

Her belly was tight and full of tension and pain. I could hardly touch it, especially the area around the scar. I worked very softly around the navel and opened the Wind Gates. She felt her circulation to be stronger than it was last week. She had only done a little homework during the last week.

e. Fifth Session

She became more responsible and really did do her homework, and gradually she became less dependent on me. She had a very weak body, but if she kept working on herself, she should get better.

She commented, "I feel like my body is getting stronger. I have regular bowel movements now, which hasn't happened in years; I have always taken laxatives. Since I do the Inner Smile and self-massage in the morning, my whole day feels light and easy. I sleep better when I do the Healing Sounds."

f. Sixth Session

I could see that she was practicing every day; the tensions around the scar were lessening. There was a lot more work to do on her, but I thought she had reached a point where she can help herself, and not depend so much on me. This was our last session because I left for the States. She knows all the Healing Sounds, and I told her to read Master Chia's book.

Eva told me, "I'm very grateful that you taught me this incredible technique. I'm going to miss my weekly appointment, but now I have something to do on myself that helps me. This is incredible, I've never experienced something like this. Thanks, I want to study more about this system."

8. Sharon

a. First Session

Sharon is 50. The congestion on her right side is especially pronounced and deep. It is affecting her psoas, the entire hip joint, ligament capsule, and piriformis muscle. A left knee injury is possibly causing compensating tightness. CNT and lower abdominal massage released the hip joint, and there is much more freedom of movement. The lower back is flatter and looser.

Sharon commented, "The work today released energy in the whole right side. It felt more balanced with the left. I feel very energized all over, especially around my sacrum and the top of my head."

I introduced her to the Healing Tao System, and encouraged her to take courses in the Microcosmic Orbit, Tai Chi, and Fusion I.

I also asked her to observe her energy levels during the week.

b. Second Session

I taught her the Microcosmic Orbit, detoxified her abdomen, and instructed her in Chi Self-Massage. I did lung, liver, and kidney strengthening points as well as other body work and lymphatic drainage. Although there was still tension in the right side, it was less than before.

c. Third Session

I did abdominal detoxification which increased her lung and kidney Chi. We discussed emotional issues of letting go of fear, anger, and judgments, and instead taking hold of personal power and loving herself. I encouraged her to practice Chi Self-Massage and taught her the Inner Smile. She commented that she felt peaceful and content, and that there was much less tension in her back and hips.

d. Fourth Session

I did abdominal detoxification. Her entire abdomen was much more relaxed and the energy was much more even, although the kidney and heart pulses were a little weak.

Sharon commented, "My abdomen feels great. It's not painful anymore; it feels open. My period is regular again, and there is no pain. Meditating is easier and more powerful."

e. Fifth Session

We reviewed the Healing Sounds and Inner Smile. Her stomach was upset today, so I did abdominal detoxification and opened the Wind Gates. She was releasing the emotion of sadness during the entire session. I didn't feel it was appropriate to spend much time on the Healing Sounds, and I just let her experience and release her sadness and grief. Her heart and spleen pulses were weak, so I balanced those meridians.

Sharon told me that she felt clearer, more at peace, and was learning to let go of control and trust more. She feels that the abdominal work has helped her to come to this point of letting go. I think that she needs more detoxification and wind work.

9. John

John is a young man in his early 30's. He is conscious of fitness and well-being. His complaint includes poor digestion for the past few months, bloated feelings in the stomach, poorly formed stools and weak appetite. John has been driving a taxicab for the past few months and relates his problems to the sitting position, aggravated by the stress of driving in heavy traffic throughout the city all day long. The sessions lasted four months.

a. First Session

John was developing a little potbelly. The skin two inches around the navel was swollen. I spent most of the first session doing skin detoxification.

I found a tender spot in the lower right quadrant that radiated a pain in the left chest. There was another tight spot in the lower left quadrant that would give pain under the rib cage on the right side. The right side of the abdomen was much more congested than the left side. There was a rod-like feeling between the lower right side of the rib cage and the navel. When pressed, the extremity of that tension, which was about one-half to one inch long, would stabilize the navel in a round and relaxed manner.

I sent him home with a lot of skin detoxification to do every day until the next session the following week.

b. Second Session

John reported working faithfully every day on his belly. He felt better from his first session; it had a positive effect on his digestion and elimination.

The tensions were lighter but still there. I worked at length on his right side, liver area, lungs, kidneys, bladder, and small and large intestine. When I applied pressure to the abdomen, the pain in his chest was gone. He reported that his breathing was easier.

c. Third Session

His condition was stationary. John reported working hard on his belly. Stools had a stronger shape and the constipation was gone. His appetite was better. The tension, however, was still there, especially that rod-like feeling on the right side.

d. Fourth Session

His condition was unchanged.

e. Fifth Session

Again, his condition remained unchanged.

f. Sixth, Seventh, Eighth, and Ninth Sessions

Throughout each of these sessions, spaced two weeks apart, John's condition remained unchanged.

g. Tenth Session

John came to the session with a great big smile. Something had happened during the week. He said, "This week I gave up coffee. I haven't been drinking coffee for five days. The first two days were terrible because of withdrawal symptoms and headaches. But on the third day, as I was doing my daily routine on my stomach, the big tension on my right side cleared out."

When I touched him, I felt immediately that he was right. The rod-like tension on the right side was not there anymore and after a few minutes of deep massage in the guts, everything else cleared out.

John was happy. He came back for a last session and check-up one week later, and everything was fine. He looked like he had lost some weight.

10. A Testimony

The following testimony was received by a CNT practitioner from his student, a woman, who received weekly sessions for one year.

"The most obvious change I have experienced since I have been receiving Chi Nei Tsang session is with my digestive system. I used to be constipated or have loose bowels constantly and a lot of gas. It is now very regular, even when I travel. That didn't use to be the case.

My whole abdomen has always felt bloated, swollen, and uncomfortable. My upper abdomen looks and feels completely different. It is not bloated anymore; my waist is a lot smaller.

I have had horribly painful cramps since the first time I had my period. I no longer experience them. My sexual organs are much more alive and sensitive. My sternum feels looser. My shoulders are where they should be, not stuck higher than their natural position. The thoracic vertebrae are looser. My lower back is not as curved as it used to be. My legs are lighter; I used to get pins and needles often. My whole body feels elongated, lighter, stronger, alive. Everybody asks me if I have lost weight, I haven't—I am just not bloated anymore.

I am now totally aware of what is happening in my body. I know if it is a nerve feeling, or if it comes from a movement in my intestine, or if it comes from a muscle. I can differentiate very easily. It has been a wonderfully exciting experience. I knew all along I was going to get great results. I trusted you completely. I didn't know that the changes would be so great and would make me a different person. We got rid of tensions that had been accumulating in my abdomen since I was born, probably. I would probably have been a perfect candidate for endometriosis.

I learned a lot about myself during the sessions. Most pains that have occurred during the sessions were familiar. Some had been forgotten. I forgot to mention that I had PMS. It's nothing now compared to what it was. My sex life is better also. Everything has improved; I am a new person. Thanks a million."

Chi Nei Tsang

Bibliography and Recommended Books

Barral, Jean-Peirre and Mercier, Pierre, *Visceral Manipulation* (Eastland Press, Seattle, 1988).

Blofeld, John, *Taoism, The Quest for Immortality*, (Mandala Books, London, 1979).

Chopra, Deepak, M.D., *Quantum Healing*, (Bantam Books, New York, 1989).

Connelly, Dianne M., *Traditional Acupuncture: The Law of Five Elements*, (The Centre [sic] for Traditional Acupuncture, Inc., Columbia, MD, 1979).

Flaws, Bob and Wolfe, Honora Lee, *Prince Wen Hui's Cook* (Paradigm Publications, Brookline, MA, 1983).

Hammer, Leon, M.D., *Dragon Rises, Red Bird Flies*, (Station Hill Press, Inc., Barrytown, NY, 1990).

Kapit, Wynn and Elson, Lawrence M., *The Anatomy Coloring Book* (Harper and Row, New York, NY, 1987).

Kapit, Wynn, Macey, Robert I., and Meisami, Esmail, *The Physiology Coloring Book* (Harper and Row, New York, NY, 1987).

Kaptchuk, Ted J., *The Web That Has No Weaver*, (Congdon & Weed, New York, 1983).

Keleman, Stanley, *Emotional Anatomy*, (Center Press, .Berkeley. CA, 1985).

Kushi, Michio, *Oriental Diagnosis: What Your Face Reveals*, (Sunwheel Publications, London, 1981).

Low, Royston, *The Secondary Vessels of Acupuncture*, (Thorsons Publishers, Inc., New York, 1983).

Maciocia, Giovanni, *The Foundations of Chinese Medicine*, (Churchill Livingstone, London & New York, 1989).

Maciocia, Giovanni, *Tongue Diagnosis in Chinese Medicine*, (Eastland Press, Seattle, 1987).

Maspero, Henri, *Taoism and Chinese Religion*, (The University of Massachusetts Press, Amherst, 1981).

Matsumoto, Kiiko and Birch, Stephen, *Hara Diagnosis: Reflections on the Sea*, (Paradigm Publications, Brookline, MA, 1988).

Rauch, Erich, *Diagnostik Nade F.X. Mayr*, (Haug-Verlag, Heidelberg, 1077).

Veith, Ilza (trans.), *The Yellow Emperor's Classic of Internal Medicine*, (U. of California, Berkeley, 1949).

Weiss, Helmut, Dr. Med., *Kranker Darm—Kranker Voerper*, Haug-Verlad, Heidelberg, 1988).

Williams, P.L., Warwick, R., Dyson, M., Bannister, L. H., *Gray's Anatomy*, 37th Edition, (Churchill Livingstone, New York, 1989).

Worsley, J.R., *Traditional Chinese Acupuncture, Vol. 1, Meridians and Points* (Element Books, Witshire, England, 1982).

Yang Jwing-Ming, *Muscle/Tendon Changing and Marrow/Brain Washing Chi Kung*; and *The Root of Chinese Chi Kung* (Yang's Martial Arts Association, Jamaica Plain, MA, 1989).

Sucessful mastery of Chi Nei Tsang is contingent upon your sucessful development using the techniques and meditations of the entire Healing Tao system. A complete listing of the available tapes and books follows this section.

THE
INTERNATIONAL
HEALING TAO SYSTEM

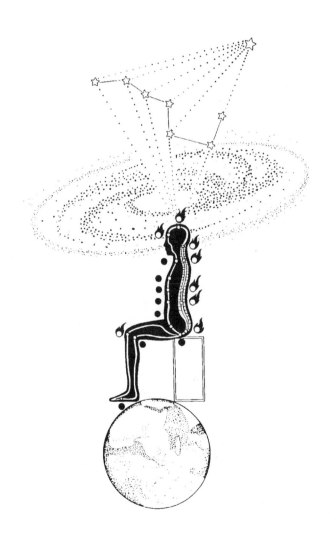

The Goal of the Taoist Practice

The Healing Tao is a practical system of self-development that enables the individual to complete the harmonious evolution of the physical, mental, and spiritual planes the achievement of spiritual independence.

Through a series of ancient Chinese meditative and internal energy exercises, the practitioner learns to increase physical energy, release tension, improve health, practice self-defense, and gain the ability to heal oneself and others. In the process of creating a solid foundation of health and well-being in the physical body, the basis for developing one's spiritual independence is also created. While learning to tap the natural energies of the Sun, Moon, Earth, and Stars, a level of awareness is attained in which a solid spiritual body is developed and nurtured.

The ultimate goal of the Tao practice is the transcendence of physical boundaries through the development of the soul and the spirit within man.

International Healing Tao Course Offerings

There are now many International Healing Tao centers in the United States, Canada, Bermuda, Germany, Netherlands, Switzerland, Austria, France, Spain, India, Japan, and Australia offering personal instruction in various practices including the Microcosmic Orbit, the Healing Love Meditation, Tai Chi Chi Kung, Iron Shirt Chi Kung, and the Fusion Meditations.

Healing Tao Warm Current Meditation, as these practices are also known, awakens, circulates, directs, and preserves the generative life-force called Chi through the major acupuncture meridians of the body. Dedicated practice of this ancient, esoteric system eliminates stress and nervous tension, massages the internal organs, and restores health to damaged tissues.

Outline of the Complete System of The Healing Tao

Courses are taught at our various centers. Direct all written inquiries to one central address or call:

The Healing Tao Center
P.O. Box 1194
Huntington, NY 11743

To place orders please call: 1-800-497-1017
or for overseas customers: 1-717-325-9380
Fax: 1-717-325-9357

INTRODUCTORY LEVEL I: Awaken Your Healing Light

Course 1: (1) Opening of the Microcosmic Channel; (2) The Inner Smile; (3) The Six Healing Sounds; and (4) Tao Rejuvenation—Chi Self-Massage.

INTRODUCTORY LEVEL II: Development of Internal Power

Course 2: Healing Love: Seminal and Ovarian Kung Fu.

Course 3: Iron Shirt Chi Kung; Organs Exercise and Preliminary Rooting Principle. The Iron Shirt practice is divided into three workshops: Iron Shirt I, II, and III.

Course 4: Fusion of the Five Elements, Cleansing and Purifying the Organs, and Opening of the Six Special Channels. The Fusion practice is divided into three workshops: Fusion I, II, and III.

Course 5: Tai Chi Chi Kung; the Foundation of Tai Chi Chuan. The Tai Chi practice is divided into seven workshops: (1) Original Thirteen Movements' Form (five directions, eight movements); (2) Fast Form of Discharging Energy; (3) Long Form (108 movements); (4) Tai Chi Sword; (5) Tai Chi Knife; (6) Tai Chi Short and Long Stick; (7) Self-Defense Applications and Mat Work.

Course 6: Taoist Five Element Nutrition; Taoist Healing Diet.

INTRODUCTORY LEVEL III: The Way of Radiant Health

Course 7: Healing Hands Kung Fu; Awaken the Healing Hand—Five Finger Kung Fu.

Course 8: Chi Nei Tsang; Organ Chi Transformation Massage. This practice is divided into three levels: Chi Nei Tsang I, II, and III.

Course 9: Space Dynamics; The Taoist Art of Energy Placement.

INTERMEDIATE LEVEL: Foundations of Spiritual Practice

Course 10:
Lesser Enlightenment Kan and Li: Opening of the Twelve Channels; Raising the Soul, and Developing the Energy Body.

Course 11: Greater Enlightenment Kan and Li: Raising the Spirit and Developing the Spiritual Body.

Course 12: Greatest Enlightenment: Educating the Spirit and the Soul; Space Travel.

ADVANCED LEVEL: The Immortal Tao (The Realm of Soul and Spirit)

Course 13: Sealing of the Five Senses.

Course 14: Congress of Heaven and Earth.

Course 15: Reunion of Heaven and Man.

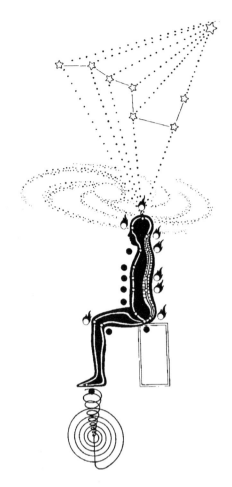

Course Descriptions of The Healing Tao System

INTRODUCTORY LEVEL I: Awaken Your Healing Light
Course 1:

A. The first level of the Healing Tao system involves opening the Microcosmic Orbit within yourself. An open Microcosmic Orbit enables you to expand outward to connect with the Universal, Cosmic Particle, and Earth Forces. Their combined forces are considered by Taoists as the Light of Warm Current Meditation.

Through unique relaxation and concentration techniques, this practice awakens, circulates, directs, and preserves the generative life-force, or Chi, through the first two major acupuncture channels (or meridians) of the body: the Functional Channel which runs down the chest, and the Governor Channel which ascends the middle of the back.

Dedicated practice of this ancient, esoteric method eliminates stress and nervous tension, massages the internal organs, restores health to damaged tissues, increases the consciousness of being alive, and establishes a sense of well-being. Master Chia and certified instructors will assist students in opening the Microcosmic Orbit by passing energy through their hands or eyes into the students' energy channels.

B. The Inner Smile is a powerful relaxation technique that utilizes the expanding energy of happiness as a language with which to communicate with the internal organs of the body. By learning to smile inwardly to the organs and glands, the whole body will feel loved and appreciated. Stress and tension will be counteracted, and the flow of Chi increased. One feels the energy descend down the entire length of the body like a waterfall. The Inner Smile will help the student to counteract stress, and help to direct and increase the flow of Chi.

C. The Six Healing Sounds is a basic relaxation technique utilizing simple arm movements and special sounds to produce a cooling effect

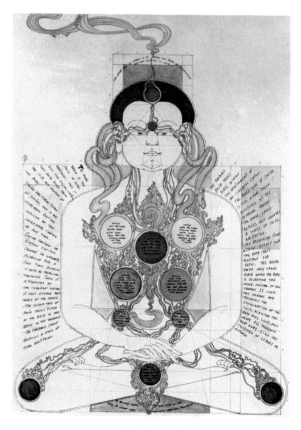

Catalog-5

upon the internal organs. These special sounds vibrate specific organs, while the arm movements, combined with posture, guide heat and pressure out of the body. The results are improved digestion, reduced internal stress, reduced insomnia and headaches, and greater vitality as the Chi flow increases through the different organs.

The Six Healing Sounds method is beneficial to anyone practicing various forms of meditation, martial arts, or sports in which there is a tendency to build up excessive heat in the system.

D. Taoist Rejuvenation—Chi Self-Massage is a method of hands-on self-healing work using one's internal energy, or Chi, to strengthen and

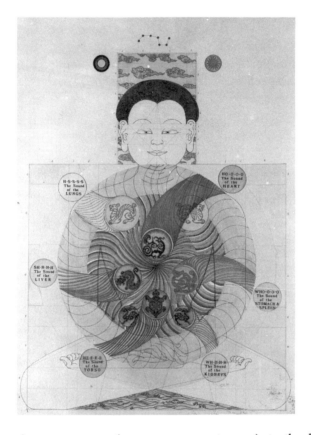

rejuvenate the sense organs (eyes, ears, nose, tongue), teeth, skin, and inner organs. Using internal power (Chi) and gentle external stimulation, this simple, yet highly effective, self-massage technique enables one to dissolve some of the energy blocks and stress points responsible for disease and the aging process. Taoist Rejuvenation dates back 5000 years to the Yellow Emperor's classic text on Taoist internal medicine.

Completion of the Microcosmic Orbit, the Inner Smile, the Six Healing Sounds, and Tao Rejuvenation techniques are prerequisites for any student who intends to study Introductory Level II of the Healing Tao practice.

INTRODUCTORY LEVEL II: Development of Internal Power

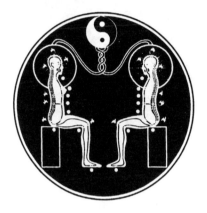

Course 2: *Healing Love: Seminal and Ovarian Kung Fu; Transforming Sexual Energy to Higher Centers, and the Art of Harmonious Relationships*

For more than five thousand years of Chinese history, the "no-outlet method" of retaining the seminal fluid during sexual union has remained a well-guarded secret. At first it was practiced exclusively by the Emperor and his innermost circle. Then, it passed from father to chosen son alone, excluding all female family members. Seminal and Ovarian Kung Fu practices teach men and women how to transform and circulate sexual energy through the Microcosmic Orbit. Rather than eliminating sexual intercourse, ancient Taoist yogis learned how to utilize sexual energy as a means of enhancing their internal practice.

The conservation and transformation of sexual energy during intercourse acts as a revitalizing factor in the physical and spiritual development of both men and women. The turning back and circulating of the generative force from the sexual organs to the higher energy centers of the body invigorates and rejuvenates all the vital functions. Mastering this practice produces a deep sense of respect for all forms of life.

In ordinary sexual union, the partners usually experience a type of orgasm which is limited to the genital area. Through special Taoist techniques, men and women learn to experience a total body orgasm without indiscriminate loss of vital energy. The conservation and transformation of sexual energy is essential for the work required in advanced Taoist practice.

Seminal and Ovarian Kung Fu is one of the five main branches of Taoist Esoteric Yoga.

Course 3: *Iron Shirt Chi Kung;*
Organs Exercises and
Preliminary Rooting
Principle

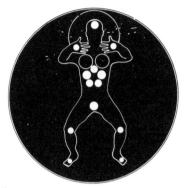

The Iron Shirt practice is divided into three parts: Iron Shirt I, II, and III.

The physical integrity of the body is sustained and protected through the accumulation and circulation of internal power (Chi) in the vital organs. The Chi energy that began to circulate freely through the Microcosmic Orbit and later the Fusion practices can be stored in the fasciae as well as in the vital organs. Fasciae are layers of connective tissues covering, supporting, or connecting the organs and muscles.

The purpose of storing Chi in the organs and muscles is to create a protective layer of interior power that enables the body to withstand unexpected injuries. Iron Shirt training roots the body to the Earth, strengthens the vital organs, changes the tendons, cleanses the bone marrow, and creates a reserve of pure Chi energy.

Iron Shirt Chi Kung is one of the foundations of spiritual practices since it provides a firm rooting for the ascension of the spirit body. The higher the spirit goes, the more solid its rooting to the Earth must be.

Iron Shirt Chi Kung I—Connective Tissues' and Organs' Exercise: On the first level of Iron Shirt, by using certain standing postures, muscle locks, and Iron Shirt Chi Kung breathing techniques, one learns how to draw and circulate energy from the ground. The standing postures teach how to connect the internal structure (bones, muscles, tendons, and fasciae) with the ground so that rooting power is developed. Through breathing techniques, internal power is directed to the organs, the twelve tendon channels, and the fasciae.

Over time, Iron Shirt strengthens the vital organs as well as the tendons, muscles, bones, and marrow. As the internal structure is strengthened through layers of Chi energy, the problems of poor posture and circulation of energy are corrected. The practitioner learns the importance of being physically and psychologically rooted in the Earth, a vital factor in the more advanced stages of Taoist practice.

Iron Shirt Chi Kung II—Tendons' Exercise: In the second level of Iron Shirt, one learns how to combine the mind, heart, bone structure, and Chi flow into one moving unit. The static forms learned in the first level of Iron Shirt evolve at this level into moving postures. The goal of Iron Shirt II is to develop rooting power and the ability to absorb and discharge energy through the tendons. A series of exercises allow the student to change, grow, and strengthen the tendons, to stimulate the vital organs, and to integrate the fasciae, tendons, bones, and muscles into one piece. The student also learns methods for releasing accumulated toxins in the muscles and joints of the body. Once energy flows freely through the organs, accumulated poisons can be discharged out of the body very efficiently without resorting to extreme fasts or special dietary aids.

Iron Shirt Chi Kung I is a prerequisite for this course.

Bone Marrow Nei Kung (Iron Shirt Chi Kung III)—Cleansing the Marrow: In the third level of Iron Shirt, one learns how to cleanse and

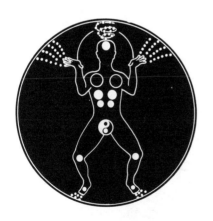

grow the bone marrow, regenerate sexual hormones and store them in the fasciae, tendons, and marrow, as well as how to direct the internal power to the higher energy centers.

This level of Iron Shirt works directly on the organs, bones, and tendons in order to strengthen the entire system beyond its ordinary capacity. An extremely efficient method of vibrating the internal organs allows the practitioner to shake toxic deposits out of the inner structure of each organ by enhancing Chi circulation. This once highly secret method of advanced Iron Shirt, also known as the Golden Bell System, draws the energy produced in the sexual organs into the higher energy centers to carry out advanced Taoist practices.

Iron Shirt Chi Kung is one of the five essential branches of Taoist Esoteric Practice.

Prior study of Iron Shirt Chi Kung I and Healing Love are prerequisites for this course.

Course 4: ***Fusion of the Five Elements,***
Cleansing of the Organs, and
Opening of the Six Special Channels

Fusion of the Five Elements and Cleansing of the Organs I, II, and III is the second formula of the Taoist Yoga Meditation of Internal Alchemy. At this level, one learns how the five elements (Earth, Metal, Fire, Wood,

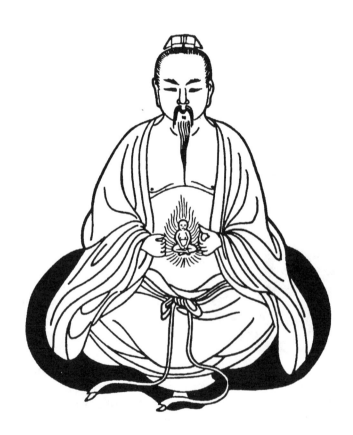

and Water), and their corresponding organs (spleen, lungs, heart, liver, and kidneys) interact with one another in three distinct ways: producing, combining, and strengthening. The Fusion practice combines the energies of the five elements and their corresponding emotions into one harmonious whole.

Fusion of the Five Elements I: In this practice of internal alchemy, the student learns to transform the negative emotions of worry, sadness, cruelty, anger, and fear into pure energy. This process is accomplished by identifying the source of the negative emotions within the five organs of the body. After the excessive energy of the emotions is filtered out of the organs, the state of psycho/physical balance is restored to the body. Freed of negative emotions, the pure energy of the five organs is crystallized into a radiant pearl or crystal ball. The pearl is circulated in the body and attracts to it energy from external sources—Universal Energy, Cosmic Particle Energy, and Earth Energy. The pearl plays a central role in the development and nourishment of the soul or energy body. The energy body then is nourished with the pure (virtue) energy of the five organs.

Fusion of the Five Elements II: The second level of Fusion practice teaches additional methods of circulating the pure energy of the five organs once they are freed of negative emotions. When the five organs are cleansed, the positive emotions of kindness, gentleness, respect, fairness, justice, and compassion rise as a natural expression of internal balance. The practitioner is able to monitor his state of balance by observing the quality of emotions arising spontaneously within.

The energy of the positive emotions is used to open the three channels running from the perineum, at the base of the sexual organs, to the top of the head. These channels collectively are known as the Thrusting Channels or Routes. In addition, a series of nine levels called the Belt Channel is opened, encircling the nine major energy centers of the body.

Fusion of Five Elements III: The third level of Fusion practice completes the cleansing of the energy channels in the body by opening the positive and negative leg and arm channels. The opening of the Microcosmic Orbit, the Thrusting Channels, the Belt Channel, the Great Regulator, and Great Bridge Channels makes the body extremely permeable to the circulation of vital energy. The unhindered circulation of energy is the foundation of perfect physical and emotional health.

The Fusion practice is one of the greatest achievements of the ancient Taoist masters, as it gives the individual a way of freeing the body of negative emotions, and, at the same time, allows the pure virtues to shine forth.

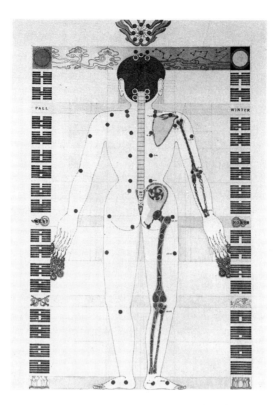

Course 5: *Tai Chi Chi Kung; The Foundation of Tai Chi Chuan*

The Tai Chi practice is divided into seven workshops: (1) the Original Thirteen Movements' Form (five directions, eight movements); (2) Fast Form of Discharging Energy; (3) Long Form (108 movements); (4) Tai Chi Sword; (5) Tai Chi Knife; (6) Tai Chi Short and Long Stick; (7) Self-Defense Applications and Mat Work.

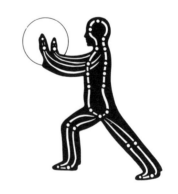

Through Tai Chi Chuan the practitioner learns to move the body in one unit, utilizing Chi energy rather than muscle power. Without the circulation of Chi through the channels, muscles, and tendons, the Tai Chi Chuan movements are only physical exercises with little effect on the inner structure of the body. In the practice of Tai Chi Chi Kung, the increased energy flow developed through the Microcosmic Orbit, Fusion work, and Iron Shirt practice is integrated into ordinary movement, so that the body learns more efficient ways of utilizing energy in motion. Improper body movements restrict energy flow causing energy blockages, poor posture, and, in some cases, serious illness. Quite often, back problems are the result of improper posture, accumulated tension, weakened bone structure, and psychological stress.

Through Tai Chi one learns how to use one's own mass as a power to work along with the force of gravity rather than against it. A result of increased body awareness through movement is an increased awareness of one's environment and the potentials it contains. The Tai Chi practitioner may utilize the integrated movements of the body as a means of self-defense in negative situations. Since Tai Chi is a gentle way of exercising and keeping the body fit, it can be practiced well into advanced age because the movements do not strain one's physical capacity as some aerobic exercises do.

Before beginning to study the Tai Chi Chuan form, the student must complete: (1) Opening of the Microcosmic Orbit, (2) Seminal and Ovarian Kung Fu, (3) Iron Shirt Chi Kung I, and (4) Tai Chi Chi Kung.

Tai Chi Chi Kung is divided into seven levels.

Tai Chi Chi Kung I is comprised of four parts:

a. Mind: (1) How to use one's own mass together with the force of gravity; (2) how to use the bone structure to move the whole body with very little muscular effort; and (3) how to learn and master the thirteen movements so that the mind can concentrate on directing the Chi energy.

b. Mind and Chi: Use the mind to direct the Chi flow.

c. Mind, Chi, and Earth force: How to integrate the three forces into one unit moving unimpeded through the bone structure.

d. Learn applications of Tai Chi for self-defense.

Tai Chi Chi Kung II—Fast Form of Discharging Energy:

a. Learn how to move fast in the five directions.

b. Learn how to move the entire body structure as one piece.

c. Discharge the energy from the Earth through the body structure.

Tai Chi Chi Kung III—Long Form Tai Chi Chuan:

a. Learn the 108 movements form.

b. Learn how to bring Chi into each movement.

c. Learn the second level of self-defense.

d. Grow "Chi eyes."

Tai Chi Chi Kung IV—the Tai Chi Sword.
Tai Chi Chi Kung V—Tai Chi Knife.
Tai Chi Chi Kung VI—Tai Chi Short and Long Stick.
Tai Chi Chi Kung VII—Application of Self-Defense and Mat Work.
Tai Chi Chuan is one of the five essential branches of the Taoist practice.

Course 6: *Taoist Five Element Nutrition; Taoist Healing Diet*
Proper diet in tune with one's body needs, and an awareness of the seasons and the climate we live in are integral parts of the Healing Tao. It is not enough to eat healthy foods free of chemical pollutants to have good health. One has to learn the proper combination of foods according to the five tastes and the five element theory. By knowing one's predominant element, one can learn how to counteract imbalances inherent in one's nature. Also, as the seasons change, dietary needs vary. One must know how to adjust them to fit one's level of activity. Proper diet can become an instrument for maintaining health and cultivating increased levels of awareness.

INTRODUCTORY LEVEL III: The Way of Radiant Health

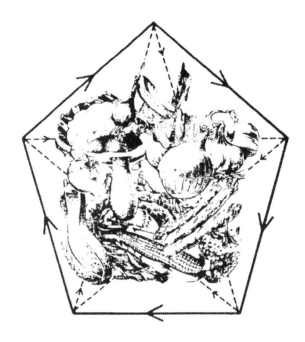

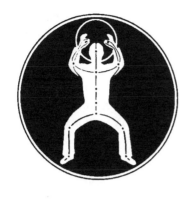

Course 7: *Healing Hands Kung Fu; Awaken the Healing Hand—Five Finger Kung Fu*

The ability to heal oneself and others is one of the five essential branches of the Healing Tao practice. Five Finger Kung Fu integrates both static and dynamic exercise forms in order to cultivate and nourish Chi which accumulates in the organs, penetrates the fasciae, tendons, and muscles, and is finally transferred out through the hands and fingers. Practitioners of body-centered therapies and various healing arts will benefit from this technique. Through the practice of Five Finger Kung Fu, you will learn how to expand your breathing capacity in order to further strengthen your internal organs, tone and stretch the lower back and abdominal muscles, regulate weight, and connect with Father Heaven and Mother Earth healing energy; and you will learn how to develop the ability to concentrate for self-healing.

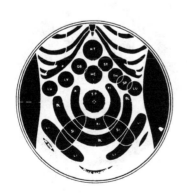

Course 8: *Chi Nei Tsang; Organ Chi Transformation Massage*

The practice is divided into three levels: Chi Nei Tsang I, II, and III.

Chi Nei Tsang, or Organ Chi Transformation Massage, is an entire system of Chinese deep healing that works with the energy flow of the five major systems in the body: the vascular system, the lymphatic system, the nervous system, the tendon/muscle system, and the acupuncture meridian system.

In the Chi Nei Tsang practice, one is able to increase energy flow to specific organs through massaging a series of points in the navel area. In Taoist practice, it is believed that all the Chi energy and the organs, glands, brain, and nervous system are joined in the navel; therefore, energy blockages in the navel area often manifest as symptoms in other parts of the body. The abdominal cavity contains the large intestine, small intestine, liver, gall bladder, stomach, spleen, pancreas, bladder, and sex organs, as well as many lymph nodes. The aorta and vena cava divide into two branches at the navel area, descending into the legs.

Chi Nei Tsang works on the energy blockages in the navel and then follows the energy into the other parts of the body. Chi Nei Tsang is a very deep science of healing brought to the United States by Master Mantak Chia.

Course 9: *Space Dynamics; The Taoist Art of Placement*

Feng Shui has been used by Chinese people and emperors for five thousand years. It combines ancient Chinese Geomancy, Taoist Metaphysics, dynamic Psychology, and modern Geomagnetics to diagnose energy, power, and phenomena in nature, people, and buildings. The student will gain greater awareness of his own present situation, and see more choices for freedom and growth through the interaction of the Five Elements.

INTERMEDIATE LEVEL: Foundations of Spiritual Practice

Course 10: *Lesser Enlightenment (Kan and Li); Opening of the Twelve Channels; Raising the Soul andDeveloping theEnergy Body*

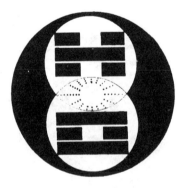

Lesser Enlightenment of Kan and Li (Yin and Yang Mixed): This formula is called *Siaow Kan Li* in Chinese, and involves a literal steaming of the sexual energy (Ching or creative) into life-force energy (Chi) in order to feed the soul or energy body. One might say that the transfer of the sexual energy power throughout the whole body and brain begins with the practice of Kan and Li. The crucial secret of this formula is to reverse the usual sites of Yin and Yang power, thereby provoking liberation of the sexual energy.

This formula includes the cultivation of the root (the Hui-Yin) and the heart center, and the transformation of sexual energy into pure Chi at the navel. This inversion places the heat of the bodily fire beneath the coolness of the bodily water. Unless this inversion takes place, the fire simply moves up and burns the body out. The water (the sexual fluid) has the tendency to flow downward and out. When it dries out, it is the end. This formula reverses normal wasting of energy by the highly advanced method of placing the water in a closed vessel (cauldron) in the body, and then cooking the sperm (sexual energy) with the fire beneath. If the water (sexual energy) is not sealed, it will flow directly into the fire and extinguish it or itself be consumed.

This formula preserves the integrity of both elements, thus allowing the steaming to go on for great periods of time. The essential formula is to never let the fire rise without having water to heat above it, and to never allow the water to spill into the fire. Thus, a warm, moist steam is produced containing tremendous energy and health benefits, to regrow all the glands, the nervous system, and the lymphatic system, and to increase pulsation.

The formula consists of:
1. Mixing the water (Yin) and fire (Yang), or male and female, to give birth to the soul;
2. Transforming the sexual power (creative force) into vital energy (Chi), gathering and purifying the Microcosmic outer alchemical agent;
3. Opening the twelve major channels;
4. Circulating the power in the solar orbit (cosmic orbit);
5. Turning back the flow of generative force to fortify the body and the brain, and restore it to its original condition before puberty;
6. Regrowing the thymus gland and lymphatic system;
7. Sublimation of the body and soul: self-intercourse. Giving birth to the immortal soul (energy body).

Course 11: *Greater Enlightenment (Kan and Li); Raising the Spirit and Developing the Spiritual Body*

This formula comprises the Taoist Dah Kan Li (Ta Kan Li) practice. It uses the same energy relationship of Yin and Yang inversion but increases to an extraordinary degree the amount of energy that may be

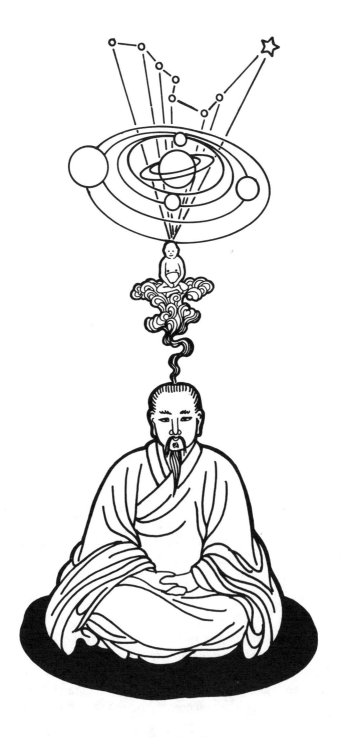

drawn up into the body. At this stage, the mixing, transforming, and harmonizing of energy takes place in the solar plexus. The increasing amplitude of power is due to the fact that the formula not only draws Yin and Yang energy from within the body, but also draws the power directly from Heaven and Earth or ground (Yang and Yin, respectively), and adds the elemental powers to those of one's own body. In fact, power can be drawn from any energy source, such as the Moon, wood, Earth, flowers, animals, light, etc.

The formula consists of:

1. Moving the stove and changing the cauldron;
2. Greater water and fire mixture (self-intercourse);
3. Greater transformation of sexual power into the higher level;
4. Gathering the outer and inner alchemical agents to restore the generative force and invigorate the brain;
5. Cultivating the body and soul;
6. Beginning the refining of the sexual power (generative force, vital force, Ching Chi);
7. Absorbing Mother Earth (Yin) power and Father Heaven (Yang) power. Mixing with sperm and ovary power (body), and soul;
8. Raising the soul;
9. Retaining the positive generative force (creative) force, and keeping it from draining away;
10. Gradually doing away with food, and depending on self sufficiency and universal energy;
11. Giving birth to the spirit, transferring good virtues and Chi energy channels into the spiritual body;
12. Practicing to overcome death;
13. Opening the crown;
14. Space travelling.

Course 12: *Greatest Enlightenment (Kan and Li)*

This formula is Yin and Yang power mixed at a higher energy center. It helps to reverse the aging process by re-establishing the thymus glands and increasing natural immunity. This means that healing energy is radiated from a more powerful point in the body, providing greater benefits to the physical and ethereal bodies.

The formula consists of:

1. Moving the stove and changing the cauldron to the higher center;
2. Absorbing the Solar and Lunar power;
3. Greatest mixing, transforming, steaming, and purifying of sexual

power (generative force), soul, Mother Earth, Father Heaven, Solar and Lunar power for gathering the Microcosmic inner alchemical agent;

4. Mixing the visual power with the vital power;
5. Mixing (sublimating) the body, soul and spirit.

ADVANCED LEVEL: The Immortal Tao
The Realm of Soul and Spirit
Course 13: *Sealing of the Five Senses*

This very high formula effects a literal transmutation of the warm current or Chi into mental energy or energy of the soul. To do this, we must seal the five senses, for each one is an open gate of energy loss. In other words, power flows out from each of the sense organs unless there is an esoteric sealing of these doors of energy movement. They must release energy only when specifically called upon to convey information.

Abuse of the senses leads to far more energy loss and degradation than people ordinarily realize. Examples of misuse of the senses are as follows: if you look too much, the seminal fluid is harmed; listen too much, and the mind is harmed; speak too much, and the salivary glands are harmed; cry too much, and the blood is harmed; have sexual intercourse too often, and the marrow is harmed, etc.

Each of the elements has a corresponding sense through which its elemental force may be gathered or spent. The eye corresponds to fire; the tongue to water; the left ear to metal; the right ear to wood; the nose to Earth.

The fifth formula consists of:

1. Sealing the five thieves: ears, eyes, nose, tongue, and body;
2. Controlling the heart, and seven emotions (pleasure, anger, sorrow, joy, love, hate, and desire);
3. Uniting and transmuting the inner alchemical agent into life-preserving true vitality;
4. Purifying the spirit;
5. Raising and educating the spirit; stopping the spirit from wandering outside in quest of sense data;
6. Eliminating decayed food, depending on the undecayed food, the universal energy is the True Breatharian.

Course 14: *Congress of Heaven and Earth*

This formula is difficult to describe in words. It involves the incarnation of a male and a female entity within the body of the adept. These two entities have sexual intercourse within the body. It involves the mixing of the Yin and Yang powers on and about the crown of the head, being totally open to receive energy from above, and the regrowth of the pineal gland to its fullest use. When the pineal gland has developed to its fullest potential, it will serve as a compass to tell us in which direction our aspirations can be found. Taoist Esotericism is a method of mastering the spirit, as described in Taoist Yoga. Without the body, the Tao cannot be attained, but with the body, truth can never be realized. The practitioner of Taoism should preserve his physical body with the same care as he would a precious diamond, because it can be used as a medium to achieve immortality. If, however, you do not abandon it when you reach your destination, you will not realize the truth.

This formula consists of:
1. Mingling (uniting) the body, soul, spirit, and the universe (cosmic orbit);
2. Fully developing the positive to eradicate the negative completely;
3. Returning the spirit to nothingness.

Course 15: *Reunion of Heaven and Man*

We compare the body to a ship, and the soul to the engine and propeller of a ship. This ship carries a very precious and very large diamond which it is assigned to transport to a very distant shore. If your ship is damaged (a sick and ill body), no matter how good the engine is, you are not going to get very far and may even sink. Thus, we advise against spiritual training unless all of the channels in the body have been properly opened, and have been made ready to receive the 10,000 or 100,000 volts of super power which will pour down into them. The Taoist approach, which has been passed down to us for over five thousand years, consists of many thousands of methods. The formulae and practices we describe in these books are based on such secret knowledge and the author's own experience during over twenty years of study and of successively teaching thousands of students.

The main goal of Taoists:
1. This level—overcoming reincarnation, and the fear of death through enlightenment;
2. Higher level—the immortal spirit and life after death;
3. Highest level—the immortal spirit in an immortal body. This body functions like a mobile home to the spirit and soul as it moves through the subtle planes, allowing greater power of manifestation.

Healing Tao Books

THE INNER STRUCTURE OF TAI CHI: Tai Chi Chi Kung I

This book is designed for Tai Chi practitioners of all levels. Stripping away the unnecessary mystery surrounding Tai Chi, Taoist Master Mantak Chia demonstrates, with the help of hundreds of drawings and detailed illustrations by Juan Li, the relationship of the inner structure of Tai Chi to the absorption, transformation, and circulation of the Three Forces, or energies—the Universal Force, the Cosmic Force, and the Earth 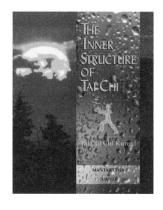 Force— that enliven us. The Inner Structure of Tai Chi is an indespensable resource for anyone who now practices or wants to learn a form of Tai Chi. Illustrated by Juan Li. Softbound. 182 pages.

$14.95 plus $3.95 for postage & handling
(Foreign Shipping: Please see page Catalog-38)
Order by Item No. B12

AWAKEN HEALING LIGHT *Of The Tao*

This book contains procedures that have been refined with over ten years of teaching experience at hundreds of workshops and feedback from thousands of students. *Awaken Healing Light of the Tao* clearly presents the most comprehensive instructions (basic and advanced) for realizing and developing our inherent energetic potentials. It explains in simple terms how to use the power of the mind to refine, transform, and 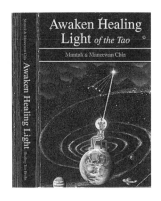 guide energy through the two primary acupuncture channels of the body which comprise the Microscomic Orbit. Practical methods for strengthening the immune system, recycling stressful energies, and restoring vibrant health are included. Illustrated by Juan Li. Softbound. 640 pages.

$16.95 plus $3.95 for postage & handling
(Foreign Shipping: Please see page Catalog-38)
Order by Item No. B11

TAOIST SECRETS OF LOVE:
CULTIVATING MALE SEXUAL ENERGY

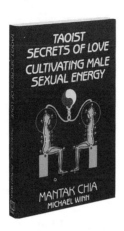

Master Mantak Chia reveals for the first time to the general public the ancient sexual secrets of the Taoist sages. These methods enable men to conserve and transform sexual energy through its circulation in the Microcosmic Orbit, invigorating and rejuvenating the body's vital functions. Hidden for centuries, these esoteric techniques make the process of linking sexual energy and transcendent states of consciousness accessible to the reader.

This revolutionary book teaches: Higher Taoist practices for alchemical transmutation of body, mind, and spirit; The secret of achieving and maintaining full sexual potency;

The Taoist "valley orgasm"—pathway to higher bliss;

How to conserve and store sperm in the body;

The exchange and balancing of male and female energies within the body, and with one's partner;

How this can fuel higher achievement in career, personal power, and sports.

This book, co-authored with Michael Winn, is written clearly, and illustrated with many detailed diagrams. Softbound. 250 pages.

$16.00 plus $3.95 for postage & handling
(Foreign Shipping: Please see page Catalog-38)
Order by Item No. B02

HEALING LOVE THROUGH THE TAO: CULTIVATING FEMALE SEXUAL ENERGY

This book outlines the methods for cultivating female sexual energy. Master Mantak Chia and Maneewan Chia introduce for the first time in the West the different techniques for transforming and circulating female sexual energy. The book teaches: The Taoist internal alchemical practices to nourish body, mind, and spirit;

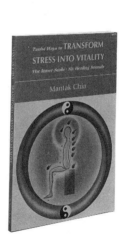

How to eliminate energy loss through menstruation;

How to reduce the length of menstruations;

How to conserve and store ovary energy in the body;

The exchange and balance of male and female energies within the body, and with one's partner;

How to rejuvenate the body and mind through vaginal exercises.

Written in clear language by Master Mantak Chia and Maneewan Chia. Published by Healing Tao Books. Softbound. 328 pages.

$14.95 plus $3.95 for postage & handling
(Foreign Shipping: Please see page Catalog-38)
Order by Item No. B06

TAOIST WAYS TO TRANSFORM STRESS INTO VITALITY

The foundations of success, personal power, health, and peak performance are created by knowing how to transform stress into vitality and power using the techniques of the Inner Smile and Six Healing Sounds, and circulating the smile energy in the Microcosmic Orbit.

The Inner Smile teaches you how to connect with your inner organs, fall in love with them, and smile to them, so that the emotions and stress can be transformed into creativity, learning, healing, and peak performance energy.

The Six Healing Sounds help to cool down the system, eliminate trapped energy, and clean the toxins out of the organs to establish organs that are in peak condition. By Master Mantak Chia. Published by Healing Tao Books. Softbound. 156 pages.

$10.95 plus $3.95 for postage & handling
(Foreign Shipping: Please see page Catalog-38)
Order by Item No. B03

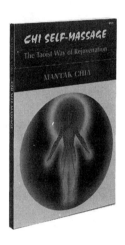

CHI SELF-MASSAGE: THE TAOIST WAY OF REJU- VENATION

Tao Rejuvenation uses one's internal energy or Chi to strengthen and rejuvenate the sense organs (eyes, ears, nose, tongue), the teeth, the skin, and the inner organs. The techniques are five thousand years old, and, until now, were closely guarded secrets passed on from a Master to a small group of students, with each Master only knowing a small part. For the first time the entire system has been pieced together in a logical sequence, and is presented in such a way that only five or ten minutes of practice daily will improve complexion, vision, hearing, sinuses, gums, teeth, tongue, internal organs, and general stamina. (This form of massage is very different from muscular massage.)

By Master Mantak Chia. Published by Healing Tao Books. Softbound. 176 pages.

$10.95 plus $3.95 for postage & handling
(Foreign Shipping: Please see page Catalog-38)
Order by Item No. B04

IRON SHIRT CHI KUNG I: INTERNAL ORGANS EXERCISE

The main purpose of Iron Shirt is not for fighting, but to perfect the body, to win great health, to increase performance, to fight disease, to protect the vital organs from injuries, and to lay the groundwork for higher, spiritual work. Iron Shirt I teaches how to increase the performance of the organs during sports, speech, singing, and dancing.

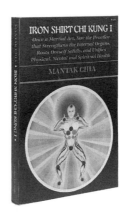

Learn how to increase the Chi pressure throughout the whole system by Iron Shirt Chi Kung breathing, to awaken and circulate internal energy (Chi), to transfer force through the bone structure and down to the ground. Learn how to direct the Earth's power through your bone structure, to direct the internal power to energize and strengthen the organs, and to energize and increase the Chi pressure in the fasciae (connective tissues).

By Master Mantak Chia. Published by Healing Tao Books. Softbound. 320 pages.

$14.95 plus $3.95 for postage & handling
(Foreign Shipping: Please see page Catalog-38)
Order by Item No. B05

BONE MARROW NEI KUNG: IRON SHIRT CHI KUNG III

Bone Marrow Nei Kung is a system to cultivate internal power. By absorbing cosmic energy into the bones, the bone marrow is revitalized, blood replenished, and the life-force within is nourished. These methods are known to make the body impervious to illness and disease. In ancient times, the "Steel Body" attained through this practice was a coveted asset in the fields of Chinese medicine and martial arts. Taoist methods of "regrowing" the bone marrow are crucial to rejuvenating the body, which in turn rejuvenates the mind and spirit. This system has not been revealed before, but in this ground-breaking work Master Chia divulges the step-by-step practice of his predecessors.

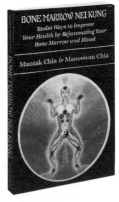

By Master Mantak Chia and Maneewan Chia. Published by Healing Tao Books. Softbound. 288 pages.

$14.95 plus $3.95 for postage & handling
(Foreign Shipping: Please see page Catalog-38)
Order by Item No. B08

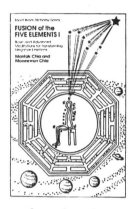

FUSION OF THE FIVE ELEMENTS I

Fusion of the Five Elements I, first in the Taoist Inner Alchemy Series, offers basic and advanced meditations for transforming negative emotions. Based on the Taoist Five Element Theory regarding the five elemental forces of the universe, the student learns how to control negative energies and how to transform them into useful energy. The student also learns how to create a pearl of radiant energy and how to increase its power with additional internal energy (virtue energy) as well as external sources of energy—Universal, Cosmic Particle, and Earth. All combine in a balanced way to prepare the pearl for its use in the creation of an energy body. The creation of the energy body is the next major step in achieving the goal of creating an immortal spirit. Master Mantak Chia leads you, step by step, into becoming an emotionally balanced, controlled, and stronger individual as he offers you the key to a spiritual independence.

$12.95 plus $3.95 for postage & handling
(Foreign Shipping: Please see page Catalog-38)
Order by Item No. B09

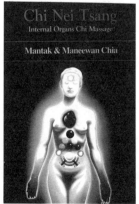

CHI NEI TSANG
(Internal Organ Chi Massage)

Chi Nei Tsang presents a whole new understanding and approach to healing with detailed explanations of self-healing techniques and methods of teaching others to heal themselves. Also included are ways to avoid absorbing negative, sick energies from others.

The navel's center is where negative emotions, stress, tension, and sickness accumulate and congest. When this occurs, all vital functions stagnate. Using Chi Nei Tsang techniques in and around the area of the navel provides the fastest method of healing and the most permanent results.

By Master Mantak Chia and Maneewan Chia. Published by Healing Tao Books. Softbound. 448 pages.

$16.95 plus $3.95 for postage & handling
(Foreign Shipping: Please see page Catalog-38)
Order by Item No. B10

AWAKEN HEALING ENERGY THROUGH THE TAO
Learn how to strengthen your internal organs and increase circulation through the flow of Chi energy. By Master Mantak Chia. Softbound. 193 pages.

$12.50 plus $3.95 for postage & handling
Order by Item No. B01

HEALING TAO INSTRUCTORS' BOOKS

LIVING IN THE TAO by THE PROFESSOR
This book is a Healing Tao instructor's accumulation of knowledge and wisdom from a volume of books and life experiences attained through his practice and instruction. An insider's view at life in the Tao.

- $9.95 plus $3.95 for postage & handling—**Order by Item No. IB01**

THE TAO AND THE TREE OF LIFE by Eric Yudelove
Using the basic structure of the Shamanic Universe, this book provides a context in which to examine the concepts, philosophy, and practical work of Taoist Internal Alchemy. Revealing parallels between Hebrew and western traditions, and long-lost sexual and alchemical secrets, hidden in the Zohar and Sepher Yetzirah.

- $14.95 plus $3.95 for postage & handling–**Order by Item No. IB02**

THE TAO OF NATURAL BREATHING by Dennis Lewis

- $17.95 plus $3.95 for postage & handling–**Order by Item No. IB03**

FORTHCOMING PUBLICATIONS

Cosmic Chi Kung—Techniques developing healing hands and ability to heal from a distance.

Five Element Nutrition—Ancient Chinese cooking based on the Five Elements Theory.

Fusion of the Five Elements II—Thrusting and Belt Channels. Growing positive emotions, psychic and emotional self-defense.

COSMIC COMIC BOOKS

Join us for some enlightened humor. Our first theme comic book—$5.95, add $3.95 for shipping and handling.

Item	Title
CB01	The Inner Smile (Energy Medicine of the Future)

VHS VIDEOS

Invite Master Chia into your living room.

Guided videos 30-60 minutes long $29.95 per tape. Please order by Item Number. Our videos are available in PAL System. **Add postage and handling as follows: 1 video—$3.95, 2 videos—$5.75, 3 or more videos—$6.50. (Foreign Shipping**: Please see page Catalog-38)

Item	Title
V40-G	Home Basic Sitting Meditation (complements V61)
V41-G	Home Basic Standing Meditation
V42-G	Inner Smile
V43-G	Six Healing Sounds

Workshop videos 60-120 minutes long, one tape $39.95; 2 tapes set $69.95 .

Item	Title
V50-TP	Tai Chi Chi Kung I (set of 2 tapes)
V51-TP	Tai Chi Chi Kung II (set of 2 tapes)
V52-TP	Chi Self Massage
V57-TP	Iron Shirt Chi Kung I
V58- TP	Iron Shirt III—Bone Marrow Nei Kung (2 tapes)
V59- TP	Iron Shirt II—Tendons exercises (set of 2 tapes)
V60-TP	Cosmic Chi Kung (Basic and Advanced Buddha Palm)

V61-TM   Awaken Healing Light (set of 2 tapes)
V63-TP   Healing Love through The Tao (set of 2 tapes)
V64-TM   Fusion of Five Elements I (set of 2 tapes)
V65-TM   Fusion of Five Elements II (set of 2 tapes)
V66-TM   Fusion of Five Elements III (set of 2 tapes)
V67-TP   Chi Nei Tsang (set of 2 tapes)
V68-P   Chi Nei Tsang's Healing Power Practice
V69-TP   Tao-In: Regaining a Youthful Body (set of 2 tapes)

CASSETTE TAPES

Guided Practice Tapes C09-C18 are guided by Master Mantak Chia.
$9.95 each, add $3.95 for shipping and handling.
  (**Foreign Shipping**: Please see page Catalog-38)

Item	Title
C09	Inner Smile
C10	Six Healing Sounds
C11	Microcosmic Orbit
C11a	Healing Love
C12	Tai Chi Chi Kung I
C13	Iron Shirt Chi Kung I
C14	Sitting Meditation for Home Instruction
C15	Standing Meditation for Home Instruction
C16	Fusion of the Five Elements I
C17	Fusion of the Five Elements II
C18	Fusion of the Five Elements III

BONE MARROW NEI KUNG (IRON SHIRT III) EQUIPMENT

Only sold as listed!

Item No.	Title	Price	Postage & Handling
62C	Untreated Drilled Jade Egg	$15.95	$3.95
62DG	Chi Weight-Lifting Bar and Silk Cloth	25.95	7.25
62EF	Wire Hitter, Rattan Hitter, Bag for Equipment	39.95	7.25

CARDS

✦Eight Immortal Greeting cards sold in sets of 2 (16 cards in all). Full color, depicting the Eight Immortals with a short history of each one. Ideal for sharing with family and friends! **$9.95 per set.**
✦ Instructional formulas Chi Cards. Now also available in French. **$9.95 each.**
Add $3.95 for shipping and handling.

Item	Title
GC01	Eight Immortal Greeting Cards Set
CC01	Chi Cards - Level 1 (20 cards/set)
CC02	Chi Cards - Level 2 (18 cards/set)
CC03	Chi Cards - Level 3 (18 cards/set)

THE INTERNATIONAL HEALING TAO CENTERS:

AMERICA
• *BERMUDA*
• *CANADA*
Ontario
British Columbia
Quebec
• *UNITED STATES*
Alabama
Arizona
California
    Los Angeles
    San Francisco
Colorado
Connecticut
Delaware
Florida
Hawaii
Illinois

Kansas
Massachusetts
Michigan
Minnesota
New Hampshire
New Jersey
New Mexico
NewYork
North Carolina
Oklahoma
Oregon
Pennsylvania
South Dakota
Virginia

ASIA
• *INDIA*
• *JAPAN*

• *THAILAND*

AUSTRALIA

EUROPE
• *AUSTRIA*
• *ENGLAND*
• *FRANCE*
• *GREECE*
• *HOLLAND*
• *SWITZER-LAND*
• *NETHER-LANDS*
• *SPAIN*
• *GERMANY*
• *ITALY*

Our new center in Thailand holds retreats during the winter and summer seasons, and is located in Chiang Mai. For more information, please call, fax, or write to: The Healing Tao Center
274 Moo 7, Laung Nua
Doi Saket, Chiang Mai 50220
Phone: (66, 53) 495-596 through 599—Fax: (66, 53) 495-852

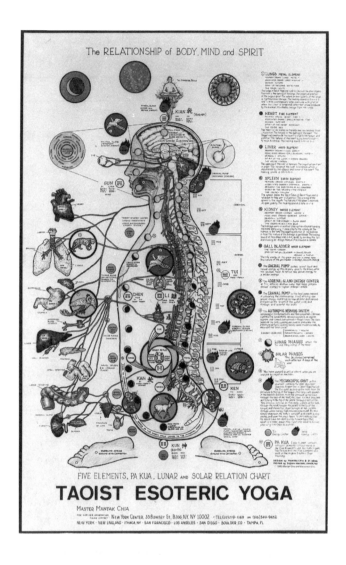

BODY/MIND/SPIRIT CHART 23" x 35", full-color chart by Susan McKay.

$7.50 per copy plus $3.95 for postage and handling
(Foreign Shipping: Please see page Catalog-38)
Order by Item No. C H47

POSTERS

18 x 22", four-color process posters were created by artist Juan Li. Please order by item number.

Sold as Poster set of 12 for $59.95
(Foreign Shipping: Please see page Catalog-38)
Order by Item No. 45.

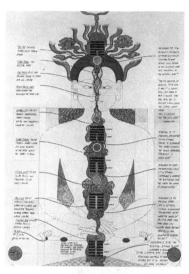

The Microcosmic Orbit—Small Heavenly Cycle—The Functional Channel (Yin). The Microcosmic Orbit Meditation is the key to circulating internal healing energy, and is the gateway to higher Taoist Meditations.
Item No. P31

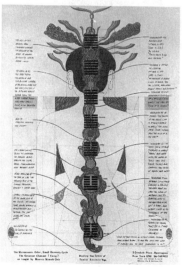

The Microcosmic Orbit—Small Heavenly Cycle—The Governor Channel (Yang). The Governor Channel of the Microcosmic Orbit Meditation allows the Yang (hot) energy to flow from the base of the spine to the brain.
Item No. P32

Healing Love and Sex—Seminal Kung Fu. By conserving their seeds during lovemaking, men can transform sexual energy into spiritual love, and, at the same time, enjoy a higher orgasm. The main purpose of Seminal and Ovarian Kung Fu is to utilize sexual energy for attaining higher levels of consciousness so that the sexual urge does not control the person.
Item No. P35

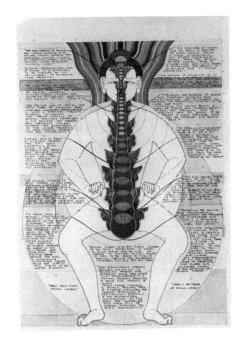

Healing Love and Sex—Ovarian Kung Fu. The Taoists teach women to regulate their menstrual flow and transmute sexual orgasm into higher spiritual love. The techniques of Seminal and Ovarian Kung Fu allow the practitioner to harness sexual impulses so that sex does not control the person. By controlling sexual impulses, people are able to move from the mortal level into higher levels of consciousness.
Item No. P36

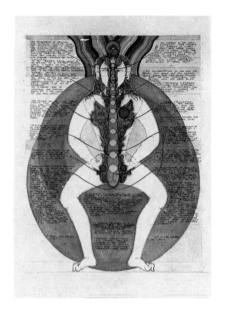

Fusion of the Five Elements I—Cleansing, Clearing, and Harmonizing of the Organs and the Emotions. Each organ stores a separate emotional energy. When fused into a single balanced Chi at the navel, the opening of the six special channels becomes possible.

Item No. P37

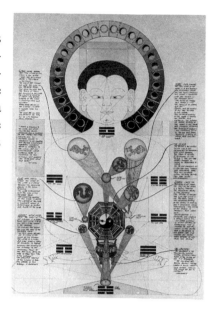

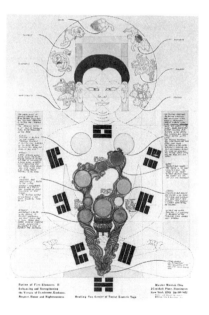

Fusion of the Five Elements II—Enhancing and Strengthening the Virtues. Fusion of the Five Elements II strengthens positive emotions, balances the organs, and encourages in men and women the natural virtues of gentleness, kindness, respect, honor, and righteousness.

Item No. P38

Fusion of the Five Elements II—Thrusting Channels. Running through the center of the body, the Thrusting Routes allow the absorption of cosmic energies for greater radiance and power.
Item No. P39

Fusion of the Five Elements II—Nine Belt Channel. The Taoist Belt Channel spins a web of Chi around the major energy vortexes in the body, protecting the psyche by connecting the power of Heaven and Earth. **Item No. P40**

The Harmony of Yin and Yang. "Yin cannot function without the help of Yang; Yang cannot function without the help of Yin." —Taoist Canon, 8th century A.D. **Item No. P41**

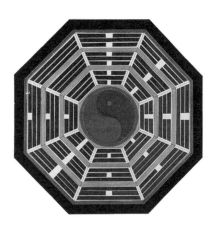

Pa Kua. The Cauldron of Fusing the Energy and Emotions. *Also sold separately, $7.50 each copy, add $3.95 for shipping and handling.*
Item No. P42➤

Fusion of the Five Elements III—Yin Bridge and Regulator Channels. Fusion of the Five Elements III uses special meridians to cleanse the aura and regulate high-voltage energy absorbed by the body during meditation. **Item No. P43**

Fusion of the Five Elements III—Yang Bridge and Regulator Channels. Fusion of the Five Elements III teaches the yogic secrets of safely

regulating the release of the kundalini power using special meridians.
Item No. P44

NEW PRODUCTS

POSTERS
$9.50 each add $3.95 shipping and handling.

The Inner Alchemy of the Tao. Beautifully illustrated chart. Instructional pamphlet is included. Item No. CH48

The Eight Immortal Forces. The legendary figures of the Eight Immortals are depicted in this chart with full explanations of their mysteries. Instructional pamphlet is included. **Item No. CH49**

BOOKS

THE MULTI-ORGASMIC MAN

In this book co-written by Master Mantak Chia and Doug Arava, and published by Harper Collins, you'll learn the amazing facts about the multi-orgasmic capabilities of men. By learning to separate orgasm and ejaculation—two distinct physical processes—men can transform a momentary release into countless peaks of whole body orgasms without losing an erection. In addition to becoming better sexual partners, multi-orgasmic men enjoy increased vitality and longetivity because they minimize the fatigue and depletion that follow ejaculation.

$20 plus $3.95 for postage & handling
(Foreign Shipping: Please see page Catalog-38)
Order by Item No. B13
Harper Collins Publisher
ISBN# 0-06-251335-4

HOW TO ORDER

Prices and Taxes:
Subject to change without notice. New York State residents please add 8.25% sales tax.

Payment:
Send personal check, money order, certified check, or bank cashier's check to:

The Healing Tao Center
P.O. Box 1194
Huntington, NY 11743
To place orders please call: 1-800-497-1017
or for overseas customers: 1-717-325-9380
Fax: 1-717-325-9357
All foreign checks must be drawn on a U.S. bank. Mastercard,
Visa, and American Express cards accepted.

Shipping

Domestic Shipping: via UPS, requires a complete street address.   Allow 3-4 weeks for delivery.

Foreign Shipping: *European countries only: Worldmail by DHL, surface mail ($7.95 per book), air mail ($15.95 per book).* Courier service by air, as an alternative for traceable shipments or heavy orders, is also available as a collect service. For other products please see chart below.

Order Total	Domestic Zone 1-6	Domestic Zones 7 & 8	Foreign by Surface	Foreign by Air
$20.00 or less	$ 3.95	$ 3.95	$ 7.95	$15.95
20.01 - 40.00	6.95	7.25	17.95	30.95
40.01 - 60.00	8.50	9.25	27.50	45.95
60.01 - 80.00	9.75	10.75	37.95	60.95
80.01 - 100.00	11.00	12.75	47.95	75.95
100.01 - 120.00	12.25	14.50	57.95	90.95
120.01 - 140.00	13.50	16.25	67.95	105.95
140.01 - 200.00	16.50	21.50	97.95	150.95
Over 200.00	add $4.95/every$50		add $20.95 /every $50	add $40.95 /every $50

Zones 7 & 8—Zip codes with the first 3 digits:
577, 586 - 593, 677 - 679, 690, 693
733, 739, 763 - 772, 774 - 774, 778 - 797, 798 - 799
800 - 899, 900 - 994
All other Zip codes are Zones 1 - 6

❖**Please call or write for additional information in your area**❖

NOTES

NOTES